BUSINESS AND
LEGAL ESSENTIALS FOR
NURSE PRACTITIONERS

FROM NEGOTIATING YOUR FIRST JOB
THROUGH OWNING A PRACTICE

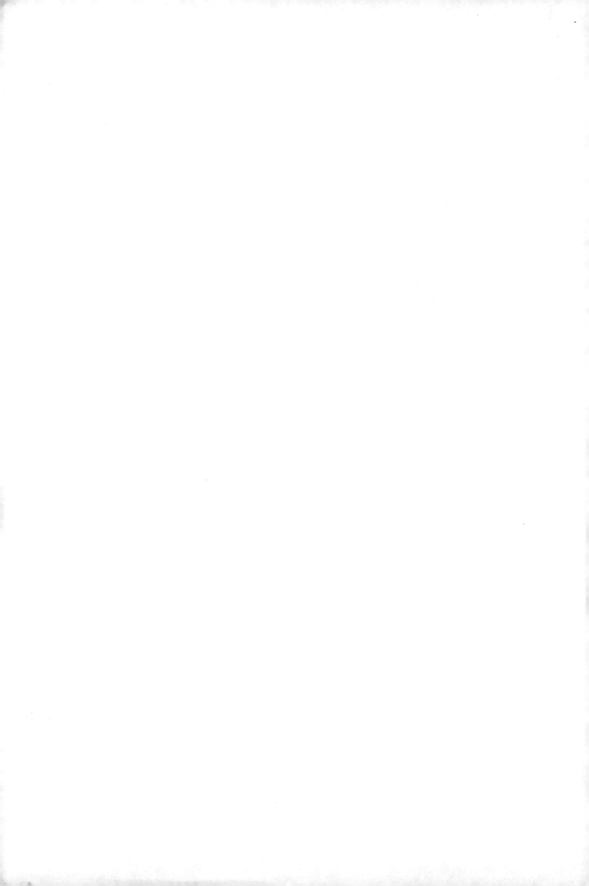

BUSINESS AND LEGAL ESSENTIALS FOR NURSE PRACTITIONERS

FROM NEGOTIATING YOUR FIRST JOB THROUGH OWNING A PRACTICE

SALLY J. REEL, PHD, APRN, BC, CFNP, FAAN, FAANP
Associate Dean for Academic Practice and Clinical Professor
Director, Arizona AHEC
University of Arizona College of Nursing
Tucson, Arizona

IVO L. ABRAHAM, PHD, RN, FAAN, CS

Principal
Matrix 45, LLC
Earlysville, Virginia

Adjunct Professor
University of Pennsylvania
Center for Health Outcomes
  and Policy Research, School of Nursing
Leonard Davis Institute of
  Health Economics,
  Wharton School of Business
Philadelphia, Pennsylvania

Adjunct Clinical Professor
College of Nursing
University of Arizona
Tucson, Arizona

Clinical Professor
School of Nursing
University of Virginia
Charlottesville, Virginia

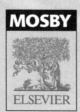

MOSBY

ELSEVIER

MOSBY
ELSEVIER

11830 Westline Industrial Drive
St. Louis, Missouri 63146

Business and Legal Essentials for Nurse Practitioners: ISBN-13: 978-0-323-03610-8
From Negotiating Your First Job Through Owning a Practice   ISBN-10: 0-323-03610-4

NOTICE

Neither the publisher nor the author assumes any liability for any injury and/or damage to persons or property arising from this publication. It is the responsibility of the treating practitioner, relying on independent expertise and knowledge of the patient, to determine the best treatment and method of application for the patient.

This publication is designed to provide accurate and authoritative information in regard to the subject matter covered. In publishing this book, neither the Editor nor the Publisher is engaged in rendering legal, accounting, or other professional service. If legal advice or other expert assistance is required, the services of a competent professional should be sought.

The Publisher

ISBN-13: 978-0-323-03610-8
ISBN-10: 0-323-03610-4

Acquisitions Editor: Sandra Clark Brown
Senior Developmental Editor: Cindi Anderson
Publishing Services Manager: Gayle May
Project Manager: Tracey Schriefer
Senior Designer: Jyotika Shroff

Printed in the United States of America

Last digit is the print number: 9 8 7 6 5 4 3 2 1

We dedicate this book to the clinician and entrepreneur in every nurse practitioner:

*—Committed to the best for patients and families, using today's
knowledge and open to tomorrow's new insights;*

*—Realistic about the business and legal ramifications of our decision
to be dedicated clinicians in a regulatory and financially
complex healthcare system;*

*—Seeking ultimately to develop innovative and sustainable ways of
providing healthcare to all those who need it*

Ivo L. Abraham, PhD, RN, FAAN, CS
Principal
Matrix 45, LLC
Earlysville, Virginia
Adjunct Faculty
University of Pennsylvania
University of Arizona
University of Virgina

Gail P. Barker, MBA, PhD
Clinical Assistant Professor, Pathology
Assistant Professor, College of Public Health
University of Arizona
Tuscon, Arizona

Mona Counts, PhD, CRNP, FNAP, FAANP
Elouise Ross Eberly Professor
School of Nursing
The Pennsylvania State University
University Park, Pennsylvania
Clinical Director
Primary Care Center of Mt. Morris
Mt Morris, Pennsylvania

Saowapa Dedkhard, MS, RN
Doctoral Candidate, Graduate Assistant
Department of Nursing
The University of Arizona
Tucson, Arizona

Jane M. Dyer, MS, RN, CNM, FNP, MBA
Director,
Nurse Midwifery Program
University of Utah College of Nursing
Salt Lake City, Utah

Alison Hughes, MPA
Director
Rural Health Office
Mel and Enid Zuckerman College of Public Health
Tuscon, Arizona

David W. Kelly, PhD, MS, RN
Former Nurse Consultant
Health Resources and Services Administration
Department of Health and Human Services
Rockville, Maryland

Susan Bragg Leight, EdD, RNCS, CRNP, FAANP
Associate Professor
Department of Nursing
West Virginia Wesleyan College
Buckhannon, West Virginia

Valerie Light, MBA
Clinical Practice Administrator
University of Arizona/University Physicians Healthcare
Department of Radiology
Tucson, Arizona

Karen M. MacDonald, PhD, RN
Principal
Matrix 45, LLC
Earlysville, Virginia

Donna Behler McArthur, PhD, APRN, BC, FAANP
Clinical Professor
Director DNP Program
University of Arizona College of Nursing
Tucson, Arizona

Regina Mayolo
Technical Assistance Specialist
Center for Excellence in Disabilities
West Virginia University
Assistive Technology Demonstration Clinics
Morgantown, West Virgnia

Deborah M. Nadzam, PhD, RN
Executive Director, The Quality Institute
The Cleveland Clinic Foundation
Cleveland, Ohio

Julie C. Novak, DNSc, RN, CPNP, FAANP
Professor and Head
Purdue School of Nursing
Associate Dean
Schools of Pharmacy, Nursing, and Health Sciences
West Lafayette, Indiana

Sally J. Reel, PhD, APRN, BC, CFNP, FAAN, FAANP
Associate Dean for Academic Practice and Clinical Professor
Director, Arizona AHEC
University of Arizona College of Nursing
Tucson, Arizona

Mariann T. Shinoskie, CNM, MS, JD
Staff Attorney
Office of the General Counsel
University of Arizona
Tuscon, Arizona

Jan Towers, PhD, NP-C, CRNP, FAANP
Director of Health Policy
The American Academy of Nurse Practitioners
Office of Health Policy
Washington, DC

Carolyn Zaumeyer, MSN, ARNP
President
Women's Health Watch, Inc.
West Milford, New Jersey

Priscilla Lee, MD, FNP-C
Nurse Practitioner II
UCLA Gonda Vascular Surgery Center
UCLA School of Nursing
Los Angeles, California

Shelly Anderson Wells, BSN, MSN, MBA, PhD
Assistant Professor of Nursing
The University of Oklahoma College of Nursing: Tulsa Campus
Tulsa, Arizona

Theresa Pluth Yeo, BSN, MSN, MPH, ACNP, ANP
Adjunct Assistant Professor
Johns Hopkins University
School of Nursing
Baltimore, Maryland

One of the most significant shifts in healthcare is the ever-growing prominence of nurse practitioners (NPs) in practices ranging from acute to long-term care. Increasingly, patients and families are recognizing that many of their healthcare needs may be met accurately and economically by NPs— a perspective that significantly expands conventional healthcare. As providers at the interface of primary and specialty care and at the center of most healthcare processes, NPs are infusing American healthcare (and increasingly healthcare abroad) with a unique paradigm of care.

Healthcare is very big business, regardless of how much one would like to emphasize its altruistic nature and benefit to humanity. Too often, the lack of money makes it impossible for healthcare providers to pursue the missions of quality and well-being. This book attempts to close a small portion of this gap. ***Business and Legal Essentials for Nurse Practitioners*** emerged from many years of practice and service by Dr. Reel as a nurse practitioner educator, including development and direction of a nurse-managed center, and the long-standing mentorship of knowledge development and business processes by Dr. Abraham. The book cuts across settings and markets—rural and urban, independent and interdependent NP practices, integration of NP practice into other health care practices, as well as academic practice, including faculty practice and nursing centers. This book is for clinical practitioners, educators, and students. While health professionals are oriented to the legalities associated with practice—particularly risk management and malpractice, at some point in every NP's career, usually at the first supervised clinical practicum, practice collides with business.

Most NP programs do not focus heavily, if at all, on the business side of practice simply because the need to educate a sound, safe clinician is paramount. An NP's first reality check with the business side of practice may be when he or she is asked to sign an employment contract, and shortly thereafter when he or she receives (or does not receive) the first productivity bonus. Later, when confident as a clinician and ready to strike out into independent practice, the NP finds a completely new set of legal and business issues to contend with.

This is a pragmatic book with a conceptual foundation. While this book provides practical information about advanced practice, its greater strength is that it is not a series of "how to's" but that it raises the bar for thinking about "how to do." Thus, this is a book relevant to academics and practitioners, written to raise questions and to direct the reader to seek out additional information and resources.

The four chapters in **Part I** provide information and raise questions that an NP should consider when going into advanced practice. Whether a novice or expert NP, questions about employment, scope-of-practice, business planning, etc. are bi-directional. For an NP just entering practice, understanding the terms of employment and the types of questions to ask can translate into a better salary and benefits package. For an NP employer, understanding the terms an NP will expect on employment is good for business—such knowledge lays the groundwork for productivity expectations and good business outcomes. A successful advanced practice is not only about quality and safety; it is also about clearing the books. For NPs to navigate this successfully, sound business knowledge is as essential as clinical knowledge. *Chapter 1* provides information about defining the role of the NP, outlines key terms (such as credentialing and scope-of-practice, prescriptive authority, collaborative agreements, common employment law terms, elements of an employment contract, benefits, performance evaluation), and opens a dialogue about what to consider when thinking about starting an independent practice. *Chapter 2* discusses scope-of-practice issues. *Chapter 3* outlines what NPs need to know about prescriptive authority as they start their practices. *Chapter 4* delves into the myriad of terms and complexities of credentialing.

Part II addresses the pragmatics of owning an independent practice. *Chapters 5* and *6* describe what to think about before going into business and describe the advantages and disadvantages of owning a business. *Chapter 7* discusses the development of the business plan. *Chapter 8* describes many nuances of practice operations, including the legal structure of the practice, how to manage collaborative agreements when the NP is the practice owner, policy and procedure manuals, insurances, hiring employees, and managing practice finances. *Chapter 9* focuses on the realties of NPs getting reimbursement for services rendered. *Chapter 10* delves into marketing strategy for the practice as this relates to assuring solid, quality services. *Chapter 11* addresses the importance of location and physical space considerations for designing the work environment. *Chapter 12* is an overview of the electronic practice—electronic health records, health information technologies, and HIPAA (Health Insurance Portability and Accountability Act of 1996). *Chapter 13* introduces the challenges of managing business growth.

Part III describes academic nursing practices, the role of the federal government in the development of nursing centers, faculty practice, the impact of alternative care delivery models that often employ NPs, and the rural health clinic. *Chapter 14* provides background information about academic practice. *Chapter 15* describes the historical and current role of the federal government, particularly the Division of Nursing of the Health Resources Services Administration, Bureau of Health Professions, as a major funding agency of academic nursing centers. *Chapter Sixteen* presents a more detailed description of academic practice, specifically faculty practice. Several examples of faculty practice are provided and a discussion of the Doctor of Nursing Practice is introduced as well. *Chapter 17* focuses on rural health clinics, including community health centers, and the role these clinics have with respect to providing care to rural populations.

Part IV describes special considerations that impact an NP practice, including telemedicine, quality, and risk management issues. *Chapter 18* highlights electronic innovations in health care practice, particularly telemedicine and informatics. *Chapter 19* introduces several concepts related to quality of care and quality management. *Chapter 20* addresses several legal, business, and regulatory issues related to advanced practice.

This book is the result of people's belief and confidence in the role of the NP in American healthcare—and as time passes, in other parts of the world as well. The challenges facing NPs are not only clinical, assuring the highest quality of care to patients and their families, but these challenges also encompass the myriad of business and legal issues that come with practicing independently and interdependently. Whether running an independent business or being a critical part of a larger business, getting money in on time so that staff, personnel, and operating expenses can be paid on time is critical to your success. As the editors of this book, we are the first ones to advocate the mission. Our experience over the past couple decades has also taught us that without money, there is no mission.

Sally J. Reel
Ivo L. Abraham

*T*he editors acknowledge and express their sincere thanks to Jennifer Zuniga, Program Coordinator, Senior, University of Arizona College of Nursing, for her many efforts during the development, writing and production of this book.

I. Advanced Practice

1. **Entering Advanced Practice, 3**
   Sally J. Reel

2. **Scope of Practice, 25**
   Sally J. Reel

3. **Nurse Practitioners and Prescriptive Authority, 37**
   Jan Towers

4. **Credentialing, 45**
   Mona Counts and Regina Mayolo

II. Owning a Practice

5. **What to Think About Before Going Into Business: Personal and Professional Planning, 61**
   Carolyn Zaumeyer

6. **Advantages and Disadvantages to Owning a Business: Feasibility and Finance, 71**
   Carolyn Zaumeyer

7. **The Business Plan: A Development and Management Tool, 83**
   Ivo L. Abraham, Karen M. MacDonald, and Sally J. Reel

8. **Practice Management, 99**
   Sally J. Reel and Ivo L. Abraham

9. **Reimbursement, 123**
   Gail P. Barker and Valerie Light

10. **Marketing: Understanding Strategies to Build an NP Practice, 137**
    Sally J. Reel and Ivo L. Abraham

11. **Physical Practice Space Considerations, 149**
    Sally J. Reel

12. **The Electronic Practice: Electronic Health Records, Health Information Technologies, and HIPAA Considerations, 163**
    Sally J. Reel

13. **Managing Growth, Thinking Beyond the Box: The (Not-So-Obvious) Opportunities and the (Not-So-Hidden) Dangers, 175**
    Ivo L. Abraham and Karen M. MacDonald

III. Academic Practices and Alternate Business Forms

14. Academic Practice and Academic Nursing Centers, 181
    Donna Behler McArthur

15. The Academic Nursing Center: A History of Federal Support, 191
    David W. Kelly

16. Faculty Practice, 203
    Julie C. Novak

17. Rural Health Centers, 215
    Alison Hughes

IV. Special Considerations

18. The Electronic Nurse Practitioner: Supporting Innovations in Care, 225
    Susan Bragg Leight

19. Managing Quality of Care by Measuring Performance, 233
    Ivo L. Abraham, Deborah M. Nadzam, and Karen M. MacDonald

20. Risk Management, 245
    Jane M. Dyer, Mariann T. Shinoskie, and Donna Behler McArthur

Appendices

A. Contact Information for State Boards of Nursing and the District of Columbia, 265
    Compiled by Saowapa Dedkhard

B. Collaborative Agreements, 271

C. Sample Employment Contract, 285

D. Contract Negotiation for Nurse Practitioners, 291

E. Sample Advanced Practice Nurse Contract, 299

F. Sample Business Plan, 303

G. Glossary of Terms for Reimbursement, 311
    Gail P. Barker and Valerie Light

H. Practice Start-Up Timeline, 315

I. Resources for the Nurse Practitioner, 319

J. National Provider Identifier (NPI), 331

K. National Provider Identifier (NPI) Application/Update Form, 333

Business and Legal Essentials for Nurse Practitioners

From Negotiating Your First Job Through Owning a Practice

PART I

ADVANCED PRACTICE

Entering Advanced Practice

SALLY J. REEL

ntering advanced nursing practice is an exciting and challenging experience. It encompasses a raised level of sophistication in nursing practice, along with new legal and business pitfalls one should be aware of and the subsequent possible economic consequences. Understanding the legal and business aspects of advanced practice is important in regard to the goals of improving patient outcomes and competing successfully in the health care market. Today's health care market provides many employment opportunities for nurse practitioners (NPs), as well as opportunities for self-employment. The business environment for advanced practice is complex, and NPs may find employment opportunities that are different from those available in the past. Practice environments today include hospital settings, nursing homes, group practices, specialty practices, multispecialty group practices, and solo practice, in addition to independent NP-owned practices. Each of the health care environments has its own set of strengths and weaknesses that NPs must consider.[1]

Some basic things you need to know when going into advanced practice include knowing how to meet regulatory and licensing requirements and how to maintain those requirements, understanding and complying with scope of practice laws and prescriptive authority requirements, and becoming savvy about things such as collaborative practice agreements and employment contracts. This chapter provides background information needed for entering advanced practice as an NP. The nurse practitioner role, credentialing and certification, scope of practice, employment rights, negotiation of employment agreements, and some parameters to think about concerning developing an independent practice are described. Regulatory and scope of practice issues are discussed in greater detail in Chapters 2 and 3.

DEFINING THE ROLE OF THE NURSE PRACTITIONER

NPs are advanced practice nurses. Although advanced practice roles can vary, one defining feature of advanced practice is the central competency of direct clinical practice.[2] The American Academy of Nurse Practitioners (AANP) defines NPs as follows:

> Nurse practitioners are primary care providers who practice in ambulatory, acute and long-term care settings. According to their practice specialty these providers provide nursing and medical services to individuals, families and groups. In addition to diagnosing and managing acute episodic and chronic illnesses, nurse practitioners emphasize health promotion and disease prevention. Services include, but are not limited to, ordering, conducting, supervising, and interpreting diagnostic and laboratory tests, and prescription of pharmacologic agents and nonpharmacologic therapies. Teaching and counseling individuals, families and groups are a major part of nurse practitioner practice. Nurse practitioners practice autonomously and in collaboration with health care professionals and other individuals to diagnose, treat and manage the patient's health problems. They serve as health care researchers, interdisciplinary consultants and patient advocates.[3]

States may define the role of NPs within the state nurse practice act or scope of practice laws. Federal law also defines nurse practitioners. In addition to state and federal law, NPs are also sometimes referred to, especially outside the disciplines of nursing, as advanced practice nurses, mid-level providers, and physician extenders.[4]

Nurse practitioners are involved in a wide variety of specialization practices. According to a United States *Nurse Practitioner Workforce Data Survey* published by the American Academy of Nurse Practitioners,[5] current characteristics of NPs include the following:

- 88% have graduate degrees

- 92% are nationally certified

- 39% have hospital privileges

- 20% practice in rural or frontier settings

Approximately 106,000 NPs are practicing in the United States, and 5000 to 6000 new NPs are prepared each year. Types of practice are diverse among NPs—the greatest percentage being prepared as family nurse practitioners (FNPs), 41.2%; followed by adult nurse practitioners (ANPs), 19.5%; women's health nurse practitioners (WHNPs), 11.3%; and pediatric nurse practitioners (PNPs), 10.9%. The majority of all NPs prescribe medications (96.5%) and two thirds practice in at least one primary care site and another 31% practice in nonprimary care sites such as inpatient units, emergency units, or other specialty services.[5] These data indicate the nurse practitioner role is well established in the health care industry.

NURSE PRACTITIONER CREDENTIALING, LICENSURE, AND NATIONAL CERTIFICATION

Credentialing and national certification reflect standardization of nurse practitioner practice. Credentialing may refer to the process of licensure, registration, certification, accreditation, and recognition. However, when the term *credentialing* is used by a hospital or managed care organization, credentialing refers to the process of obtaining, verifying, and analyzing the eligibility and qualifications of the practitioner to execute health care services.[6] The process of credentialing is described in Chapter 4, and national certification linked with scope of practice is described in Chapter 2. Because both processes are essential for entering advanced practice, highlights of both are presented.

Credentialing and delineation of clinical privileges for health care providers is mandated by the Joint Commission on Accreditation of Healthcare Organizations (JCAHO) and recognized by other agencies such as the National Committee for Quality Assurance (NCQA) and managed care organizations (MCOs). Credentialing is about assuring that professionals within an institution are competent and practicing within their scope of practice. Credentialing and privileging are distinct processes that have unique meanings and purposes. In the past, credentialing and privileging applied usually to physicians, but because nurse practitioners are employed in many institutions now, it is necessary to credential NPs as well.[7]

Terms associated with credentialing include the following[7]:

- *Credentials*: proof of applicant's background and experience

- *Credentials verification*: process of reviewing an applicant's background and verifying information to corroborate accuracy and completeness of information

- *Privileges*: delineates applicant's scope of practice, ensures competencies required by accrediting bodies, and averts both institutional and professional liability issues; also determines what impact the practitioner will have on the institution's financial status; usually granted on an individual basis

- *Privileging*: process by which an institution grants specific authority to the practitioner to provide designated clinical activities

Credentials are usually periodically reviewed and renewed as a means of assuring continued quality.[7]

Licensure is the process by which a state governmental agency grants permission to an individual to engage in a given occupation upon finding that the applicant meets the minimum degree of competency necessary to reasonably protect public health and safety. The purpose of licensure is to regulate nursing practice by the state to, again, protect the health, safety, and welfare of the public. State licensing laws usually also establish the minimal educational criteria for entry into practice.[8]

Certification, on the other hand, is the process by which a nongovernmental agency grants recognition to an individual who has met certain predetermined qualifications. Such qualifications may include graduation from an accredited or approved program, acceptable performance on a qualifying examination, and/or completion of a given amount of work experience. Many states require national certification as part of the process for licensure as a nurse practitioner. Certification validates nurse practitioner specialty knowledge and demonstrates that an NP meets nationally recognized standards. Certification also is required by many third-party payers for reimbursement, and as an example, the Center for Medicare and Medicaid Services (CMS) requires national certification for reimbursement. Although certification can be used as a requirement for entry into practice and for licensure, it also may be used as the standard for validating competence, particularly beyond basic licensure; for recognizing nurses whose practice may be directly reimbursable; and for recognizing excellence or otherwise regulating practice quality.[6,9]

Eligibility for certification usually requires holding an active, unrestricted registered nurse (RN) license, holding a master's degree or higher in nursing, and completing a formal education program in the area of practice in which you are seeking certification (e.g., family, adult, acute care NP). Most certifying agencies also require NP programs to be accredited and meet certain educational standards before someone can take the examination. For example, both the American Nurses Credential Center (ANCC) and the American Academy of Nurse Practitioners (AANP) require that NP programs be offered by an approved and/or accredited graduate-level institution. Further, these programs must include both didactic and clinical components and a minimum of 500 hours of supervised clinical practice in the specialty area and role.

National certification is granted for a specified period of time, often 5 years, upon successfully passing the examination. To maintain certification beyond this period requires recertification. Recertification involves documenting current knowledge and practice through a specified number of continuing education options and a minimum number of documented practice hours within your NP specialty. ANCC, for example, requires 1000 hours of practice within the 5-year certification period and a minimum of 75 contact hours of continuing education credits. Failure to maintain certification could lead to loss of licensure in states that require certification for licensing. Agencies that certify nurse practitioners are shown in Table 1-1.

SCOPE OF PRACTICE

Professional nursing and state governments recognize the need to describe and recognize the responsibilities of nurse practitioners and other advanced practice nurses. Scope of practice may be described as those functions performed by a nurse practitioner and the minimum competencies needed to perform those functions. Each state has legislated regulatory parameters for nurse practitioner practice.

TABLE 1-1

Types of Nurse Practitioner and Certifying Agencies

TYPE OF NP	AMERICAN ACADEMY OF NURSE PRACTITIONERS (AANP)	AMERICAN NURSES CREDENTIALING CENTER (ANCC)	NATIONAL CERTIFICATION BOARD OF PEDIATRIC NURSE PRACTITIONERS AND NURSES (NAPNP)	NATIONAL CERTIFICATION CORPORATION FOR THE WOMEN'S HEALTH, OBSTETRIC, AND NEONATAL NURSING SPECIALTIES (NCC)
Family NP	X	X		
Adult NP	X	X		
Gerontologic NP		X		
Adult Psychiatric Mental Health NP		X		
Family Psychiatric Mental Health NP		X		
Pediatric NP		X	X	
Women's Health NP				X
Acute Care NP		X		

These state legislated rules and regulations define legal scope of practice including privileges for diagnosis, prescriptive authority, and reimbursement.[9]

The scope of practice for nurse practitioners can be found in the Nurse Practice Act for each state and the District of Columbia. Scope of practice statements are often written broadly and may not involve the delineation of specific tasks. Whereas state laws and rules provide the legal authority for nurse practitioner practice, the nursing profession plays a pivotal role in establishing the context of practice and the standards of practice—on which legislatures, government agencies, and courts often base their actions.[10]

It is important for NPs to understand the rights, privileges, and limitations of their practice within the state they intend to practice because scope of practice rules and regulations are not uniform across all states. It is a wise strategy to get a copy of the Nurse Practice Act that governs state practice and become very familiar with that state's scope of practice laws. Contact information for each state board of nursing is found in Appendix A. In addition, many state boards of nursing publish the Nurse Practice Act on their website.

PRESCRIPTIVE AUTHORITY

Every state also allows some degree of prescriptive authority for nurse practitioners.[11] The American Academy of Nurse Practitioners (AANP) advocates for nurse practitioners to have unlimited prescriptive authority and dispensing privileges within their scope of practice. AANP supports NPs being able to prescribe, without limitation, legend and controlled drugs, devices, adjunct health/medical services, durable medical goods, and other equipment as important parameters needed for NPs to facilitate the provision of cost-effective, quality health care.[12] Although NPs have some capacity to prescribe or otherwise arrange for a patient to get prescription medication, prescriptive authority varies widely from state to state. Some states allow NPs to prescribe without any physician involvement requirement. However, many other states require some type of collaborative agreement with a physician for NPs to be granted prescriptive authority. And although some states require formal written agreements, others do not.[4, 11]

Many states allow NPs to prescribe controlled substances as well; however, states vary on the nature of what controlled substances NPs may prescribe. Controlled substances include narcotics, depressants, stimulants, and hallucinogenic drugs that are covered under the federal Controlled Substances Act. The five established schedules of controlled substances are known as schedules I, II, III, IV, and V. Table 1-2 describes each schedule and provides examples of drugs under each schedule. A complete listing of drugs controlled under the Controlled Substances Act may be found online at the U.S. Drug Enforcement Administration website under the heading *Title 21, Food and Drugs • Chapter 13, Drug Abuse Prevention and Control • Subchapter I, Control and Enforcement • Part B, Authority to Control; Standards and Schedules* (http://www.usdoj.gov/dea/pubs/csa.html).

To prescribe controlled substances, NPs must register with the federal Drug Enforcement Administration (DEA) and obtain a DEA number. Federal registration is based on the NP's compliance with state and local laws. New applicants can apply to the DEA on DEA Form 224, which is available online at https://www.deadiversion.usdoj.gov/webforms/app224Login.jsp. The application fee at the time of this writing is $390. States also may have separate fees related to prescriptive authority applications and DEA registration.

COLLABORATIVE PRACTICE AGREEMENTS

Collaboration is based on a fundamental assumption that quality patient care is achieved through the contributions of all care providers. Ideally, good collaboration is based on the knowledge and expertise brought to the situation rather

TABLE 1-2

Controlled Substance by Drug Classification

Controlled Substance Schedule Classification*	Description of Schedule*	Example of Drugs included in Schedule[†]
Schedule I	Drug or substance has high potential for abuse Drug or substance has no accepted medical use in the USA Drug or substance lacks accepted safety for use under medical supervision	Gamma hydroxybutyric acid (GHB) Heroin LSD Marijuana Mescaline Psilocybin (magic mushrooms) Thiofentanyl (China white)
Schedule II	Drug or substance has a high potential for abuse Drug or substance has a currently accepted medical use in USA and use is severely restricted Drug or substance abuse may lead to psychological or physical dependence	Amphetamine (Dexedrine) Codeine Hydromorphone (Dilaudid) Meperidine (Demerol) Methadone Methamphetamine (Desoxyn) Methylphenidate (Ritalin) Morphine Oxycodone (OxyContin, Percocet) Pentobarbital (Nembutal)
Schedule III	Drug or substance has potential for abuse less than those in schedules I and II Drug or substance has a currently accepted medical use in the USA Abuse of drug or substance may lead to moderate or low physical dependence or high psychological dependence	Anabolic steroids Butalbital (Fiorinal) Codeine combination product 90 mg/du (APAP w/codeine) Hydrocodone combination product less than 15 mg/du (Lorcet) Opium combination product 25 mg/du (Paregoric) Thiopental (Pentothal)
Schedule IV	Drug or substance has a low potential for abuse relative to the drugs or other substances in schedule III Drug or substance has a currently accepted medical use in the USA Abuse of the drug or other substance may lead to limited physical dependence or psychological dependence relative to the drugs or other substances in schedule III	Alprazolam (Xanax) Chloral hydrate (Noctec) Dextropropoxyphene (Darvon) Diazepam (Valium) Flurazepam (Dalmane) Lorazepam (Ativan) Phenobarbital (Luminal) Zolpidem (Ambien) Zopiclone (Lunesta)

Continued

TABLE 1-2		

Controlled Substance by Drug Classification—cont'd

CONTROLLED SUBSTANCE SCHEDULE CLASSIFICATION*	DESCRIPTION OF SCHEDULE*	EXAMPLE OF DRUGS INCLUDED IN SCHEDULE[†]
Schedule V	Drug or substance has a low potential for abuse relative to the drugs or other substances in schedule IV Drug or substance has a currently accepted medical use in the USA Abuse of the drug or substance may lead to limited physical dependence or psychological dependence relative to the drugs or other substances in schedule IV	Codeine preparations—200 mg/100 ml or 100 g Difenoxin preparations—0.5 mg/25 µg AtSO4/du (Motofen) Dihydrocodeine preparations—10 mg/100 ml or 100 g (Cophene-S) Diphenoxylate preparations 2.5 mg/25 µg AtSO4 (Lomotil)

*Data from U.S. Drug Enforcement Agency: Title 21, Food and Drugs/Chapter 13, Drug Abuse Prevention and Control/ Subchapter I, Control and Enforcement/Part B, Authority to Control; Standards and Schedules (website): http://www. usdoj.gov/dea/pubs/csa/812.htm
[†]Data from DEA Office of Diversion Control: Controlled Substance Schedules (website): http://www.deadiversion.usdoj. gov/schedules/schedules.htm

than on a hierarchy.[13] Collaboration is an inherent component of nurse practitioner practice and in many states a collaborative relationship is mandated by law. Collaboration generally does not mean "delegatory" or "supervisory." However, collaboration is regulated and varies by state law from having a physician available for consultation or referral to submitting a signed written agreement to some of the state boards of nursing—sometimes for approval and sometimes for recording and documenting the parties' agreement to participate in a collaborative agreement. Some states still require specific information such as lists or categories of medications that the nurse practitioners may prescribe. Yet, collaboration is changing in the United States, with some states, including the District of Columbia, no longer requiring collaborative agreements with physicians.[11] Although collaborative practice arrangements vary in terms of formality, you do need to understand and comply with collaborative practice regulations within the state where you practice.[4]

A written collaborative practice agreement defines the relationship between an NP and the collaborative physician. Some states limit written agreements to prescriptive authority only, whereas others require that the written agreement identify the services to be provided within the scope of each practitioner's expertise. Written agreements may require identification of supervision and at what point NPs may not proceed on their own to provide treatment. Some states also require the identification of established protocols to guide NP practice and specific information about how emergencies will be managed. Some states also require actions such as periodic review of charts and cosignatures on charts or prescriptions. Other states may require the identification of a collaborative relationship but no written agreement is required. You must understand and comply with your state's requirements for collaborative practice. Sample collaborative agreements are shown in Appendix B. Many boards of nursing have sample agreements that you may request to help you draft an appropriate agreement.

EMPLOYMENT LAW: GENERAL CONSIDERATIONS RELEVANT TO NP PRACTICE

Both states and the federal government have many statues related to employment. All states have workers' compensation laws, for example, and many have other statutes on health and safety in the workplace such as OSHA (Occupational Safety and Health Act of 1970). Employment legislation is about protecting the health and safety of workers and fosters a workplace free from discrimination and disruptive labor management, among many other things such as provision of a minimum level of economic support to workers.[14]

Title VII of the Civil Rights Act of 1964 is the most important statute on discriminatory employment practices. Title VII and other federal statutes are enforced under the Equal Employment Opportunity Commission (EEOC) Act of 1972 and subsequent amendments. In addition to Title VII, several other statutes prohibit discrimination in specific areas of employment. Some of the important statutes include the Equal Pay Act of 1963, the Age Discrimination in Employment Act of 1967, the Americans with Disabilities Act of 1990, and the Pregnancy Discrimination Act of 1978. These statutes protect job health and safety, provide income protection, and protect against job discrimination.[14]

Types of Employment

In the United States the majority of nurse practitioners are employed by others. In most states employment is "at-will." Many nurse practitioners, however, are offered employment contracts.[4] NPs should know the terms under which they are offered employment and the implications of being hired with or without a written contract.

"At-Will" Employment

"At-will" employment has been practiced in the United States since the latter 19th century and means that an employee or employer may terminate employment for any reason whatsoever. An at-will employee does not have a set term for employment and can quit at anytime and for any reason. The at-will doctrine more simply means that when an employee does not have a written contract and the employment is of an indefinite duration, the employer can fire the employee at any time and for any reason (e.g., for good cause, bad cause, or no cause at all). The at-will doctrine today is qualified by modern antidiscrimination laws and the doctrine of abusive discharge.[14,15]

Independent Contractor

An alternative to at-will employment is that of being an independent contractor. Independent contractors are contracted by another to do something, but are not controlled by the other. Whether a nurse practitioner is considered an employee or independent contractor is important from a liability perspective. A nurse practitioner that is considered an employee has some protection under the doctrine of respondeat superior when alleged to have committed some act of negligence. Under respondeat superior the employer incurs liability for acts of employees when those acts are within the scope of employment. Independent contractors generally do not have respondeat superior protection.[16]

Employment by Contract

An employment contract is a legally enforceable contract that describes the requirements of both the employer and employee. An employment contract can be complex, and it is important that you understand what it contains before you sign it.

Legal language can be difficult to understand, and an NP may want to consider hiring an attorney familiar with employment law and nurse practitioner practice to review a contract before agreeing to it. The following section briefly describes what a contract is.

Contract Defined

A contract is a legally enforceable agreement that can be either implied or expressed. A legally valid contract contains four key elements[14]:

1. Capacity of all the parties

2. Mutual agreement or a meeting of the minds (e.g., a valid offer and acceptance of the offer)

3. Consideration (e.g., something of value that is given in exchange for some promise)

4. Legality of the subject matter of the contract

A contract is an enforceable rule.[14] It does not matter that the rule to be enforced is derived from voluntary agreements between two individuals. This voluntary agreement does not make the rule any less enforceable.[14]

Contracts are binding upon the parties just as is any statute or other law once a contract is made. One party cannot withdraw without agreement by the other.[14] Most legal contracts are reached through negotiation. Negotiation may be formal or informal. Once there is an agreement, or meeting of the minds, on the fundamental elements of that agreement, the parties are bound by the contract. Agreements are defined by the Uniform Commercial Code. Under this code "agreements" are defined as *the bargain of the parties*. This bargain is derived from mutual agreement.[14]

Mutual agreement (assent) of the parties to a contract is usually manifested through the legal concept of the offer and the acceptance. A formal offer is a straightforward way to form an express contract. Generally, an express contract is a formal process because the contract itself usually is communicated in more formally expressed language. This contract may be transmitted by acts or words, spoken or written, directly to the person being offered the contract (the offeree). This may be done through conversation, mail, wire, or by any medium whatsoever. The offer should contain the fundamental elements of the contract.[14]

The deal is bound when the offeree accepts this offer. An acceptance of the offer should be clear and unqualified. When the offeree modifies the offer or attempts to get a better offer, this is treated as a counteroffer. A counteroffer is a rejection of the original offer. However, an offeree must accept in any manner stipulated by the offer. For example, if the offer stipulates that the answer must be received by 12:00 noon on Wednesday, March 20th, failure to have an answer by the defined deadline may void the offer. Additionally, an offer can generally be revoked or withdrawn any time before it is accepted unless the contract includes an option clause.[14]

Elements of an Employment Contract

A written contract can be brief or it can be a lengthy and detailed document. Monarch[16] describes and defines the following minimum terms that need to be included in a written contract:

- *Scope*: describes the activities governed by the written agreement and the services provided by the parties are identified. Services may be stated broadly or listed individually.

- *Effective date*: defines the date when the agreement commences. Dates throughout the written agreement need to be clearly written, with numbers and other symbols used sparingly to avoid confusion.

- *Relationship and responsibilities of the parties*: describes the working relationship of the parties. In this section the nurse practitioner should be identified as either an employee or an independent contractor. If the NP is described as an independent contractor, then this has implications for how the rest of the contract will read. An independent contractor, for example, would not have a contract that dictates when, where, and how the service would be performed. The NP would also not accrue sick leave, annual leave, health insurance, or other company benefits unless those benefits are clearly addressed in the contract. The responsibilities of each party are also defined, and this section may again be brief or lengthy.

- *Confidentiality:* describes how information and documents that are considered confidential will be treated. Although a written contract may contain a simple statement that confidential, proprietary, and trade secret information shall not be disclosed to third parties, if there are any questions about what specific information is protected, it may be important to include that in the contract.

- *Conflict of interest:* statements provided to ensure that both parties are acting in the best interest of the relationship. The clause usually requires the party to disclose the conflict as soon as he or she becomes aware of a potential conflict.

- *Compensation:* describes the payment that will be given once agreed-to services are provided. Compensation may be stated simply, such as in the form of an annual amount to be paid and the dates payments will occur. If productivity payments will be made, the NP should know what formulas are used to determine how bonus payments are determined.

- *Indemnification and subrogation:* indemnification is a statement extended from one party to another, a promise to hold each other harmless for the wrongdoings of the other party. Subrogation in health care matters permits the health care facility, for example, to recover from the NP monetary losses sustained after the agency is found liable for negligence of the NP or other individual to whom the NP delegated any aspect of care or treatment.

- *Dispute resolution:* describes the process to be followed when there is a disagreement between the parties.

- *Term, renewal, and termination:* statements that specify the length of the contract and the process used to renew and terminate the agreement.

- *Remedies for breach:* statements that describe the remedies or consequences of breeching the contract or failing to perform the services as detailed in the contract.

- *Notices:* a statement that identifies the persons who are to receive notice from the other party and includes contact information.

- *Modifying and assigning the agreement:* provisions that describe how the terms of the agreement may be modified without having to implement a new contract.

- *Severability:* a statement that details the noncontested and enforceable provision of the contract in effect.

- *Conflict of laws:* identifies the jurisdiction where the agreement was executed and what jurisdiction governs contractual disputes that may arise.

- *Legal authority:* acknowledges that the parties to the agreement have the authority to enter into the agreement.

- *Force majeure:* ensures that the agreement will not be considered breeched in situations where an act of God prohibits one party from performing in accordance with the terms of the contract.

- *Covenant not to compete:* such covenants limit an NP's ability to enter into any ventures that compete with the interests of the organization with whom the NP is contracting.

- *Signatures:* section wherein the parties sign and date the contract. Once all parties have signed the document, it is considered executed and that a mutual agreement has been reached.

Important Clauses to Understand

Buppert[4] describes three clauses commonly found in employment contracts that can be challenging for NPs to interpret and also can have significant impact on an NP's life. These clauses are (1) restrictive covenants, (2) bonus formulas, and (3) termination clauses.

Restrictive covenants are promises not to compete.[4] In an employment contract such a clause may restrict an employee from practicing within a set number of miles from an employer's business for a set period of time after the employee leaves the employer's business. Such a clause protects the employer, for example, in situations where an NP leaves the practice and a patient follows the NP to the next position. A restrictive covenant is legal in many states. A restrictive covenant clause may be determined unreasonable when the restraint is greater than necessary to protect the employer's legitimate business interests. Sometimes courts consider restrictive covenants unreasonable when the effect is potential harm to the public.[4] It is important to understand the terms of any noncompete agreement because failure to understand the terms may significantly impact your ability to relocate if the job does not work out.[17]

Bonus formulas for NPs vary considerably. It is important that both the employer and employee understand the formula and that it be consistent with quality patient care.[4] The written language for the formula needs to be clearly stated to avoid being interpreted in different ways by different people. Formulas may be productivity-based, quality-based, profit-based, or patient satisfaction–based. Each has its own strengths and weaknesses.[4]

Productivity-based formulas are based on the number of patients seen per year and are a good choice for fee-for-service practices.[4] In this type of productivity arrangement, NPs that see large numbers of patients are considered productive and deserving of a salary bonus. A productivity-based formula is a disadvantage in capitated practices. In a capitated reimbursement arrangement, practices are paid a set fee per patient per month regardless of the number of patient visits. In capitated arrangements, the goal is delivery of quality patient care in as few visits as possible.[4]

Quality measures are a better reflection of productivity than patient numbers in capitated fee arrangements. Under quality productivity formulas, an NP would receive a productivity bonus based on meeting or exceeding some quality standard set by the health plan. This type of productivity is more challenging to track than number of patient visits. Examples of quality measures may include meeting a certain rate of immunization or other preventive screening standards.[4]

Profit-based and patient satisfaction formulas are productivity options too. Profit-based formulas usually reflect some type of profit-sharing plan between employers and NPs. The caveat is to describe clearly beforehand the methods for determining profits. NPs need to understand the accounting method used because these methods can maximize or minimize profits. Profits also are affected by terms such as gross profit or net profit, which in the end means the difference between a bonus and no bonus. Patient satisfaction formulas are sometimes implemented too but have the challenge of being difficult to measure because patient satisfaction is subjective and open to conflicting interpretations.[4]

A *termination-without-cause statement* basically states that an employer can terminate an employee at any time, without cause, with 30 days notice.[4] Such a clause effectively defeats the purpose of an employment contract and also places an NP in a disadvantaged position in regard to assuring other provisions of the contract are adhered too. For example, if an NP protests too much, the employer can simply terminate the NPs employment. One reason to consider a termination-without-cause statement, however, is a situation in which you cannot commit to a full year's employment.[4]

Employment Contracts and Nurse Practitioners

So, what does all of this mean as you negotiate an employment deal? First, you need to know the terms and what to expect. Many new NPs focus on salary and benefits, but there are many professional benefits and nonmonetary aspects of the job to consider.[4] Your first job as an NP also may be the first time you are asked to sign an employment contract. Finch[18] notes:

> The two most important things to remember about employment contracts are: Everything is negotiable; and put it in writing. Both parties should remember that a so-called 'offer of employment' letter may constitute an employment contract. Also, each side should understand to which commitments, if any, each party has agreed. Because of the rights, duties and liabilities that are at stake, the company or the individual would be penny-wise and pound-foolish to enter into an employment contract without the advice of legal counsel.

Terms of your employment translate into benefits (or the lack of them) for you. As a nurse practitioner you bring productivity value to a practice that translates into money and profits and direct income for your employer. Understanding how this works has employment contract considerations for you.

As you negotiate employment, keep in mind the basic terms. Know how you will be employed, such as at-will versus an employment contract. As noted, at-will employment generally means that an employer can fire you for no reason. The exceptions to at-will employment include things such as having a union contract, an individual employment contract with a termination-for-cause stipulation; an implied contract such as an employee handbook; a public policy violation such as termination for jury duty, military reserve service, refusing to perform an illegal act, or whistle blowing; or violation of civil rights laws.[18]

Employment contracts also may include minimum employment term, termination-for-cause stipulations, job title, higher guaranteed salary, performance bonuses, and many other conditions such as medical and life insurance options, tuition reimbursements, car allowance, moving expenses, cell phones, laptops, parking, housing allowances, severance pay, and outplacement.[18] Your employment contract prevents having to negotiate terms of employment on a piecemeal basis and avoids having to reach agreement on issues as the issues arise rather than anticipating many possible issues in advance.[4] So, it is wise to know what the parameters of employment negotiation for NPs are all about.

You want to develop and maintain a good long-term relationship with an employer. One way to do this is to avoid surprises later on, which is one benefit of an employment contract. Although most of us know to review issues such as salary, vacation time, sick days, and insurance coverage, sometimes seemingly minor issues can lead to significant disagreement. For example, you might want to spell out whether sick time or annual leave can be bought out or whether you can roll over unused sick time or annual leave. You also should know whether you can add future family members to your insurance coverage. For example, what happens if you marry after employment? Will your spouse be covered by your insurance? If maternity and child coverage is needed, can it be added?[19]

You also need to know how salary and, as noted, productivity will be handled. Salary usually reflects both the amount of income that you will bring into the practice and the associated costs to the practice. General guidelines to keep in mind when determining what compensation you may expect include understanding what percentage of practice income goes into overhead expenses, what percentage the practice will want to take for net profit, and what percentage of your gross receipts are expected to be used for physician consultation.[20]

Because most employers will want to keep a percentage of your earnings as profit, knowing your monetary contribution minus operational expenses, consultation, and profits is important to understanding how you are paid. To illustrate, overhead expenses include things such as rent, material costs, staff salaries, taxes and benefits, insurance fees, legal fees, and cleaning fees. In a small practice, expenses can be 40% to 50% of the income, whereas in a large practice, expenses are often lower at 20% to 30% of income.[4]

Bupert notes that physician consultation time also varies by the level of experience you bring to the practice. A new nurse practitioner usually has a greater physician consultation time need than a more experienced one. Part of this is simply driven by practice laws requiring collaborative practice agreements, and because of these agreements, most nurse practitioners should expect to pay something for physician consultation. An experienced NP may pay physician consultation at 10% to 15% of their net income; however, a new NP may expect to pay 15% to 25% of net earnings for physician consultation. Both seasoned and new NPs may pay 10% to 15% of net earnings to an employer as profit.[4]

Common salary arrangements also may reflect "straight salary," a "percentage salary," or a "base salary plus a percentage" arrangement. A *straight salary arrangement* means that you are paid a set amount of money to perform according to the job description. In a *percentage arrangement* you are paid the amount you bill minus accounts receivable and minus your portion of practice expenses including physician consultation. In a *base salary plus a percentage arrangement* you are usually guaranteed a certain set salary level but can make more salary if your practice generates income over same set amount. In addition to these types of salary arrangements, some NPs also may be paid on an hourly basis. Generally straight salary arrangements are more common than percentage-based arrangements. The advantage of a percentage-based arrangement is that you can have some control over your earnings, particularly if you are an experienced and productive NP.[4]

How then do you document your monetary contribution to the practice? Income is usually generated as fee-for-service or per-member-per-month basis (in managed care/capitated arrangements). Understanding your income generation on a fee-for-service basis is done by multiplying the number of patient visits by the fee collected per visit. Capitated income is calculated by multiplying the number of patients on your panel by the per-member-per-month fee coming into the practice. An employer's cost for maintaining you in the practice can then be calculated by adding practice expenses and the cost of physician consultation. [4]

One other way of projecting salary is to become familiar with the salary range for the position you are seeking within the community where you are seeking employment. A position with a low salary in the community may reflect financial instability or an undervaluing of your potential contribution. A position with a high salary on the community scale may indicate a job that is undesirable for some reason and consequently hard to fill.[17]

Knowing how salary is determined and knowing the prevailing salary rates within the community are important factors in negotiating a salary with which you will be satisfied. Negotiating is also about strategy. Burke suggests that if a salary range is discussed, such as a range from $65,000 to $70,000, one response might be to simply state that the $70,000 would be acceptable. She also advises against quoting a specific figure unless the limits of the salary range for the job are known because the employer might be willing to offer more than requested. You can always make a counteroffer if the salary quoted is too low.[17] Sometimes getting the salary you want or need boils down to asking for that salary.

Benefits

Negotiating benefits should not be taken lightly. A good benefits package can be worth 20% to 40% of your salary. Burke lists the following benefit items to negotiate:[17]

- Full family medical and dental insurance
- Indemnity plan or managed care
- Acceptable panel of providers

- Point-of-service clause
- Prescription plan
- Vision plan
- Orthodontics
- Preexisting condition clause
- Annual leave
- Sick leave
- Retirement benefits
- Time required for vesting
- Safety of investments in the pension plan
- Optional short-term disability
- Optional long-term care insurance
- Dependent-care reimbursement account
- Health care reimbursement account
- Tax-deferred annuities
- Malpractice insurance
- Opportunities for advancement and career development
- Corporate cellular phone rates
- E-mail access
- Tuition waivers
- Continuing education including travel and registration fee
- Professional dues
- Payment of consulting physician
- Provision of office space, supplies, personnel, and computers
- Payment of answering service and/or pagers

Performance Evaluation

If you have a written employment contract, having a clause concerning how performance evaluation will be measured is also important to avoid unpleasant surprises later on. Employers vary on how performance is measured. Some use highly structured methods such as the number of patients seen per month or quarter, income generated, or implementation of other detailed evaluation tools. Other employers may use no performance measures. Knowing in advance how your performance will be measured affords you a better opportunity to meet employer expectations.[4]

Sample employment contracts are shown in Appendixes C through E.

MOVING TOWARD AN INDEPENDENT PRACTICE: GENERAL CONSIDERATIONS

A successful NP practice, whether it is one in which you are an employee or in which you are the owner, combines specialized graduate education and hard work. Managing that practice also takes research and planning to maximize personal benefits. A major difference for the independent practitioner is that the NP seeking an independent practice also must acquire business knowledge. It takes business talent and skill to get a market advantage. Although you gain clinical skills through graduate education and employment as an NP, and some practical experience concerning how productivity relates to salary and patient outcomes, independent practice success starts with decisive and correct business moves.

At some point you may begin to think about owning a practice. Just as you consider what type of practice environment is right for you, you also must take time up front to explore and evaluate how starting an independent practice will impact your business and personal goals. This careful evaluation is essential for building a comprehensive and well-thought-out business plan that will help you reach these goals.[21] The process of developing a business plan is discussed in Chapter 7. That process will help you think through some important issues that you may not have considered and will become a valuable tool as you set out to raise money for your business. It should also provide milestones by which to gauge your success. The U.S. Small Business Administration details several key questions that should be explored as you get started with a new business.[21] These include knowing something about why you want to go into business, and make no bones about it, operating your own practice is a business. You also need to think about what type of business is right for you and what kind of income you need from that business because that will impact time and resources needed for success. You also need to determine whether your practice will fill a particular business niche. Is there a particular unmet health need or population you will target? Do you have the professional skills for this market? Will it fit a community need and is it practical? Who is your competition and what advantage might your practice have over your competitor? With this in mind, can you deliver a better-quality service and create demand for your practice?

You will need to evaluate realistically what experience you could bring to the practice. Being an excellent health care provider is essential from a quality perspective. And understanding how business works is crucial for practice economic success. This means you will need to explore legal business structures and determine how these fit your practice model. You will need to determine how patient and business records will be maintained. You will need to understand how to manage risks—not just malpractice, but business risks as well. You will need to understand capital resources, where these are generated, and how these resources flow. You may need to learn the language of business financing. You will need to learn about practice space and location and how this impacts practice success. You also have to learn about naming a business. These issues are just a few of the many considerations you will face.

Starting an independent practice is not an endeavor for the faint-hearted! There are many ups and downs of practice ownership. Financial success may come incrementally because it may take awhile to reach a daily patient load that supports higher personal salary and covers all practice expenses. It takes work and good marketing to keep the appointment book filled. Financial difficulties may be a realty until the practice becomes profitable, which could take months or years. New businesses can be hard on family life. You may need to adjust to a lower standard of living or place family assets at risk short-term as the practice is started. You will need the support of your family during this time, and they will need to know what to expect from you.[22]

It will not be possible to remove all the risks associated with starting your own practice. Because *you* are the brains behind the practice, you need to critically analyze your ability to develop practice initiatives, organize your time, and follow through on details. You need to be able to work with many different people including a practice staff, vendors, bankers, attorneys, accountants, and other contractors. You need skills for dealing with the demanding patient as well as skills for dealing with demanding staff, vendors, and other business people. You also must be able to make decisions quickly and maybe while under pressure.[22]

Poor planning is responsible for most business failures. Success depends primarily on foresight and organization. These reasons have been identified as why small businesses fail: lack of experience, insufficient capital, poor location, poor inventory management, overinvestment in fixed assets, poor credit arrangement management, personal use of business funds, and unexpected growth.[23] Failure to seek legal help at critical development stages of the business is another central reason businesses fail.[23]

That said, there are advantages to having and owning an independent practice. You decide on the length of time spent with a patient. You decide how the practice is run. You choose your employees. You control practice quality. You control referrals. You titrate workload to income and keep practice profits.[4]

There are also barriers that must be managed when starting an NP practice. You may need a collaborating physician if your state's scope of practice laws or Medicare requires this. You will need to be on third-party payer panels to get reimbursed for services. You may need hospital privileges. You also may need the authority to admit patients to nursing homes, to order home care, or to direct hospice services.[4]

CONCLUSION

Careful planning is *essential* for practice success. Many of the issues you will encounter as you enter advanced practice and/or think about establishing an independent practice are discussed throughout this book. Ultimately, you must evaluate your clinical confidence and determine what additional education or training you need for the type of advanced practice that best suits you.

REFERENCES

1. Letz K: *Business essentials for nurse practitioners*, Ft Wayne, IN, 2003, PreviCare.
2. Hanson C, Hamric A: Reflections on the continuing evolution of advanced practice nursing, *Nurs Outlook* 51(5):203-211, 2003.
3. American Academy of Nurse Practitioners: *Scope of practice for nurse practitioners*, revised 2002 (website): http://www.aanp.org/NR/rdonlyres/edhltucoxqd2xnrfwbve26d3cowleh5rqqcfmhlc oi3sp7ihpzxry7rdqtkezw5zvpggxsuc7z4iao/scope%2bof%2bpractice%2bv2.pdf. Accessed July 21, 2005.
4. Buppert C: *Nurse practitioner's business practice and legal guide*, ed 2, Boston, 2004, Jones and Bartlett.
5. American Academy of Nurse Practitioners: *Nurse practitioner workforce data survey 2004* (website): http://www.aanp.org/Practice+Policy+and+Legislation/Practice/NP+Workforce+Dat a±Survey+2004.htm. Accessed September 20, 2005.
6. Smolenski MC: Credentialing, certification, and competence: issues for new and seasoned nurse practitioners, *J Am Acad Nurse Pract* 17(6):201-204, 2005.
7. Magdic KS, Hravnak M, McCartney S: Credentialing for nurse practitioners: an update, *AACN Clin Issues* 16(1):16-22, 2005.
8. Waddle F: Licensure: achievements and limitations. In American Nurses Association Committee for the Study of Credentialing in Nursing: *The study of credentialing in nursing: a new approach*, vol II, Kansas City, MO, 1979, American Nurses Association, pp 126-164.
9. Dunphy L, Youngkin E, Smith N: Advanced practice nursing: doing what had to be done, radicals, renegades, and rebels. In Joel L, editor: *Advanced practice nursing: essentials for role development*, Philadelphia, 2004, FA Davis, pp 3-30.
10. Betts V, Keepnews D, Monarch K: The law, the courts, and the advanced practice nurse. In Joel L, editor: *Advanced practice nursing: essentials for role development*, Philadelphia, 2004, FA Davis, pp 612-638.
11. Towers J: Where are we now? The status of nurse practitioner practice in statute and regulation December of 2002, *J Am Acad Nurse Pract* 15(2):50-55, 2003.
12. American Academy of Nurse Practitioners: *Position statement on nurse practitioner prescriptive privilege*, revised 2002 (website): http://www.aanp.org/NR/rdonlyres/esrot7i3abwldz6cennkxif maks2tnlhfgvl7w63xpj67nq6zuj3xwtu5qfpiyyyrmb3lrujkbhjlk/Prescriptive%2bAuthority.pdf. Accessed September 2, 2005.
13. Smith T, Vezina M: Mediated roles: working through other people. In Joel L, editor: *Advanced practice nursing: essentials for role development*, Philadelphia, 2004, FA Davis, pp 455-474.
14. Emerson R: *Business law*, ed 4, Hauppauge, NY, 2004, Barrons.
15. Muhl C: The employment-at-will doctrine: three major exceptions, *Monthly Labor Review* (serial online), January 2001, pp 3-11: http://www.bls.gov/opub/mlr/2001/01/ art1full.pdf. Accessed July 21, 2005.
16. Monarch K: The advanced practice nurse as employee or independent contractor: it makes a difference. In Joel L, editor: *Advanced practice nursing: essentials for role development*, Philadelphia, 2004, FA Davis, pp 534-552.

17. Burke C: Marketing the role: formulating, articulating, and negotiating advanced practice nursing positions. In Stanley J: *Advanced practice nursing: emphasizing common roles*, ed. 2, Philadelphia, 2005, FA Davis, pp 226-254.
18. Finch G: Employment contracts: more than just a handshake, *Consulting-Specifying Engineer* (serial online), June 1, 2005, p 50: http://www.csemag.com/article/CA609776.html?text=employment+and+contracts. Accessed June 2, 2005.
19. Allen C: Associate employment contracts: scrutinize them prior to signing, *DVM Newsmagazine* (serial online), October 1, 2004, pp 38-39:http://www.dvmnews.com/dvm/article/articleDetail.jsp?id=126506. Accessed June 2, 2005.
20. American Academy of Nurse Practitioners Committee on Practice: *Contract negotiation for nurse practitioners* (website): http://www.aanp.org/NR/rdonlyres/eo7k3vikpbqsxrkvlsvvl6w7zozvk5u55x3kgera3nsioplavoqhaas2sc2c3h2kwx7rahdl3fe6pg/NP%252bContract2.pdf. Accessed June 2, 2005.
21. United States Small Business Administration: *Starting Your Business, Startup Basics* (website): http://www.sba.gov/starting_business/startup/basics.html. Accessed June 2, 2005.
22. United States Small Business Administration: *Starting Your Business, Startup Basics, Are you ready?*(website): http://www.sba.gov/starting_business/startup/areyouready.html. Accessed June 2, 2005.
23. United States Small Business Administration: *Starting Your Business, Legal Aspects* (website): http://www.sba.gov/starting_business/legal/buslaws.html. Accessed June 2, 2005.

Scope of Practice

SALLY J. REEL

*N*urse practitioners (NPs) are registered nurses with specialized advanced education who provide primary care, acute care, and/or long-term health care in a variety of health care settings. NPs provide care to individuals, families, and groups according to the specific NP specialty in which the NP is prepared to practice.[1] *Scope of practice* refers to the legal authority granted to a professional to provide and be reimbursed for health care services.[2] Scope of practice determines the limits and privileges of an NP's license as well as whom an NP can see and treat and under what circumstance or guidance an NP can provide care to patients.[3] Other related terms include *standards of practice* and *standards of care*.

SCOPE OF PRACTICE

The legal environment for nursing practice is derived from legislation, regula- tions, and the action of courts that interpret and enforce laws. Advanced practice, in particular, is influenced by legislation that is passed in the U.S. Congress and by state legislatures. Trotter Betts[4] notes that "Legislation defines the legal authority for practice, legal responsibilities of practitioners, many of the penalties for failing to live up to those legal responsibilities, and other critical aspects of practice, including reimbursement."

State legislatures and Congress define different responsibilities. Congress generally passes laws that relate to national or federal issues and the states address health care issues. For example, Congress votes on legislation involving use of federal funds such as Medicare and has the power to define and shape the Medicare program. States define many health care issues such as licensure requirements for health care professionals and the scope of practice of nurse practitioners and other advance practice nurses. State legislatures define issues of collaborative practice and the limits on nurse practitioner prescriptive authority.[4]

State laws and rules provide the legal authority for nursing practice. The legal scope of practice for NPs is found in the Nurse Practice Act of each state and the District of Columbia.[4] The rules governing NP practice are created by multiple stakeholders, but the regulation of practice is generally left to states. Sources of law affecting nurse practitioner practice include statutory law, administrative law, and judicial law. *Statutory law* is derived from Congress or state legislatures. Nurse practice acts are statutory laws. *Administrative law* has to do with administrative agencies, boards, and commissions legislated by Congress or state legislatures (e.g., State Board of Nursing). *Judicial law* results from judicial opinions.[5]

Nurse Practice Acts

Historically, NPs usually practiced under a physician's direction or orders, and without an order, practice was limited to traditional nursing roles. NP practice has evolved significantly, and legal authority to practice has expanded over time as well. NP roles continue to expand and change; thus issues about scope of practice often lack clearly defined parameters.[5]

Each state has a legal Nurse Practice Act that is designed to protect the public. Although it is beyond this chapter to describe legal authority for NP practice by state, Susanne Phillips[6] provided a comprehensive review of legislation affecting advanced practice for *The Nurse Practitioner*. Figure 2-1 provides a summary of advanced practice nurse legislation related to legal authority for scope of practice.

The Nurse Practice Act is the most significant law affecting practice in each state. NPs are required to practice within the limits of the Nurse Practice Act within the state they are licensed to practice. Nurse Practice Acts usually are written broadly and language varies by state.[5] Scope of practice, or the legal boundaries of professional nurse activities, is defined under the Nurse Practice Act. Whether or not an NP can diagnose, treat, prescribe medications for, or manage a patient's care is addressed in the Nurse Practice Act. Detailed descriptions are usually found in the rules and regulations publicized by state boards of nursing. Some state medical boards also have rules affecting NP practice. Nurse practice acts may be challenging to interpret because they are statutory laws; thus any amendments to the act must be accomplished through the legislative process, which can be slow. Regardless, failure to practice within these limits opens an NP to charges of violating the Nurse Practice Act for that state.[5]

State Boards of Nursing

State boards of nursing significantly influence NP practice. The state boards of nursing get their authority from the Nurse Practice Act, which creates and authorizes the board to administer and enforce the rules about the nursing profession. State boards of nursing establish requirements for obtaining an NP license. Many state boards of nursing, for example, require national certification (see Chapter 4) as a prerequisite for NP licensure.[5]

Violating the scope of practice as defined by the Nurse Practice Act or any official ruling of the State Board of Nursing may result in disciplinary action. Whenever there is a question about the board's position on a practice issue, an NP can telephone the board and ask whether there is a specific ruling about the

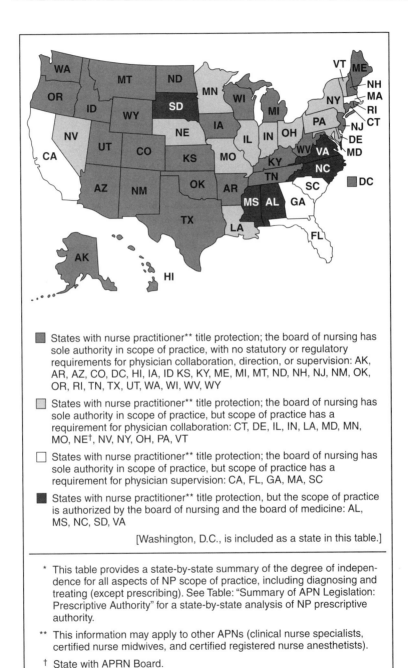

States with nurse practitioner** title protection; the board of nursing has sole authority in scope of practice, with no statutory or regulatory requirements for physician collaboration, direction, or supervision: AK, AR, AZ, CO, DC, HI, IA, ID KS, KY, ME, MI, MT, ND, NH, NJ, NM, OK, OR, RI, TN, TX, UT, WA, WI, WV, WY

States with nurse practitioner** title protection; the board of nursing has sole authority in scope of practice, but scope of practice has a requirement for physician collaboration: CT, DE, IL, IN, LA, MD, MN, MO, NE†, NV, NY, OH, PA, VT

States with nurse practitioner** title protection; the board of nursing has sole authority in scope of practice, but scope of practice has a requirement for physician supervision: CA, FL, GA, MA, SC

States with nurse practitioner** title protection, but the scope of practice is authorized by the board of nursing and the board of medicine: AL, MS, NC, SD, VA

[Washington, D.C., is included as a state in this table.]

* This table provides a state-by-state summary of the degree of independence for all aspects of NP scope of practice, including diagnosing and treating (except prescribing). See Table: "Summary of APN Legislation: Prescriptive Authority" for a state-by-state analysis of NP prescriptive authority.

** This information may apply to other APNs (clinical nurse specialists, certified nurse midwives, and certified registered nurse anesthetists).

† State with APRN Board.

Figure 2-1

Summary of advanced practice nurse (APN) legislation: legal authority for scope of practice. *From Phillips SJ: Nurse Pract 31(1):6-11, 2006.*

issue in question and what the conditions are to engage in that specific practice issue.[5] For example, in Arizona NP's may complete a death certificate, but there is a specific education module that must be completed before an NP is qualified to do so.[7] If the state board has not ruled on a particular practice issue, an NP may write the board for a ruling; however, some boards may not provide a formal ruling but may provide a decision-making algorithm to which an NP may refer to answer the question based on applicable laws and regulations.[5]

NPs may obtain a copy of the Nurse Practice Act by contacting the State Board of Nursing.[5] Scope of practice statements and advanced practice rules and regulations also may be found on the Internet site for state boards of nursing or by browsing the National Council of State Boards of Nursing (NCSBN) website at www.NCSBN.org.[8] The contact information for each State Board of Nursing is shown in Appendix A.

Stakeholders: The Role of Professional Bodies and Determining Scope of Practice

Although legislation, laws, and rules provide legal authority for nurse practitioner practice, the nursing profession itself plays a significant role in determining both the context of practice and standards of practice on which legislatures, courts, and other governmental agencies base their actions.[4] Professional organizations such as the American Academy of Nurse Practitioners (AANP) and other national nursing organizations such as the American Nurses Association (ANA) work daily to improve the practice of NPs nationwide. National organizations do impact NP practice from the global perspective and also where federal policy change is required. National organizations also may influence statutory changes at the state level as well.[6] National organizations also may publish standards of practice that influence the quality of NP practice.

STANDARDS OF PRACTICE

Standards of practice refers to a minimum set of criteria outlining practice competency and provides a standard by which others can judge the quality of care that an NP provides. Standards of care are usually found in most nurse practice acts.[5] Standards are developed nationally by stakeholder groups such as the ANA and the AANP. Standards are broad, authoritative statements that the nursing profession uses to describe the responsibilities for which members are accountable. Nurse practitioners are accountable to the standards of practice publicized by both the nursing profession and various advanced practice nursing specialties.[8]

Standards of practice are not new. Early nursing leaders called for standards as early as the 1890s, and in 1950 the ANA adopted the first *Code of Ethics for Nursing* that established written nursing standards of care.[5] The latest *Code of Ethics* may be viewed online at the American Nurses Association website (http://www.nursingworld.org/ethics/ecode.htm). The provisions and the interpretive statements are both copyrighted, and the full code with interpretive statements for practice may be purchased from the ANA at http://nursingworld.org/books/pdescr.cfm?cnum=24#CEN21.[9] ANA also publishes standards of practice for nursing. The latest version, *Nursing: Scope and Standards of Practice*, can be purchased online at http://nursingworld.org/books/pdescr.cfm?cnum=15#03SSNP. An example of standards of practice published by the AANP is shown in Box 2-1.[10]

BOX 2-1	AMERICAN ACADEMY OF NURSE PRACTITIONERS STANDARDS OF PRACTICE

I. Qualifications

Nurse practitioners are primary care providers who practice in ambulatory, acute, and long-erm care. They are registered nurses with specialized advanced education and clinical competency to provide health and medical care for diverse populations in a variety of primary care, acute, and long-term care settings. A Master's degree is required for entry level practice.

II. Process of Care

The nurse practitioner utilizes the scientific process and national standards of care as a framework for managing patient care. This process includes:

A. Assessment of health status

The nurse practitioner assesses health status by:
- Obtaining a relevant health and medical history
- Performing a physical examination based on age and history
- Performing or ordering preventive and diagnostic procedures based on the patient's age and history
- Identifying health and medical risk factors

B. Diagnosis

The nurse practitioner makes a diagnosis by:
- Utilizing critical thinking in the diagnostic process
- Synthesizing and analyzing the collected data
- Formulating a differential diagnosis based on the history, physical examination, and diagnostic test results
- Establishing priorities to meet the health and medical needs of the individual, family, or community

C. Development of a treatment plan

The nurse practitioner, together with the patient and family, establishes an evidence-based, mutually acceptable, cost-awareness plan of care that maximizes health potential. Formulation of the treatment plan includes:
- Ordering additional diagnostic tests
- Prescribing/ordering appropriate pharmacologic and nonpharmacologic interventions
- Developing a patient education plan
- Appropriate consultation/referral

Continued

BOX 2-1	AMERICAN ACADEMY OF NURSE PRACTITIONERS STANDARDS OF PRACTICE—cont'd

D. Implementation of the plan

Interventions are based upon established priorities.
Actions by the nurse practitioners are:
- Individualized
- Consistent with the appropriate plan of care
- Based on scientific principles, theoretical knowledge, and clinical expertise
- Consistent with teaching and learning opportunities

Actions include:
- Accurately conducting, supervising, and interpreting diagnostic tests
- Prescribing/ordering pharmacologic agents and nonpharmacologic therapies
- Providing relevant patient education
- Making appropriate referrals to other health professionals and community agencies

E. Follow-up and evaluation of the patient status

The nurse practitioner maintains a process for systematic follow-up by:
- Determining the effectiveness of the treatment plan with documentation of patient care outcomes
- Reassessing and modifying the plan with the patient and family as necessary to achieve health and medical goals

III. Care Priorities

The nurse practitioner's practice model emphasizes:

A. Patient and family education

The nurse practitioner provides health education and utilizes community resource opportunities for the individual and/or family.

B. Facilitation of patient participation in self care

The nurse practitioner facilitates patient participation in health and medical care by providing information needed to make decisions and choices about:
- Promotion, maintenance, and restoration of health
- Consultation with other appropriate health care personnel
- Appropriate utilization of health care resources

C. Promotion of optimal health

D. Provider of continually competent care

E. Facilitation of entry into the health care system

F. The promotion of a safe environment

IV. Interdisciplinary/Collaborative Responsibilities

The nurse practitioner participates as a team member in the provision of health and medical care, interacting with professional colleagues to provide comprehensive care.

V. Accurate Documentation of Patient Status and Care

The nurse practitioner maintains accurate, legible, and confidential records.

Continued

BOX 2-1	AMERICAN ACADEMY OF NURSE PRACTITIONERS STANDARDS OF PRACTICE—cont'd

VI. Responsibility as Patient Advocate

Ethical and legal standards provide the basis of patient advocacy. As an advocate, the nurse practitioner participates in health policy activities at the local, state, national, and international levels.

VII. Quality Assurance and Continued Competence

Nurse practitioners recognize the importance of continued learning through:
- Participation in quality assurance review, including systematic review of records and treatment plans on a periodic basis
- Maintenance of current knowledge by attending continuing education programs
- Maintenance of certification in compliance with current state law
- Applying standardized care guidelines in clinical practice

VIII. Adjunct Roles of Nurse Practitioner

Nurse practitioners combine the roles of provider, mentor, educator, researcher, manager, and consultant. The nurse practitioner interprets the role of the nurse practitioner to individuals, families, and other professionals.

IX. Research as Basis for Practice

Nurse practitioners support research by developing clinical research questions, conducting or participating in studies, and disseminating and incorporating findings into practice.

© American Academy of Nurse Practitioners, 1993; revised 1998, 2002.

STANDARDS OF CARE

Standards of care differ from standards of practice. Standards of care also may be referred to as *practice guidelines*. Practice guidelines provide a basis for health care providers to administer patient care and are the standards by which safety and competent care are judged. Practice guidelines may crosscut health care disciplines, and this means that standards used to evaluate NP practice are often the same as the standards used to review medical practice. Practice guidelines are derived from evidence-based practice. Agencies such as the Agency for Healthcare Research and Quality and the Centers for Disease Control and Prevention (CDC), as well as medical and nursing specialty organizations, put out practice guidelines.[8]

Practice standards have significant legal implications because the basis for malpractice lawsuits centers on the allegation that an NP failed to meet certain standards of care and that failing to meet these standards resulted in harm to the patient. In legal proceedings, the plaintiff must present evidence through means such as expert witnesses to support the contention that the standard of care was breeched, and the NP also must present evidence that the standards were *not* breeched. The court may consider written standards when standards of care are reviewed and may seek information about national standards as well as information about the policies of the NP's employer. National standards are usually the recognized standards in legal cases, and ANA's standards, for example, are likely to be more influential than local standards. Additionally, NP's who perform the same medical services as physicians are subject to the same practice standards and liabilities as physicians.[5]

Sometimes practice guidelines are used to refer to a collaborative practice agreement between an NP and a physician to define the parameters of practice for the NP. A collaborative agreement may vary from a short, one-page document to a more detailed agreement that spells out specifically prescribed protocols for specific functions based on state statutes defining NP practice. Hanson[8] notes:

> The term *protocol* in relation to advanced nursing practice was common several years ago as a physician-directed, specified guideline for the medical aspects of practice that defined each patient problem and the care directive. Some states used this "cookbook" approach to NP practice as a way to oversee prescriptive and other treatment modalities. For the most part, specific protocols for care are no longer used in most settings because it is difficult to update them and tailor them to the individual needs of patients and practices. More importantly, advanced nursing practice has evolved. As APNs [advanced practice nurses] have proven their ability to provide competent care with positive outcomes, protocols have been replaced by evidenced-based practice guidelines and collaborative practice agreements.

Some current NPs may have practiced under protocols.

SCOPE OF PRACTICE CHALLENGES

NP specialty practice often produces questions about who is qualified to practice in certain settings or who may provide care to certain patients. Scope of practice is usually legally explicated for each advanced practice nursing specialty group (see Box 2-2).[8] This is an important criteria to remember when considering whether to open an independent NP practice or when considering a specific job offer because practicing outside the scope of practice is one of the most significant liability issues for NPs. Scope of practice breeches may occur, for example, when a pediatric nurse practitioner (PNP) assesses and treats an ear infection in an adult and potentially misdiagnoses the case because the disease process may differ between a child and an adult. Another example of practicing beyond one's scope of practice is that of an NP who is not familiar with the Nurse Practice Act in the state where the NP is currently practicing orders a treatment or performs a procedure that is legal in one state but illegal in another state.[11]

As scope of practice has evolved for NPs over time, the current standards of collaborative relationships, prescriptive authority, and reimbursement issues are increasingly providing greater practice autonomy for NPs. For example, NPs are experiencing increased collaboration and autonomy with less direct supervision, increased prescriptive authority privileges, and greater recognition by third-party

| BOX 2-2 | AMERICAN ACADEMY OF NURSE PRACTITIONERS SCOPE OF PRACTICE FOR NURSE PRACTITIONERS |

Professional Role

Nurse practitioners are primary care providers who practice in ambulatory, acute, and long-term care settings. According to their practice specialty, these providers provide nursing and medical services to individuals, families, and groups. In addition to diagnosing and managing acute episodic and chronic illnesses, nurse practitioners emphasize health promotion and disease prevention. Services include, but are not limited to, ordering, conducting, supervising, and interpreting diagnostic and laboratory tests, and prescription of pharmacologic agents and nonpharmacologic therapies. Teaching and counselling individuals, families, and groups are a major part of nurse practitioner practice.

Nurse practitioners practice autonomously and in collaboration with health care professionals and other individuals to diagnose, treat, and manage the patient's health problems. They serve as health care researchers, interdisciplinary consultants, and patient advocates.

Education

Entry level preparation for nurse practitioner practice is a master's degree. Didactic and clinical courses prepare nurses with specialized knowledge and clinical competency to practice in primary care, acute care, and long-term care. Self-directed continued learning and professional development beyond the formal advanced education is essential to maintain clinical competency.

Accountability

The autonomous nature of the nurse practitioner's advanced clinical practice requires accountability for health care outcomes. Ensuring the highest quality of care requires certification, periodic peer review, clinical outcome evaluations, a code for ethical practice, evidence of continuing professional development, and maintenance of clinical skills. Nurse practitioners are committed to seeking and sharing knowledge that promotes quality health care and improves clinical outcomes. This is accomplished by leading and participating in both professional and lay health care forums, conducting research, and applying findings to clinical practice.

Responsibility

The role of the nurse practitioner continues to evolve in response to changing societal and health care needs. As leaders in primary and acute health care, nurse practitioners combine the roles of provider, mentor, educator, researcher, and administrator. Members of the profession are responsible for advancing the role of the nurse practitioner and ensuring that the standards of the profession are maintained. This is accomplished through involvement in professional organizations and participation in health policy activities at the local, state, national, and international levels.

© American Academy of Nurse Practitioners, 1993; revised, 1998, 2002.

payers for reimbursement of services. All of these gains in scope of practice open an NP to increased liability as well, especially in the areas of diagnostic responsibilities and prescriptive authority. As noted, under earlier nurse practice acts, all nurses worked under the supervision of physicians, but as NP practices are evolving, many NPs work under a collaborative agreement instead of working for a physician in a complementary role.[11] Every state also has some degree of prescriptive authority for nurse practitioners,[12] and all but four states allow NPs to prescribe controlled substances (Figure 2-2).[6]

A point of clarification is that *collaboration* generally does not mean "delegatory" or "supervisory," but in a few states these terms do persist. Regulated collaboration ranges from having a physician available for consultation or referral to submitting a signed written agreement to some of the state boards of nursing—sometimes for approval and sometimes for recording and documenting the parties' agreement to participate in a collaborative agreement. Some states still require specific information such as lists or categories of medications that the nurse practitioners may prescribe.[12] Yet, collaboration is changing because 27 states, including the District of Columbia, no longer require statutory or regulatory requirements for physician collaboration, direction, or supervision (see Figure 2-1).[6]

Scope of practice breeches also may occur when practice crosses specialty roles. State boards of nursing and credentialing bodies are raising questions about appropriateness of some practice opportunities with respect to one's NP specialty preparation. For example, historically the NP role evolved within primary care settings, but more opportunities have emerged allowing NPs to practice in acute-care and subspecialty settings. Where this gets "sticky" is determining appropriateness of the primary care NP to practice with specialized populations. Additionally, an NP prepared as an acute care NP (ACNP) is usually not prepared to practice in a primary care setting. Breeching scope of practice may occur if a geriatric nurse practitioner (GNP) assesses and treats a 25-year-old adult or if an adult nurse practitioner (ANP) assesses and treats a child. Conversely, having a physician supervise, cosign, or otherwise endorse a practice or procedure does not make the practice or procedure legal unless such practice or procedure is allowed by the state's legal scope of practice.[3]

CONCLUSION

As NP practice continually evolves, so too will scope-of-practice and related regulatory issues. Because variance exists among the states with respect to what constitutes an NP's legal scope of practice, it is imperative that one understands the Nurse Practice Act and legislative rules that govern in the state where an NP intends to practice. As practice boundaries blur, it is also imperative to know the State Board's position regarding whether a certain practice or procedure falls within the legal NP scope of practice. When in question, contact the advanced practice consultant at the State Board of Nursing for information and direction about the legality of the practice.

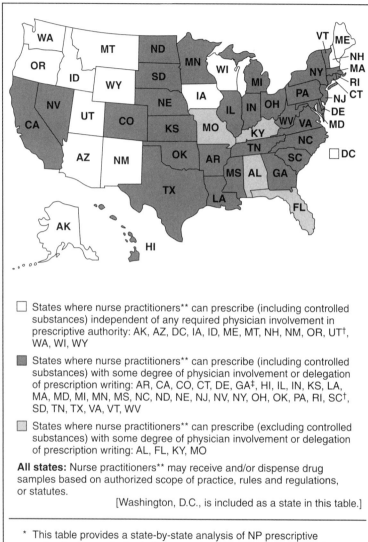

States where nurse practitioners** can prescribe (including controlled substances) independent of any required physician involvement in prescriptive authority: AK, AZ, DC, IA, ID, ME, MT, NH, NM, OR, UT†, WA, WI, WY

States where nurse practitioners** can prescribe (including controlled substances) with some degree of physician involvement or delegation of prescription writing: AR, CA, CO, CT, DE, GA‡, HI, IL, IN, KS, LA, MA, MD, MI, MN, MS, NC, ND, NE, NJ, NV, NY, OH, OK, PA, RI, SC†, SD, TN, TX, VA, VT, WV

States where nurse practitioners** can prescribe (excluding controlled substances) with some degree of physician involvement or delegation of prescription writing: AL, FL, KY, MO

All states: Nurse practitioners** may receive and/or dispense drug samples based on authorized scope of practice, rules and regulations, or statutes.

[Washington, D.C., is included as a state in this table.]

* This table provides a state-by-state analysis of NP prescriptive authority. For analysis of other aspects of the NP scope of practice (including diagnosing and treating), see Table: "Summary of APN Legislation: Legal Authority for Scope of Practice."

** The information may apply to other APNs (clinical nurse specialists, certified nurse midwives, and certified registered nurse anesthetists).

† Schedule IV and/or V controlled substances only.

‡ Nurse practitioners do not have written prescribing or dispensing authority; the process falls under delegated medical authority.

Figure 2-2

Summary of APN legislation: prescriptive authority. *From Phillips SJ: Nurse Pract 31(1):6-11, 2006.*

REFERENCES

1. American Academy of Nurse Practitioners: *Scope of Practice* (website): http://www.aanp.org/Publications/AANP+Position+Statements/Position+Statements+and+Papers.asp. Accessed February 10, 2006.
2. Hamric A: A definition of advanced practice nursing. In Hamric AB, Spross JA, Hanson CH: *Advanced practice nursing: an integrative approach*, ed 3, Philadelphia, 2005, Saunders, pp 85-108.
3. Klein T: Scope of practice and the nurse practitioner: regulation, competency, expansion, and evolution, *Topics Adv Pract Nurs eJournal* 5(2), 2005 (serial online): http://www.medscape.com/viewprogram/4188_pnt. Accessed February 9, 2006.
4. Trotter Betts V: The law, the courts, and the advanced practice nurse. In Joel L: *Advanced practice nursing: essentials for role development*, Philadelphia, 2004, FA Davis, pp 612-638.
5. *Nurse Practitioner's Legal Reference*, Springhouse, PA, 2001, Springhouse.
6. Phillips SJ:A comprehensive look at the legislative issues affecting advanced nursing practice, *Nurse Pract* 31(1):6-11, 2006.
7. Arizona State Board of Nursing: *Death Certificate Education* (website): http://www.azbn.org/DeathCertificates.asp. Accessed February 22, 2006.
8. Hanson CH: Understanding regulatory, legal, and credentialing requirements. In Hamric AB, Spross JA, Hanson CH: *Advanced practice nursing: an integrative approach*, ed 3, Philadelphia, 2005, Saunders, p 781.
9. American Nurses Association: *Code of Ethics* (website): http://nursingworld.org/books/pdescr.cfm?cnum=24#CEN21. Accessed February 24, 2006.
10. American Academy of Nurse Practitioners: *Standards of Practice* (website): http://www.aanp.org/Publications/AANP+Position+Statements/Position+Statements+and+Papers.asp. Accessed February 10, 2006.
11. NSO Risk Advisor: *Navigating the legal waters of specialty practices*, vol 13, 2005 (serial online): http://www.nso.com/newsletters/advisor/2005/NSO05_NP.pdf. Accessed February 10, 2006.
12. Towers J: Where are we now? The status of nurse practitioner practice in statute and regulation December of 2002, *J Am Acad Nurse Pract* 15(2):50-55, 2003.

Nurse Practitioners and Prescriptive Authority

JAN TOWERS

*A*lthough prescribing drugs is only one component of the role of the nurse practitioner, it has become one of the central practice activities with which nurse practitioners have had to struggle over the years. Currently nurse practitioners prescribe legend drugs under their own signature in 49 states and the District of Columbia. They prescribe controlled drugs under their own signature in all but five states. In 37 states, nurse practitioners have no limitations or are authorized to prescribe schedules II through V controlled drugs. They have been found to be safe prescribers and thorough in their evaluations of patients who are candidates for prescription medications.[1] Multiple studies have found nurse practitioners to be as safe as and often safer than physicians when comparisons are made within the nurse practitioners' scope of practice.[2]

In studies conducted by the American Academy of Nurse Practitioners,[3-5] nurse practitioner prescribing patterns followed the scope of practice of the specialty of the nurse practitioner—that is, family nurse practitioners and adult nurse practitioners most often prescribed antimicrobials, antiinflammatories, analgesics, antihypertensive bronchodilators, diabetic agents, and cardiovascular drugs. Women's health nurse practitioners most often prescribed contraceptives and gynecologic antimicrobials. Pediatric nurse practitioners most often prescribed antimicrobials and respiratory medications.

The mean daily number of prescriptions written by nurse practitioners is 19.[4,5] Family nurse practitioners and nurse practitioners practicing in emergency rooms prescribe the highest number of drugs per day (23 and 26, respectively), and neonatal nurse practitioners and nurse practitioners practicing in schools and occupational health settings prescribe the fewest (6, 8, and 9, respectively).[5] Adult, family, gerontologic, and psychiatric–mental health nurse practitioners have been found to prescribe controlled drugs at least once a week.[4] In Goolsby's 2004 survey,[5] approximately half of the nurse practitioners were prescribing or recommending herbal agents as well.

ESTABLISHING PRESCRIBING ACTIVITIES IN PRACTICE

Although nurse practitioners' prescribing patterns are consistent within the professional scope of practice for their specialty, there are some variations in state regulatory parameters. It is important, when establishing a practice, to understand the parameters for prescribing in the state in which the practice is to be located. Although the majority of states have no limitations, a few states limit the schedules of controlled drugs (Figure 3-1) that may be prescribed, and a few set limits on the number of pills or tablets and/or the number of refills of controlled drugs that may be prescribed by a nurse practitioner.

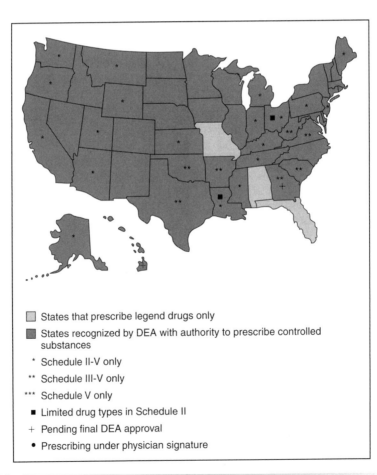

☐ States that prescribe legend drugs only

■ States recognized by DEA with authority to prescribe controlled substances

* Schedule II-V only

** Schedule III-V only

*** Schedule V only

■ Limited drug types in Schedule II

\+ Pending final DEA approval

• Prescribing under physician signature

Figure 3-1

Nurse practitioner prescriptive authority. *From American Academy of Nurse Practitioners, 2006.*

As the inappropriateness of these limitations is discovered, state statutes and regulations are being changed. However, when establishing a practice, it will be important to know the legal parameters for prescribing in the state and make arrangements for patient needs that exceed those limitations. This usually means making an arrangement with a collaborating/consulting physician for assistance with prescribing for those patients. Some state statutes and administrative rules require a formal collaborative agreement with a physician, others do not. It is important for nurse practitioners to make appropriate arrangements for prescription needs of patients in those states where limitations occur.

THE GROWTH OF PRESCRIPTIVE AUTHORITY

The ability to prescribe was not granted overnight. In the early days, nurse practitioners focused on expanding their nursing roles into assessment and diagnosis, relying on physicians to provide pharmacologic prescription when it was needed. As the nurse practitioner role developed, it became clear that nurse practitioners needed to treat as well as assess, to manage acute episodic health problems as well as advocate for health promotion/disease prevention. As the role developed farther, nurse practitioners also found themselves managing patients with chronic diseases that needed to be treated. At first nurse practitioners managed "common" chronic conditions, but as their role developed both in their care of vulnerable populations and in private insured patients, they began to manage a wide range of illnesses. Thus, in addition to using their nursing expertise in the areas of health promotion/disease prevention, patient counseling, and education, they were managing acute episodic and chronic diseases in their patients, hence the creation of a hybrid clinician who brought both nursing and medical skills to patient care. Initially, the practice arena was limited to primary care. Now it has expanded to include subspecialty and acute care.

DEVELOPMENT OF EDUCATIONAL PROGRAMS

With the expansion of the role of the nurse practitioner came the expansion of educational programs to prepare them. Early programs, not then accepted by the nursing education community, were initiated in a variety of settings: hospitals, schools of medicine, planned parenthood, and continuing education programs in nursing education facilities. The majority of the early programs were post RN certificate programs of approximately one academic year that offered continuing education certificates. As the concept caught on, and the need for primary care providers increased, it became clear that nurses in expanded roles could undertake some of the care provided by primary care physicians. The interest of the federal government in enhancing this role in the 1970s stimulated schools of nursing to espouse the educational preparation of nurse practitioners by funding graduate programs that would give significant advanced educational preparation to nurses, thus preparing them for a more significant role in the provision of primary care in this country. A major component of these educational programs included the assessment and diagnosis of the undifferentiated patient and the treatment of these patients. That treatment included prescribing appropriate medications for patients coming to the nurse practitioner for treatment. The pharmacology content of these programs built on the pharmacology presented in the student's undergraduate education and prepared them for prescribing medications independently for their patients.

Over time, the gold standard for nurse practitioner educational programs became the master's degree. Certificate programs died out, and regulators began building the master's requirement into their administrative rules throughout the country. Today there are virtually no certificate programs left in the country, and the gold standard has become master's nurse practitioner preparation with national certification in their specialty. As we move into the 21st century, the concept of clinical doctoral preparation to supplant the master's preparation has begun to evolve, reinforcing the high standards that have been demonstrated in nurse practitioner education and practice over the years.

CHANGES IN THE LAW

Although the nurse practitioner role expanded and educational programs developed, it became clear that in order for nurse practitioners to prescribe medications, changes would need to take place in the laws that govern nursing practice. Some statutes had language that prohibited nurses from performing acts of medical diagnosis and prescribing therapeutics, whereas others were silent on the matter. They did not authorize nurses to practice beyond the scope laid out in the nurse practice act and its rules and regulations. In order to legitimize the prescription of "medical therapeutics," statutes and administrative rules had to be changed. Because professional licensure takes place at the state level, the changes that would give title recognition to nurse practitioners and authorize them to prescribe medications under their own signature had to occur at the state level as well. And so it began, state by state. As the role grew and a significant body of nurse practitioners began to enter practice in each state, boards of nursing, boards of medicine, and legislatures were petitioned to make changes in statutes and regulations that would legitimize the practice of a nurse practitioner and subsequently the prescribing of medications.

Initially support from the medical community assisted nurse practitioners in their bid for title recognition and prescriptive authority. The two did not always occur simultaneously, with title recognition often coming before the authority to prescribe. In many states the authorization of joint promulgation of rules and regulations for nurse practitioner practice by boards of nursing and boards of medicine opened the way for nurse practitioners to prescribe. At that time, much of the nursing community was reluctant to support nurses who wanted to cross the line into what had been strictly the arena of medicine. As a result, jointly promulgated rules were often developed that included the oversight of a physician who would supervise and delegate prescriptive authority to the nurse practitioner. Although some states used delegatory rules to allow nurse practitioners to prescribe, others such as North Carolina developed limited formularies that would be used by nurse practitioners who were authorized to prescribe. Initially only legend drugs could be prescribed, but later as the need arose, the authority to prescribed controlled drugs began to emerge.

Several patterns for authorizing nurse practitioner prescriptive authority have emerged over the years. They included the use of established formularies, exclusionary formularies, collaborative formularies, and open formularies. *Exclusionary formularies* consist of a list of drugs or drug categories developed by regulators that state what nurse practitioners can prescribe. These lists have to be periodically updated as new drugs come on the market. Oregon continues to have this system, with regular updates to keep the list current. *Negative* or *exclusionary formularies* consist of a short list of drugs or drug formularies not allowed to be prescribed by nurse practitioners. These too are traditionally developed by regulators. Oklahoma uses this type of formulary. These two formularies are often developed with guidance from advisory committees of nurse practitioners, nurse practitioners, and other advanced practice nurses or committees comprised of nurse practitioners, advanced practice nurses, and other health care professionals such as pharmacists and physicians. *Collaborative formularies* are formularies developed by a nurse practitioner and a collaborating physician. These formularies are based on the types of patients seen in the nurse practitioner's practice. Maryland State uses collaborative formularies. *Open formularies* set no limitations on prescribing. Washington State uses an open formulary. Increasingly, states are moving to open formularies.[1] Where established and collaborative formularies are still used, efforts are made to be all inclusive so that nurse practitioners may practice to their full scope of practice.

These prescribing patterns developed through one of three routes. The first included amendments to the state's nurse practice act, authorizing nurse practitioners to practice, and allowing them to prescribe medications in their practice. In these instances, willing legislators had to be found to introduce legislation that would authorize nurse practitioners to prescribe. Often these statutory changes included requirements for education, national certification, and limits on what the nurse practitioner could prescribe. Language establishing required relationships with physicians was often included. Once a statute was passed, regulators such as boards of nursing were instructed to promulgate administrative rules for the implementation of the statute. Initially, both boards of nursing and boards of medicine were authorized to jointly develop those rules. More recently, boards of nursing alone have been authorized to develop these rules. In most states these rules must pass legislative scrutiny and be signed by the governor to be implemented. Currently only five states continue to have administrative rules promulgated jointly by boards of nursing and medicine.

The second included the development of administrative rules by a regulatory body such as the board of nursing. This can be done where statutes have broad authorization with no prohibitions regarding the activities that nurse practitioners undertake. Again, in most states such regulations still must undergo legislative scrutiny such as approval by a specific legislative committee or commission appointed by the legislature and require signing by the governor. Strictly regulatory changes do not require the efforts that are needed to have legislation introduced, passed through committees of jurisdiction, and subsequently two houses in the state legislature before being signed by the governor. However, making regulatory changes can be as prolonged as the statutory process, if there are parties that would prefer that a particular regulation not be passed.

The third route is for "stand-alone" legislation to be introduced that confers prescriptive authority without amending the nurse practice act. This method avoids "opening" the state's nurse practice act whereby other undesirable amendments might be included that could create problems for passage or for the profession and would most likely cause its defeat. Stand-alone legislation is very visible and often can become an easy target for those who wish to defeat it. As with all statutes, this legislation still requires the development of administrative rules for its implementation.

The bottom line is that changing statues and administrative rules and regulations is a slow and cumbersome process at best. Because required statutory and regulatory changes for professional practice occur at the state level, the progression of conferring prescriptive authority for nurse practitioners has been uneven. In states where primary care providers are needed and the worth of nurse practitioners has been recognized, the movement toward the use of open formularies and the independent practice of nurse practitioners has moved quickly. Although in those states where bureaucratic barriers and less recognition of the valuable contribution nurse practitioners can make exists, change has occurred more slowly. Active involvement of nurse practitioners, their patients, and other interested parties helps with the passage of both legislation and regulation that allow nurse practitioners to function at the full scope of practice for which they are educationally prepared. Gradually, as nurse practitioners have demonstrated their skill and expertise, state statutes have been amended to allow nurse practitioners to practice unencumbered and at their full scope, which includes unrestricted prescriptive authority.

WHAT DO NURSE PRACTITIONERS NEED TO KNOW ABOUT PRESCRIPTIVE AUTHORITY AS THEY ESTABLISH THEIR PRACTICE?

Although the scope of the nurse practitioner's practice is consistent, statutes and administrative rules in each state may have some variation when it comes to

(1) obtaining authorization to prescribe, (2) prescribing controlled substances, and (3) relating to others in the health care community.

As nurse practitioners establish their practices, they must be cognizant of the following:

1. What the nurse practice act and administrative rules require of nurse practitioners who wish to be authorized to prescribe.

2. What needs to be done to obtain a DEA number for prescribing controlled drugs (schedules I- to V).

3. How often the license for NP practice needs to be renewed, and what certification and continuing education requirements must be met to maintain their licenses and to prescribe in the state.

4. What limitations, if any, have been placed on nurse practitioner prescribing activities.

5. If needed, what arrangements should and can be made to provide patients with prescriptions that are outside the realm of the nurse practitioners' prescribing authority.

Nurse practitioners need to meet the educational and certification requirements established by the state in order to be authorized to prescribe. In addition, they need to submit whatever information is required to authorize them to prescribe in that state. Although the scope of practice of a nurse practitioner may vary somewhat by specialty, the only variance from state to state is the relationship, if any, that is to be maintained with other health care professionals such as physicians and, for a limited number of states, which controlled drugs may be prescribed and how. It is important to know what requirements exist in the state where a nurse practitioner's practice will be established and to develop a practice that adheres to those rules.

Active participation in nurse practitioner organizations and mentoring groups will assist with establishing a safe and legal practice. It will also provide a forum for implementing changes to obstructive statutes and administrative rules that need to be changed to allow nurse practitioners to practice to their full scope and provide the high-level quality care for which they have become so well known.

CONCLUSION

The ability to prescribe medications has broadened over the years, and as nurse practitioners continue to function more independently, most limitations will be removed. The movement will move as rapidly as nurse practitioners and their colleagues educate, inform, and guide decision makers in the legislative and regulatory arena in each state.

REFERENCES

1. Towers J: Advanced practice nurses and prescriptive authority. In Joel L, editor: *Advanced practice nursing: essentials for role development,*. Philadelphia, 2004, FA Davis.
2. Office of Technology Assessment, Congress of the United States: *Nurse practitioners, nurse midwives and physician assistants (December 1986)*, NTIS order # PB87-177465, Washington, DC, 1986, Government Printing Office.
3. Towers J: Report of the national survey of the American Academy of Nurse Practitioners. Part II. Pharmacologic management practices, *J Am Acad Nurse Pract* 1(4):137-142, 1989.
4. Towers J: *Prescribing patterns of nurse practitioners,* Washington, DC, 1999, American Academy of Nurse Practitioners.
5. Goolsby MJ: 2004 AANP National nurse practitioner sample survey. Part II. Nurse practitioner prescribing, *J Am Acad Nurse Pract* 17(12):506-511, 2005.

CREDENTIALING

MONA COUNTS • REGINA MAYOLO

*T*here are a myriad of mechanisms in the health care arena that are designed to protect the public. Credentialing, diplomas, degrees, licensure, certification, regulation, privileging, and accreditation are the most common terms used to describe the procedures used today to verify professionals' abilities within their respective disciplines. Credentials communicate to the public and to organizations needing to address risk management issues that these professionals meet identified standards. This chapter explores the maze of credentialing methods and reviews historical events leading up to credentialing, provides definitions and/or clarifications of associated terms, and offers an explanatory path that may help demystify the credentialing process.

HISTORICAL BACKGROUND AND NURSING REGULATION

The history of the health care professional regulation processes sheds some light on many of the current areas of regulatory confusion. Historically, female lay healers played integral roles within their communities. Female lay healers were usually recognized as community leaders and their commitment to service was considered an obligation to the communities they served. As the predominately male medical establishment emerged in the late 19th century, lay healers gave way to nursing schools. Ehrenreich[1] noted the following as modern nursing emerged:

> Modern nursing arose as an effort on the part of women reformers to help clean up the mess the male doctors were making ... It was nurses, or rather some of the founders of nursing, who can take credit for introducing the first bar of soap to Bellevue Hospital. Strangely, the doctors, who had not yet accepted the germ theory of disease, had never noticed the absence of soap. However, instead of being grateful the doctors were terrified that nursing might represent a new source of competition, the female lay healers reincarnate. Beginning in the late nineteenth century and

continuing into the twentieth, the medical profession campaigned vigorously to put nursing in its place, or what they thought was its place. (p. xxxiv.)

Nursing, starting with the Nightingale Training School of nurses, identified two levels of students—the ordinary probationers and the Lady probationers, the latter being those who received more lectures and study time. These were the "pioneers, teachers, and regenerators in hospital management and nursing system...."[2] Physicians, however, were the first health care providers to gain legislative recognition of their practice. "The legislative definition of the practice of medicine is an all-encompassing act to diagnose or treat, or attempt to diagnose or treat, an individual with a physical injury or deformity."[3] Safriet[4] credits this all-encompassing legislative definition of medical practice as a stumbling block for any profession that has to accommodate the predominating medical practice legislative definition.

Initially, nursing regulation was based on permissive or voluntary policies. Nurses that met the requirements were allowed to "register" with the governing board (in many states, the medical board) and then were permitted to call themselves "registered nurses" (RNs). These RNs were individuals who had graduated from an approved school of nursing and were of "good moral character." Interestingly, some states still carry this good moral character requirement.

Nursing regulation truly started in 1903 when the North Carolina Legislature passed legislation that established a Board of Nursing and a Nurse Practice Act. The era of "mandatory licensure laws for the practice of nursing" soon followed in New York in 1938 and was widespread by the 1950s.[3] By the 1960s, the expanding scope of practice for the role of the advanced practice nurse (APN), developed from the previous practices of nursing, had APNs becoming "creative innovators" as described by Dr. Loretta C. Ford, one of the original founders of the nurse practitioner movement. Currently APNs are recognized and have title protection in all 50 states and have prescriptive privileges within 49 of those states. As Milstead[3] points out in her "Health Policy and Politics":

> [the] National Council of State Boards of Nursing have proposed model rules and regulations for the regulation of advance practice nurses. However, because the battles for regulation of advance practiced nurses are fought in highly political state-by-state environments, there is a patchwork of titles, definitions, criteria for practice, scopes of practice, reimbursement policies, and models of regulation that are difficult for policymakers to navigate and understand in today's rapidly changing health care delivery system.

Credentialing and its associated application are one method to assure that APNs have the knowledge and skills to ensure the safety of the public. However, the inconsistencies in regulations and rules among the various states prohibits the ability of APNs to move easily between states and retain advanced practice recognition. To address this, there is a current movement to expand the scope of APNs and to recognize APNs as licensed independent providers (LIPs) in all 50 states.

DEFINITIONS AND CLARIFICATIONS

Many of the terms related to credentialing are used interchangeably and even differently, depending on the context. The resulting confusion adds to the already perplexing process of "becoming credentialed." Mary Smolenski[5] identifies some of the misuse of terms and provides a beginning explication. For example, she notes that there is an international definition of nurse credentials and cites the International Council of Nurses (ICN)[6] umbrella concept of credentialing that is defined as follows:

> Credentialing is a term applied to processes used to designate that an individual program, institution or product has met established standards set by an agent (governmental or nongovernmental) recognized as qualified to carry out this task. The standards may be minimal and mandatory or above the minimum and voluntary. Licensure, registration, accreditation, approval, certification, recognition, or endorsement may be used to describe different credentialing processes, but this terminology is not applied consistently across different settings and countries. Credentials are marks or "stamps" of quality and achievement communicating to employers, payers, and consumers what to expect from a "credentialed" nurse, specialist, course or program of study, intuition of higher education, hospital or health service, or healthcare product, technology, or device. Credentials must be periodically renewed as a means of assuring continued quality, and they may be withdrawn when standards of competence or behavior are no longer met. (p. 201.)

The umbrella nature of this explanation encompasses the essence of credentialing. Coupled with the historical perspective, the ICN definition allows one to see an evolution of the multiple terminologies.

Accreditation

Accreditation is a term usually applied to institutions of higher education such as colleges, universities, and schools. However, specific programs within those institutions also can be accredited, as well as organizations that provide certifying exams. In the United States, colleges and universities are accredited by one of 19 recognized institutional accrediting organizations; programs are accredited by one of approximately 60 recognized programmatic accrediting organizations. These "recognized" accrediting organizations have been reviewed for quality by the Council for Higher Education Accreditation[7] or the United States Department of Education (USDE)[8] and are private, nongovernmental organizations created for the specific purpose of reviewing higher education institutions and programs for quality. In other countries, this type of accreditation is usually carried out by government organizations.

Most universities and colleges have been accredited, and there are over 6,421 accredited institutions in the United States. Accreditors of these institutions are regional, national, and specialized.[7] The university or college that seeks accreditation does so through the appropriate regional group. Programs within institutions of higher education that are seeking accreditation are reviewed by specialized national groups.

The Council for Higher Education Accreditation (CHEA) recognizes several groups that accredit nursing programs.[7] The Commission on Collegiate Nursing Education (CCNE) and the National League for Nursing Accrediting Commission, Inc. (NLNAC) are the two major nursing program accreditors listed by the CHEA. There are also accreditors for specialty programs; one example is the Council on Accreditation of Nurse Anesthesia Educational Programs (COA)instituted by the American Association of Nurse Anesthetists (AANA). All of these organizations review nursing programs to determine the program's quality and assure program integrity to consumers. It is probably safe to assume that any individual completing a nursing program that leads to becoming an RN has experienced at least a peripheral association with this accreditation process.

Accreditation may affect a nurse's future professional endeavors. To illustrate, some graduate education admission policies require graduation from an "accredited institution." Several nurse credentialing bodies also require graduation from an "accredited institution," and this historically served as a quality control measure to assure that graduates met a certain standard of education. Seeking education at an accredited institution takes on new meaning when one realizes the effect accreditation has on one's future professional life. Prospective students should inquire about a program's accreditation status as one guide when choosing an appropriate program/school. Accreditation also curbs the development of profit-oriented "diploma mills."

An additional important accreditation organization that is usually very familiar to anyone in a health care profession is the Joint Commission on Accreditation of Healthcare Organizations (JCAHO). JCAHO is one of the most well known organizations in health care whose mission is as follows:

> To continuously improve the safety and quality of care provided to the public through the provision of health care accreditation and related services that support performance improvement in health care organizations.[9]

The impact of JCAHO's mission has led to many requirements associated with credentialing in hospitals and other health care organizations today. For example, the language disseminated by JCAHO is the language usually found in most medical staff by-laws of hospitals. These by-laws are what are generally applied by hospitals when health care professionals seek recognition and privileges at those institutions. JCAHO credentialing language historically has used the term "physician," but the term *physician* is giving way to the term of *licensed independent provider.*" This evolution of terms is in response to the increasing complexity of health care and the recognition of the multiple professions that deliver care.

Certification

Certification is a process for validating nursing specialty knowledge and demonstrates to the public and professional community that a nurse practitioner has met nationally recognized standards within a defined specialty area.[10] Many states now require national certification in order for an NP to obtain an advanced practice license. Nationally several bodies offer certification examinations in various nurse practitioner specialties. The American Academy of Nurse Practitioners Certification Program and the American Nurses Credentialing Center are two of the nationally recognized groups. Both certifying bodies are accredited by the National Commission for Certifying Agencies (NCCA) and are recognized by state boards of nursing. Agencies that offer certification examinations for nurse practitioners and are recognized by most state boards of nursing are shown in Table 4-1.

Credentialing

According to Hanson,[11] the term *credentialing* as applied to advanced practice is an umbrella term defined as follows:

> Credentialing is furnishing the documentation that one is authorized by a regulatory body to engage in certain activities and to use a certain title. Credentialing in health care is used to assure the public that the individual meets proposed standards and is prepared to perform the duties implied by the credential. (p. 787.)

Credentialing may include things like graduating from an approved nursing program, attainment of national certification, state licensure, collaborative practice with a physician, approval as a nurse practitioner, Medicare/Medicaid provider numbers, and approval of hospital privileges.[11]

Credentialing for staff or hospital privileges can be a daunting, but necessary, process for many NPs. Cary and Smolenski[12] describe categories of data required for such a credentialing application. As these authors note, the credentialing application is usually done in writing, can be a lengthy process, and must be accurate and complete to process in a timely manner. They also recommend that applicants obtain a copy of the policies and procedures for the credentialing process of the agency where the application will be submitted. It is also advisable to get the names of the credentialing committee members (in most institutions physicians constitute the majority composition of credentialing committees), dates when the credentialing committee meets, anticipated action on the application, and due process procedures. If successfully credentialed and appointed to the staff, the nurse practitioner should also get a copy of appointment and reappointment procedures so that all necessary information needed to maintain the credentials can be compiled before it is time for reappointment. The information typically needed for a credentialing application is shown in Box 4-1.

Credentialing for managed care organizations (MCOs) and third-party payers is another area NPs need to understand and is beyond the limits of this chapter. Buppert[13] notes that managed care organizations also collect and verify educational, licensure, malpractice, employment, and certification data on NPs who seek credentialing as a panel member for the MCO. Buppert also notes that contractual relationships with MCOs involve both compensation and other issues related to practice. NPs who own practices will need to negotiate managed care contracts

TABLE 4-1

Agencies Offering Certification Examinations for Nurse Practitioners

AGENCY	TYPE OF ADVANCED PRACTICE EXAMINATION OFFERED
American Academy of Nurse Practitioners The American Academy of Nurse Practitioners Certification Program Capitol Station P.O. Box 12926 Austin, TX 78711 Phone: (512)442-5202 FAX: (512) 442-5221 E-mail: certification@aanp.org	Adult Nurse Practitioner Family Nurse Practitioner
American Nurses Credentialing Center 8515 Georgia Ave, Suite 400 Silver Spring, MD 20910-3492 Phone: 1-800-284-2378 Website: http://www.ana.org/ancc/certification/	Acute Care Nurse Practitioner Adult Nurse Practitioner Family Nurse Practitioner Gerontological Nurse Practitioner Pediatric Nurse Practitioner Adult Psychiatric & Mental Health Nurse Practitioner Family Psychiatric & Mental Health Nurse Practitioner
Pediatric Nurse Certification Board 800 South Frederick Avenue, Suite 204 Gaithersburg, MD 20877-4152 Phone: (301) 330-2921 Toll Free: 1-888-641-2767 FAX: 301-330-1504 Website: http://www.pncb.org/	Pediatric Nurse Practitioner Pediatric Acute Care Nurse Practitioner
National Certification Corporation for Obstetric, Gynecological and Neonatal Nursing Specialties (NCC) P.O. Box 11082 Chicago, IL 60611-0082 Phone: 312-951-0207 FAX: 312-951-9475 Website: http://www.nccnet.org/	Women's Health Nurse Practitioner Neonatal Nurse Practitioner

BOX 4-1	CATEGORIES OF DATA REQUIRED FOR CREDENTIALING APPLICATIONS

- Personal and practice demographic information
- Education and training
- Work history
- State(s) licensure history (including state-controlled substance licenses)
- Certifications
- DEA certificates
- Liability insurance and claims history
- History of sanctions/penalties imposed on practice as well as voluntary relinquishment of licenses/certifications
- Disclosures of physical, mental, substance or criminal problems
- Attestation of information completeness and accuracy
- Authorizing statement to collect any information necessary to verify application

From Cary A, Smolenski M: Credentialing and clinical privileges and the advanced practice nurse. In Joel L: *Advanced practice nursing: essentials for role development,* Philadelphia, 2004, FA Davis, pp 137.

and Buppert suggests consulting an attorney who specializes in negotiating managed care contracts.[13]

Degrees

Controversy has beset the nursing profession regarding the degree that should be the "entry into practice" for as long as this author can remember. Registered nurses may obtain their educational preparation through a diploma program (3 years and based in a hospital setting), an associate degree program (2 years, usually based in a community college setting), a baccalaureate program (4 years, based in a college or university setting), and at the masters level as a second degree. Graduates of these various programs, if accredited by the state boards of nursing, are eligible to take the National Council of State Boards of Nursing examination (NCLEX). Upon passing the NCLEX exam and meeting requirements of the state board of nursing in the state where they intend to practice, individuals may be licensed as registered nurses (RNs).

Nurse practitioners initially experienced a similar morass of varying educational pathways to become nurse practitioners (NP) and enter advanced practice. However, a consensus on requirements by the national certifying bodies has led to the master's degree being accepted as the minimum "entry into practice" educational requirement for recognition as an NP.

Licensure

Black's Law Dictionary[14] defines licensure as "granting permission by a competent authority to do an act which, without such permission, would be illegal, a trespass, a tort, or otherwise not allowable." Licensure is equivocal to the state's regulation of a profession. The National Council of State Boards of Nursing[15] identifies that:

> Nursing regulation is the governmental oversight provided for nursing practice in each state. Nursing is regulated because it is one of the health professions that pose risk of harm to the public if practiced by someone who is unprepared and incompetent.....the government permits only individuals who meet predetermined qualifications to practice nursing. The board of nursing is the authorized state entity with the legal authority to regulate nursing.

Milstead[3] points out that licensure is the most restrictive method of credentialing. Licensure for RNs and NPs is regulated in most states and is usually under the purview and responsibility of the state board of nursing.

Clinical Privileges

Clinical privileges historically have been associated only with physician providers. With the unparalleled growth of other licensed independent providers (LIPs), however, the processes to attain clinical privileges for providers need to be expanded. Clinical privileging is the process whereby individuals are credentialed within institutions to provide specific patient care services. Credentialing may be defined as the recognition of professional and technical competence and involves establishing mechanisms to verify information and evaluate the applicant requesting privileges. An example of how agencies define clinical privileging is the Veteran's Hospital Administration (VHA) Directive 2001-005, which describes clinical privileging as follows:

> Clinical Privileging ... is the process by which a licensed practitioner is permitted by law and the facility to practice independently, to provide medical or other patient care services within the scope of the individual's license, based on the individual's clinical competence as determined by peer references, professional experiences, health status (as it relates to the individual's ability to perform the requested clinical privileges), education, training, and licensure.[16]

This definition outlines information the individual nurse practitioner must keep in order to apply for this status.

Cary and Smolenski[12] identify seven categories of privileges. Briefly these categories are *Active:* able to admit; *Courtesy:* limited admission but a active member of another medical staff; *Affiliate:* no longer active but long-standing relationship; *Outpatient:* sees patients in an outpatient setting or participates with programs associated with the institution; *Honorary:* similar to affiliate, but may admit and usually has outstanding accomplishments or reputation; *House:* admit to specialty area with approval of an active staff member; and *Allied Health Professional:* permits nonphysician health care providers to provide specified patient care services.

As delineated by these categories, the state in which the institution is located will mandate which level of staff privileges a nurse practitioner could be awarded. This process identifies the need for advanced practice nurses to achieve "licensed independent provider" status in all states.

State Licensure and Regulation

State boards of nursing have the responsibility of assuring public safety and, in that capacity, license all levels of nursing. The nurse practice acts of the various states typically (1) define the authority of the board of nursing, (2) define professional nursing and the boundaries of the scope of nursing practice, (3) identify types of licenses and titles, (4) state the requirements for licensure, (5) protect titles, and (6) identify the grounds for disciplinary action.[15]

A review of state boards of nursing roles also demonstrates the restrictive credentialing function of licensure. The scope of practice of RNs is relatively standard across states. NPs, however, have significant variation in scope of practice parameters across states. The classic example is the scope and ability to write prescriptions. Nurse practitioners in some states have no limitations and are designated as licensed independent providers. Other states, however, limit the nurse practitioner ability to write prescriptions for specific medications and may require collaboration and in some states still require supervision.

NATIONAL INFLUENCES AND REGULATIONS

Nationally several mechanisms may be considered to contribute to credentialing in the broadest scope. National certification and national provider numbers are two of the mechanisms that are part of the credentialing umbrella. As previously stated, several accreditation bodies offer certification examinations in various nurse practitioner specialties. The American Academy of Nurse Practitioners Certification Program and the American Nurses Credentialing Center both require candidates to meet certain criteria that include graduation from an approved master's level nursing program as an eligibility requirement to take national certification examinations. The certification exam is described on the AANP Certification Program website[17] as follows:

> The National Certification Examinations given by the American Academy of Nurse Practitioners Certification Program are competency-based examinations for adult and family nurse practitioners reflective of nurse practitioner knowledge and expertise for each of the specialties. The content areas of the examinations are health promotion, disease prevention and diagnosis and management of acute and chronic diseases by family and adult nurse practitioners.

As previously described, many states require national certification as a mandate for licensure as an NP in that state. Dr. Loretta C. Ford, an NP pioneer and co-founder of the first pediatric nurse practitioner program in the 1960s, was interviewed in June 2005 by Linda Pearson for Nurse Practitioner World News (NPWN) and addressed the issue of using legislation to expand the scope of practice for NPs and supported the concept for specialty credentialing to be addressed by professional nursing organizations. To clarify her position Dr. Ford stated:

> I am not a proponent of advanced licensure based on the scope of practice. Legislation is designed to protect the public, not the practitioner. My argument is that NPs will be forever fighting battles in state legislatures over each new technique, medication, and practice arrangement that arises and for which we are educationally prepared. Regardless of our educational background, we cannot practice without authorization from the state legislature. What a mistake! Also, credentialing in nursing reflects a proliferation of specialties, with many rigid boundaries and inflexible regulations that tend to limit NPs' growth, expansion, and mobility if the regulations are not properly drawn up and administered ... I also prefer that the continuing educational and specialty credentialing be handled by the professional organizations. This model would make NPs much like the other professions.[18]

Nurse practitioners would be wise to not seek national or advanced practice licensure and listen to Dr. Ford's viewpoint as NPs move forward and fulfill a role in the ever expanding and changing health care delivery system. The recognition of specialty-type practice would be analogous to the medical profession's "Board Certified in _____." Thus the scope of practice would not be legislated but would be associated with the current standards of practice of the specialty and could change as new knowledge becomes available without necessitating a legislative act.

Provider Numbers: Medicare and Universal Provider Identifying Number (UPIN)

Currently on the national level other credentials include the Medicare provider number and universal provider identifying number. The Medicare provider number is acquired through application and after a practice site is identified and national certifications examinations are completed successfully. According to Highmark Medicare Services (a contracted insurance carrier for Medicare Part B by the Centers for Medicare and Medicaid Services [CMS])website[19]:

> A physician/healthcare practitioner must have an individual provider number to submit services to Medicare Part B. A physician means doctor of medicine, doctor of osteopathy, doctor of dental surgery or dental medicine, doctor of chiropractic, a doctor of podiatric medicine, or a doctor of optometry who is licensed to practice by the state in which he or she performs services. A healthcare practitioner includes, but is not limited to, physician assistant, certified nurse-midwife, qualified psychologist, nurse practitioner, clinical social worker, physical therapist, occupational therapist, respiratory therapist, certified registered nurse anesthetist, or any other practitioner as may be specified by the Secretary as defined in 1842 (b) (4) (I) of the Social Security Act.

After receiving a Medicare number, an NP also may apply for and receive a universal provider identifying number (UPIN). This UPIN also is a national number and is used to order durable medical equipment, protheses, and other services. Some agencies have used the UPIN to track referrals and consultations.

Conceptually, if all NPs obtained and used these numbers, they would be recognized as providers of health care and not be the "hidden providers." This is one of the issues that has prevented tracking care provided by NPs; thus the data is lost that demonstrates the excellent outcomes of NP practices because the care is not documented under the NP's own provider numbers. Sadly, not all NPs have pursued the time-consuming process of acquiring individual provider numbers.

A national provider identifier (NPI) is being implemented as well and is designed to replace all other provider identifiers previously used by health care professionals. Currently this is applicable to only electronic submissions; however, it would be logical to have this number for all providers. The Administrative Simplification provisions of the Health Insurance Portability and Accountability Act of 1996 (HIPAA) mandated the adoption of standard unique identifiers for health care providers, as well as the adoption of standard unique identifiers for health plans. The purpose of these provisions is to improve the efficiency and effectiveness of the electronic transmission of health information. The Centers for Medicare and Medicaid Services (CMS) has developed the National Plan and Provider Enumeration System (NPPES) to assign these unique identifiers. An NPI is a unique 10-digit numeric identifier assigned to health care providers and organizations defined as covered entities under HIPAA. The NPI will be a permanent identifier assigned for life. There are several significant dates that are applicable for the NPI (see Appendix I). They are as follows:

- May 23, 2005: Health care providers can start applying for an NPI.

- May 23, 2007: By this date, all health care providers who utilize HIPAA standard electronic transactions must have an NPI. Providers who do not utilize HIPAA standard electronic transactions may have an NPI.

- May 23, 2007: By this date, all health plans and payers must have the capability to use the NPI to identify providers in standard electronic transactions.

Consequently, it is evident that a major national transition must ensue to identify each health care provider. Credentialing is an inherent process in obtaining these numbers.

INTERNATIONAL INFLUENCES

The impact of globalization, deregulation, privatization, health care restructuring, nursing shortages, health care needs, and the general "shrinking" of the planet have led to the need for mechanisms to validate and assure quality of health care providers. National credentialing organizations are beginning to address this need. The development of international councils and outreach programs for advance practice nurses are being started by most of the major nursing organizations.

APPLICATIONS AND IMPLICATIONS FOR PRACTICE

Credentialing, degrees, accreditation, certification, licensure, regulation, continuing education and recertification are all here to stay. The need for quality control, improved patient outcomes, and, most important, patient safety all mandate mechanisms to assure positive ends. Health care professionals all need to address and complete these processes.

The controversy surrounding the whole issue of credentialing is somewhat of a two-edged sword. On one side, credentialing allows for quality assurance and further is tied to many areas of reimbursement. Payment for services is obviously necessary to be able to continue to offer services. The other side of the sword is the inherent barrier to reimbursement for willing qualified providers. In today's world many insurance carriers refuse to recognize qualified health care providers presumably simply because they are not physicians. "Managed Care Credentialing and Reimbursements Policies: Barriers to Nurse-Healthcare Access and Consumer Choice" is an article based on a study done by the National Nursing Centers Consortium (NNCC). This summary article points out the significant barriers to nurse practitioners functioning in their full capacity and scope of practice. The entire survey can be viewed on the NNCC website at www.nncc.us. Specifically, many companies refuse to recognize nurse practitioners as primary care providers. Ironically, one large insurer that refuses to recognize nurse practitioners as primary care providers has, after years of attempts to overturn this stipulation, now recognized NP's as "specialists." There is some thought by the NP leaders that these restrictive credentialing practices are a violation of free trade.

STEP-BY-STEP APPROACH

How does one begin to navigate this morass of "credentialing?" The need for continuous documentation of experience, education, and credentials is evident within each process. That translates to KEEP GOOD RECORDS. To simplify the process the following steps are suggested:

1. **School choice:** Choose an accredited school and program. It is important to keep a record of all relevant educational experiences such as number of hours of preceptor practice, types and ages of patients seen, skills and experiences gained, and location of preceptorships and preceptors names and credentials.

2. **National certification**: Achieve national certification in the NP area of specialty as soon as possible after graduation.

3. **State licensure**: Secure state recognition as an advanced practice nurse in the state where you will be practicing (it is important to be aware of all applicable laws of the state where the NP intends to practice). Several states require a separate application for prescriptive privileges. Once you have state recognition of prescribing, you can apply for a DEA number.

4. **Credentialing and provider number**: After a practice location is identified, complete Medicare and Medicaid provider applications. Be aware that if the practice location overlaps two Medicare fiscal intermediary providers, you may have to submit applications to both intermediaries. Also start the applications for recognition with the major insurance carriers for the practice. Almost all will have separate forms in addition to the "universal application form" found in many states.

5. **Privileging**: Begin the applications appropriate for the practice in which you are participating, and within the applicable state laws. Many hospitals may need to update their "Medical Staff Bylaws" to keep pace with the changing health care provider roles.

6. **Continuing education**: Keep copies of all continuing education programs completed. It is prudent to keep the pharmacology hours separate, because these hours are required by many states for continuing prescriptive authority. All certifications and credentialing processes are self-limiting and will need to be renewed at specified intervals. This is a motivator to maintain documentation of NP practice experience, education, and continuing education efforts.

CONCLUSION

Credentialing, and all the similar processes, are intended to provide safety and quality assurance and to produce improved patient outcomes. As is evident, credentialing is a morass of effort and paperwork. However, it is also one way nurse practitioners and other advance practice nurses can document their productive and quality patient outcomes. Thus credentialing is the way in which nurse practitioners can advance from being "hidden providers" to being recognized as the quality providers of health care services.

REFERENCES

1. Ehrenreich B: Introduction: emergence of nursing as a political force. In Mason DJ, Leavitt JK, Chafee MW, editors: *Policy and politics in nursing and health care*, ed 4, Philadelphia, 2002, Saunders, pp. xxxiv.

2. Haynes L, Butcher H, Boese T: *Nursing in contemporary society: issues, trends, and transition,* New Jersey, 2004, Pearson/Prentice Hall, p 458.
3. Milstead JA: *Health policy and politics: a nurse's guide,* Boston, 2004, Jones and Bartlett.
4. Safriet BJ: Healthcare dollars and regulatory sense: the role of advanced practice nursing, *Yale Journal on Regulation* 9(2):434, 1992.
5. Smolenski MC: Credentialing, certification, and competence: issues for new and seasoned nurse practitioners, *J Am Acad Nurse Pract*17(6):201-204, 2005.
6. International Council of Nurses: *ICN on regulation: towards 21ˢᵗ century models,* Geneva, Switzerland, 1998, International Council of Nursing.
7. *Council for Higher Education Accreditation* (website): http://www.chea.org. Accessed January 22, 2006.
8. *U.S. Department of Education* (website): http://www.ed.gov. Accessed January 22, 2006.
9. *Joint Commission on Accreditation of Healthcare Organizations* (website): http://www.jcaho.org. Accessed January 22, 2006.
10. American Nurses Credentialing Center (ANCC): *Why Certify?* (website): http://www.ana.org/ancc/certification/index.html. Accessed January 22, 2006.
11. Hanson CH: Understanding regulatory, legal, and credentialing requirements. In Hamric AB., Spross JA, Hanson CH: *Advanced practice nursing: an integrative approach,* Philadelphia, 2004, Saunders, pp 781-808.
12. Cary A, Smolenski M: Credentialing and clinical privileges and the advanced practice nurse. In Joel L: *Advanced practice nursing: essentials for role development,* Philadelphia, 2004, FA Davis, pp 136-152.
13. Buppert C: *Nurse practitioner's business and legal guide,* ed 2, Boston, 2004, Jones and Bartlett.
14. Garner BA: *Black's law dictionary,* ed 6, St Paul, Minn, 1992, West.
15. National Council of State Boards of Nursing: *Nursing Regulation* (website): http://ncsbn.org/regulation/index.asp. Accessed January 22, 2006.
16. Department of Veterans Affairs: *VHA Directive 2001-055* (website): http://www1.va.gov/VHAPUBLICATIONS/ViewPublication.asp?pub_ID=127. Accessed January 22, 2006.
17. American Academy of Nurse Practitioners: *Certification Examination* (website): http://www.aanp.org/Certification/Program+Description.htm. Accessed January 22, 2006.
18. Pearson L: Opinions, ideas, & convictions: from NPs' founding mother, Dr. Loretta C. Ford, *NPWN* 10(4):11-12, 2005.
19. *Centers for Medicare and Medicaid Services (CMS)* (website): http://www.cms.hhs.gov/center/provider.asp. Accessed January 22, 2006.

PART II

OWNING A PRACTICE

What to Think About Before Going into Business

Personal and Professional Planning

CAROLYN ZAUMEYER

❧

Many nurse practitioners dream of establishing and operating an independent practice. The lure of designing the practice of your dreams that is truly your own can be very appealing. Many nurse practitioners believe that independent practice will increase their control of the future, increase their professional satisfaction, and give them the potential to increase their income.

Starting your own business is a major undertaking that should be thoroughly researched and considered carefully before you commit to the venture. Establishing your own practice will affect every facet of your life. When starting your own practice, there will be risks, sacrifices, and other hardships along the way, as well as the many rewards that come with success. Before making the commitment to start your practice, take some time to think things through.

Begin with a thorough examination of your personal strengths and weaknesses. This will help you identify unique traits that may predict your potential for success or your risk for failure. Your motivation for starting your own practice should be examined too. Is entrepreneurship your dream—or someone else's? How will it enable you to provide the best possible patient care? How many factors can you identify that propel you toward your own starting practice? When examining your motivating factors, you may identify feelings that may affect your decision to start your own practice. Do *not* ignore them but *do* examine the feelings rationally and sensitively.

Your family circumstances also should be investigated. Is your family encouraging you to start your own business? Do they understand the time commitments and responsibilities you will be facing? The support of your family and friends should not be taken for granted.

As far as lifestyle issues, are you ready to give up some of your personal time? When launching a business, you will need to put in some late hours during the week and even some week-end hours.

Your financial condition may be affected when starting your own business. If necessary, are you ready to make financial sacrifices? Do you have the resources and the financial safety net in case things are difficult early on or your venture fails? All businesses and personal situations are unique. It is difficult to predict when you will have all of your startup costs paid and be capable of covering your monthly expenses, no matter how sophisticated your financial plan may be.

You should also take some time to identify the things that make your proposed practice special or different from your competition. Why will patients come to you rather than the provider down the street? Identifying what makes you special helps you define your "niche."

Research and planning are your keys to success. If you fail to investigate up front the need for your practice and forego creating a written plan, you may be wasting valuable time, energy, and money.

Many nurse practitioner students are interested in independent practice. Although this is an exciting option, it is more important to become an experienced clinician before launching your own practice. Professional readiness should be assessed. Are you ready to present yourself and your practice to the community? Do you feel confident introducing yourself and promoting your practice? Are you confident you can deliver quality services?

Once you have completed this thorough self-assessment and you have determined that entrepreneurship is for you, go ahead! Designing your dream practice can be a fun and enlightening process. Whether you decide that starting an independent practice is or is not in your future, the self-assessment can help identify characteristics in yourself that you may not have known you possess. Identifying these qualities can help you in dealing with life situations both at home and in the workplace.

PERSONAL CONSIDERATIONS

Personal Characteristics

Much research has been done on the identification of personal characteristics of successful entrepreneurs.

The United States Small Business Administration (SBA) (www.sba.gov) has listed some of the characteristics of successful entrepreneurs. Take some time now to go through the exercise in Figure 5-1.

If you have some or all of these traits, you may be a perfect candidate for entre-preneurship. If you identify a few characteristics that really don't describe you,

Do you feel you have the following characteristics?

Characteristic	Yes	No
Persistence		
Desire for immediate feedback		
Inquisitiveness		
Strong drive to achieve		
High energy level		
Goal-oriented behavior		
Independent		
Demanding		
Self-confident		
Calculated risk taker		
Creative		
Innovative		
Vision		
Commitment		
Problem-solving skills		
Tolerance for ambiguity		
Strong integrity		
Highly reliable		
Personal initiative		
Ability to consolidate resources		
Strong management and organizational skills		
Competitive		
Change agent		
Tolerance for failure		
Desire to work hard		
Luck		

Figure 5-1

Personal characteristics of successful entrepreneurs. Modified from: *United States Small Business Administration: Do you have what it takes? © 2006, www.sba.gov/starting-business/startup/doyouhave whatittakes.html*

it doesn't necessarily mean that you will fail. By identifying your strengths and weaknesses, you will be able to determine the areas that you may want to improve upon or for which you will need to rely on the help of others.

Additionally, while identifying the positive traits of successful entrepreneurs, you should also look for negative indicators that could work against you. Some self-defeating behaviors include procrastination, obsession, self-pity, rebellion, and guilt. Are these behaviors a major part of your personality? If so, you may want to explore them and examine how you deal with them before you make the commitment to start your own practice.

If procrastination is a problem, don't worry, most people procrastinate at times. This is a behavior that can be changed. By prioritizing the items on your list of things to do, then breaking the list down into small steps, you can easily overcome this trait. If you need more motivation, try to calculate how much money you are either losing or not generating because of your procrastination. This may be enough to get you moving. If all this fails, post a visible note above your desk that says "Procrastinate Later!"

Entrepreneurs must be able to multitask. On a daily basis you may have to solve many different problems and face unique situations you may never have anticipated. Some issues will arise unexpectedly and require you to reprioritize your work for the day, the coming week, or the longer term—while all along still providing quality care for your patients.

Cultivating good work and personal habits will help you reach your goals. Take good care of yourself as well. If you are not well rested and healthy, you may not be able to handle the stresses you will encounter with independent practice. Not only must entrepreneurs work tirelessly and maintain a sense of balance in their lives but also they must learn to anticipate challenges. Just as a surgical nurse must anticipate what instruments the surgeon will need next, the business owner must always be thinking about what could possibly be the next challenge. If you have already taken the time to think things through, the next challenge may not seem so overwhelming.

Motivation

Exploring your level of motivation and what drives you can be an enlightening process. Can you envision yourself happily providing quality health care in your own dream practice? Can you see yourself dealing with unexpected challenges? What rewards, intrinsic and extrinsic, are important to you? Having this vision can help you create and control your destiny. Without creating your own vision and goals, your destiny will most likely be controlled by others.

One thing you must consider is your level of motivation and commitment. If you have a strong desire to succeed, you will have a much stronger probability of success. If you are not totally committed to your concept, you may find it easier to give up when you reach the inevitable barriers of independent practice. If you are truly committed to your venture, you will find a way to turn a problem into a challenge, and a challenge into a solution.

What motivates you? Is it:

• Helping others?

• Money?

• Learning?

• Freedom?

• Challenges?

• Power?

Are your motivating factors something you think you can use to grow your new venture?

You need to translate your motivation and commitment into personal and business goals. Setting both personal and business goals will help you formulate your game plan. Sit back and take some time to think through what you would like to accomplish in the next1, 5 and 10 years. For example, what type of work environment would you like to create? How much money would you like to make? What kind of lifestyle would you like to live? How big do you want to grow your practice? Complete the Goal Worksheet in Figure 5-2 and keep a copy of it posted within your work area. Remember to keep your goals realistic, measurable, and attainable.

Goals can be changed or adjusted in time; most likely they will be. You can break them down into monthly or weekly goals if that helps you grow your business. You can share some of your business goals with your employees so they can help you attain those goals. You should also encourage your employees to set goals of their own that will help you towards attaining yours.

Fears

Entrepreneurship and fear go hand in hand. It is normal to experience some fears when making the commitment to start your practice. Fear can be motivating for some and debilitating for others. It is important to take a few minutes to examine your fears. Are your fears related to financial failure or writing your business plan? Or are your fears more about your own capabilities or your image among your peers? Sometimes the fear of failing and having to face your friends, family, and peers can be much more frightening than the fear of losing a portion of

Goals	1 year	5 years	10 years
Personal Goal #1			
Personal Goal #2			
Personal Goal #3			
Business Goal #1			
Business Goal #2			
Business Goal #3			

Figure 5-2

Goals worksheet. *From Zaumeyer C: How to start an independent practice, Philadelphia, 2003, FA Davis.*

your savings. After you have identified and examined your fears, try to find ways to put them in perspective.

If your fears stem from financial concerns, add up the total amount of money you could potentially lose during the first year of your business. If that is totally overwhelming, maybe the risk of independent practice is not for you. Or, you may start preparing now to develop ways that could help you reduce that sum. For example, if you were to work a few days outside of the office during the first months of the start-up phase, you could reduce that scary number. Securing enough start-up capital also may help reduce those fears.

If your fears are based on personal concerns, you can work on that. You can start laying the ground work now by telling people close to you that you know you are taking a risk, but you *need* to do it, really *want* to succeed, and may want their *advice*. Enlisting their support now may help you later on down the road. Many of your peers may be envious of your plan, which is human nature. They may be very supportive or possibly react in a negative way to cover what they feel are shortcomings on their part. They may actually try to talk you out of pursuing your dream of independent practice. Alternatively, they may encourage you and assure you that they will be there for you along the way. Remember, this is your dream and your choice—if you are truly committed to your concept, keep going forward.

One way to handle fears is to mentally prepare an exit plan for yourself. For example, you may want to make an agreement with yourself for a 1-year plan. If at the end of 1 year, you are not happy, not making money, and are not providing the quality health care for your patients as you had planned, give yourself permission to make changes. Of course, you need to give the changes a lot of thought, but by setting measurable goals, you may find it easier to assess the viability of your dream practice at the end of 1 year.

Sometimes just the act of writing down your fears and evaluating whether they are reasonable or unreasonable can be of great help. After you have identified your reasonable fears, write an action plan to help alleviate them. Then, try to list any unreasonable fears and *why* they are unreasonable. The Fears Worksheet in Figure 5-3 may help you.

Do not allow the fear of potential risks of starting your own practice stop you from realizing your dream. You take risks every day of your life. The risks involved in entrepreneurship should be calculated risks—based on fact, not fancy. Your risks will be reduced by thoroughly researching and planning your practice before you open for business. Give it your best shot and you may be pleasantly surprised.

Family

Starting your own business will have an impact on your family. How easy this impact will be depends on your practice demands and how you handle them. The level of family support you receive has the potential to make or break your venture. If you have the support and understanding of your family, you will have

Reasonable Fears	Action Plan
Example: I do not know anything about bookkeeping.	1. I will take a bookkeeping course from the SBA. 2. I will hire a receptionist with good bookkeeping skills and experience. 3. I will develop a good working relationship with my CPA so I can call with questions when they arise.
1. _____	1. _____ 2. _____ 3. _____
2. _____	1. _____ 2. _____ 3. _____
3. _____	1. _____ 2. _____ 3. _____
Unreasonable Fears: Example: I can't do this on my own.	**Why the fear is unreasonable:** You don't have to. There are many people that will want to help you. All you have to do is seek them out and ask.
1. _____	_____ _____ _____
2. _____	_____ _____ _____

Figure 5-3

Fears worksheet.

a greater chance for success. The best way to achieve this support and understanding is with open communication. From the beginning, you should share your hopes and dreams of starting your own practice. It is important that your family understand how important this venture is to you. You also may want to express some of your fears so they can better understand your mindset. Share your goals with them but also share your exit plan. Alert them that you will need them even more if things do not work out.

Describe what you anticipate your schedule will be. Create a system so they will have an idea of when they will be seeing you. A large wall calendar that is updated often can help with your family's scheduling. Reassure them that they are very important to you and you will do everything you can to share in their lives as always. Also, explain that there may be times where you are needed at your practice when you would rather be with them. If you have this conversation before the opening of your practice, it may help them understand and accept the changes and challenges in all of your lives. Do all this in consideration of each family member's developmental level. Talking about all this to your spouse or partner will be different from talking to, for instance, an adolescent or a toddler. Don't ignore adult children you may have either; or your own parents. Everyone in your family will be impacted by your decision to open your independent practice.

Including your friends and family in the planning and launching of your practice is a good way to get them to support and understand your practice. Brainstorming with your family and friends can lead to creative marketing ideas and unique problem solving. It will also let them feel they are a part of your business. This inclusion may encourage them to lend their support to you. There are many ways to do this; for example, ask for their help in naming the practice, painting the office, preparing the office, cleaning, and helping with organizing supplies. Again, communication is so very important. You want your family and friends to feel that they are still a very important part of your life; you also want them to accept and support your decision.

Lifestyle Changes

What are your lifestyle goals? Have you taken the time to really quantify what you believe your ideal lifestyle would be? Remember, goals should be realistic, attainable, and measurable. You may want to list some aspects of your life and rank them for importance. Some things you may want to include could relate to your independence, daily schedule flexibility, financial goals, altruistic goals, travel, control over your life, professional autonomy, and ability to pursue interests other than your work. As you can see, the paycheck is not the only consideration when making career decisions.

Gary Shine has coined the term *lifestyle entrepreneur* in his book *How to Succeed as a Lifestyle Entrepreneur*. It demonstrates how your new practice can lead you to living your life at its best.[1] Independent practice is an opportunity to use your skills to design your own lifestyle. Many people think about entrepreneurship simply as a way to make a lot of money. You may have different goals. You can design a lifestyle that grants you the freedom to do what interests you other than work.

As an entrepreneur you have the power to choose where you will live, work, and play. You will have the flexibility to work as much or as little as you wish and have control over your own destiny. Depending on what your current activities are, you may have more or less free time than before you started your practice. One of the benefits of independent practice is that you have the ability to set your own schedule.

The responsibility to your patients and your practice will be yours and yours alone. These are not responsibilities to be taken lightly. You have to treat your patients and your practice with the most conscientious care. Your liability will inevitably increase when starting your practice. You must be aware of all the laws and regulations and follow them to the letter.

Conclusion

In summary, this chapter is intended to help you in the personal and professional decision-making process about starting your practice. You don't have to be perfect in all aspects, but you do need to know where your weaknesses are and determine how you will compensate for them. Once you have the personal and professional issues figured out and squared away, you should start addressing the feasibility and finances of your independent practice.

REFERENCES

1. Schine G: *How to succeed as a lifestyle entrepreneur: running a business without letting it run your life*, Chicago, 2003, Kaplan.

HELPFUL RESOURCES

Small Business Administration (SBA) (website): www.sba.gov.
Zaumeyer C: *How to start an independent practice: the nurse practitioner's guide to success,* Philadelphia, 2003, FA Davis.

ADVANTAGES AND DISADVANTAGES TO OWNING A BUSINESS

Feasibility and Finance

CAROLYN ZAUMEYER

❦

There are many things to consider regarding finances before starting your practice. First, you must objectively look at your personal financial standing. Creating a list of your monthly expenses will help plan how much money you will need to have available until you are receiving a monthly paycheck (realistically, think also about the possibility of paychecks in varying amounts, including no paycheck occasionally in the early months).

Perhaps we all prefer to put feasibility over finance, but the reality is that feasibility is not possible without a good financial plan. Feasibility is more exciting, especially to nurses because we are so often driven by innovation, enthusiasm, and altruism. Often we would rather not think about the financial implications. This chapter aims to help you in linking the two "f's" of feasibility and finance. Plan the finance, so you can achieve your goals.

If you find completing the Monthly Expense Worksheet in Figure 6-1 difficult, try tracking and logging everything you spend for at least 1 month. Once you have real numbers to work with, you can look for ways to reduce your spending if necessary. For example, do you really need:

- More than one vehicle?

- Cable TV?

- To eat out so often?

Rent/Mortgage _____

Utilities

    Electric _____

    Gas _____

    Water _____

Telephone

    Home _____

    Cellular _____

Cable/Satellite/DSL _____

Subscriptions

    Newspapers _____

    Magazines _____

Personal Care Items _____

Pet Care _____

Food

    Home _____

    Lunch _____

    Restaurants _____

Transportation

    Car payment _____

    Gas _____

    Maintenance _____

Insurance

    Health _____

    Car _____

    Life _____

    Home/Rental _____

Clothing _____

Entertainment _____

Credit Card Payments _____

Loan Payments _____

Gym _____

Vacation _____

Gifts

    Birthdays _____

    Christmas _____

    Misc. _____

Other _____

Contingency margin

    (10% of all of the above) _____

Total _____

Figure 6-1

Personal Monthly Expense Worksheet.

- The gym membership?

- Long vacations?

    Friedman[1] recommends that you have 1 year's salary in the bank to cover your personal expenses while starting your business. She also recommends that if you are eager to start and feel now is the time but don't have the savings, that you should consider starting your business part-time. Some people have cashed in (part of) their retirement accounts, most of them paying a 10% early withdrawal penalty and income taxes that are likely to be higher than when retired. Talk to an accountant or financial advisor before going this route.

    Writing down all of your assets and listing all of your debts will give you a clear picture of your overall financial standing. This exercise will help you when making the decision regarding taking the risk of independent practice.

    Unless you keep your fulltime job, you will definitely notice a change in your financial situation. It may take considerable time to generate your prior income from your new venture. However, your savings may help cover this deficit; supportive family and friends may be a resource as well.

    Assessing the financial potential of your proposed practice is a necessity. It is fairly easy to do. You will need to estimate your potential income and compare it to your potential expenses (Figures 6-2 and 6-3).

    Once you have an estimate of your initial and monthly costs, you are better prepared to calculate how much money you will need for start-up. You can then determine how much money you will need to borrow or access from your savings.

Using the figures from your current practice and a calculator, you can easily estimate your income:

Basic Formula:

#_____ visits per day X average $_____ per visit = $_____ one days estimated income

#_____ visits per week X average $_____ per visit = $_____ weekly estimated income

#_____ visits per month X average $_____ per visit = $_____ monthly estimated income

Other factors to add in:

Special Procedures

Laboratory Income

Injections

Other Income

Figure 6-2

Estimating the Income of Your Proposed Practice. *From Zaumeyer C: How to start an independent practice, Philadelphia, 2003, FA Davis.*

	Start-up Costs	Monthly Costs
Office Space		
First, last and security deposit		
Monthly charge		
Renovations (add counter, move walls, etc.)		
Utilities		
Water		
Garbage		
Power		
Advertising		
Association Dues		
Auto		
Bank Fees		
Building and Business Insurance		
Continuing Education		
Disability Insurance		
Entertainment and Promotions		
Hazardous Waste Disposal		
Health Insurance		
Laboratory Fees		
Liability Insurance		
Licenses		
MD Consulting Fee		
Medical Equipment		
Medical Supplies		
Office Equipment		
Office Maintenance and Cleaning		
Office Supplies		
Outdoor Signage		
Payroll		
Payroll Taxes		
Pest Control		
Printing		
Professional Fees		
Sales Tax		
Security System		
Subscriptions		
Telephone		

Figure 6-3

Estimated Expenses Worksheet. *From Zaumeyer C: How to start an independent practice, Philadelphia, 2003, FA Davis.*

There are many options for acquiring startup capital. The easiest and most convenient lender may be a friend or family member (within the investment community, often derisively referred to as FFFs; friends, families, and fools). Just because they are not a traditional lender does not mean you can treat the loan casually. In fact, you should be extra-sensitive about approaching them because you risk losing some valuable relationships in the long term. You must draw up a loan paper (forms are available at business supply stores), set up terms of repayment and interest and also detail how you will secure the loan, if required.

Sources for startup capital include:

- Savings account
- Bank loans (secured, line of credit, small business loan)
- SBA loans (www.sba.gov)
- Finance company
- Private investors (people who believe in your concept)
- Credit cards
- Grants

Building a good relationship with your local banker could be one of the best business relationships that you will forge. A banker that understands your practice may be able to suggest banking programs and packages that can help you grow your business. Don't necessarily go for the "big bank" in town; consider local banks as well. The smaller banks know the local market, have greater flexibility in terms of decision making, and will be easier to work with in case of "rainy days."

NICHE

Your "niche" is basically what makes you special, different, and appealing to potential clients. What is it about you and your practice that will inspire potential patients to pick up the telephone and call to schedule with you rather than their current provider? Refer to your research of the other providers in your area to help identify and label your niche. Start by writing down positive descriptors of you and your practice. Your niche may be related to your location, gender, philosophy of health care, special services, procedures, schedule, fees, and more. Once you have identified your niche, try to describe it in a clear concise manner. Be ready for when someone asks you why they should come to you rather than the provider down the road. A good response may be "you can usually be seen on the same day that you call, in a clean and friendly office, by a competent provider, for an affordable fee, and with your future health in mind." It is better to be prepared for these questions that having to come up with a description of your practice off the cuff. Ideally, try to come up with a moniker that you can put around your office, include on business cards, and use to enhance your advertising.

Have you noticed something about the local providers that is missing? A certain type of exam, procedure, or service that the community could use that is not currently available. This may help you find your niche. For example, diabetes education, weight loss programs, sclerotherapy, home visits, cosmetic procedures, nutritional counseling, and so forth.

RESEARCH AND PLANNING

Research and planning are the keys to success. This makes sense, without researching the need for your dream practice and making a plan for the practice to function, you cannot succeed.

If you are serious about starting a practice, start now and create a notebook of thoughts and questions. It may help to organize the notebook into sections such as the following:

- Physician of protocol

- Legal questions

- Accounting questions

- Supplies needed

- Equipment needed

Then, when you go into meetings, you can be more assured they will be productive and concise. Remember, time is money when dealing with professionals.

Before starting the research process, you must first outline your future practice. Write down the type of practice, the services and products you will provide, the desired location, growth projections, number of employees, your niche, and the need for your practice. Try to be as specific as possible in this first description of your practice. Most likely, this description will change over time. Now that you have the basic description of your practice sketched out, you will be better prepared to research your competition more efficiently.

The main reason for your research is to learn whether there is a need for your practice in the area where you would like to open your practice. In other words, what is the likelihood that you can run a profitable practice in your desired location? The research can be a simple process. Find out who your competitors are and how they run their practices. You will want to learn what services they are providing, their hours, locations, advertising methods, fees, and the major insurers in your area. Much of this information can be found in the local telephone directory, library, and on the Internet. The local hospital administrative office may have statistical information available that could be beneficial. For example, who are the top three insurers in the area? What percentage of your target market (potential patients) are unemployed? This information also may be found on the Internet, at the local library, and at the office of the U.S. Small Business Administration (www.sba.gov).

If there is a lot of competition in your area, you may want to physically map out their office locations on a local map. You may see that a section of town is not currently being served. This could help you decide on a location. You will also want to research public transportation available around your proposed location. Is it easy for people without vehicles to get to your office? Using the Competition

	Example:	#1 Competitor	#2	#3	#4
Name:	Dr. Meyer				
Location:	US1 & Main				
Telephone:	555-5555				
Hours:	9-5 M-F				
Services:	GP, School				
	Physicals				
	Sclerotherapy				
Advertising Methods:	Yellow pages only				
Cost of 1st Exam:	$150				
Insurances:	PPO only				
	No Medicare				
	No Medicaid				
	No HMO				

Figure 6-4

Competition Assessment Worksheet.*
*You can revise this form to answer the questions you would like answered about your competition. Your competition can then be easily compared.

Worksheet (Figure 6-4) as a guide, create your own chart to help you organize your research findings. This will help you when comparing the competition and identifying unmet needs in the community.

The Competition Assessment Worksheet will make it easy to see the strengths and weaknesses of the local competition. You may identify services or procedures that are missing that could become your niche. Business success depends on good decisions made from good information.

The business plan (see Appendix F) is the traditional written description of all aspects of your proposed business. Your business plan should be written clearly and concisely. The goal is to create a vision from your words for someone who knows nothing of your practice so they can understand it clearly. A business plan is traditionally used to present your concept to prospective lenders for financing. Preparing a traditional business plan can be a daunting but rewarding task. If you do not have to sell your concept to lenders, the plan can be used as a simple plan for starting and operating your business. Similar to the care plan you used for your patients in the hospital, the business plan can direct the care for your business. Taking the time to sketch out the design of your practice can be an invaluable process. You may think of things that you had not thought of before. The business plan is an inexpensive way to help you focus on the most important parts of your business. This plan can help you save a lot of time and money.

Small Business Development Centers are attached to many universities. Their mission is to strengthen small businesses in the community. They can give you advice and direction and are especially helpful when you are writing your business plan.

CLINICAL READINESS

Do you prefer to work on your own? Or do you thrive in a collaborative environment? Have you been practicing as a nurse practitioner for a number of years? Do you feel confident providing patient care in an independent setting?

When first starting your practice, you may feel very alone and vulnerable. But, just as you are not expected to know everything about business before you start your practice, you don't have to know everything about every aspect of patient care. Help is just a telephone call away. You can always shut your office door and open your books or call a colleague for guidance. One of the smartest things you can do in independent practice is to remember your limits. You will not be doing yourself or your patients any favors by keeping them in your care when their issues are clearly outside your scope of practice.

Developing a good referral network of health care providers in your area is critical. Knowing someone in each health care specialty to whom you can entrust your patient's care is invaluable over time; these colleagues may start referring patients to you. A great compliment to you is when you receive referrals from providers in your community. Once they get to know you and the quality care that you are providing, they will most likely refer patients to you.

When you identify an area of patient care that you would like to learn more about, do the research, take a course, and learn a new skill. The more you grow clinically, the more you can grow your business.

MANAGEMENT READINESS

Assessing your level of business knowledge can be a valuable process. The good news is that a good part of business can be learned as you go. Having a working knowledge of basic accounting is beneficial. Just as with patient care, realizing what you don't know is just as important as what you do know. There are experts available to help you with all aspects of business (lawyers, accountants, marketing professionals, insurance representatives, financial advisors.). Many books and resources are available to help you learn the ropes. The U.S. Small Business Administration (SBA) (www.sba.gov) has many publications and courses available to help you hone your business knowledge. Some courses you may consider include:

- Financial management
- Marketing

- Employee relations

- Business planning

- Tax planning

Just as you have built a referral network of health care providers for your patients, you must build a network of support professionals. These are relationships that can make or break your practice. Be sure to interview your professionals before hiring them. Make sure they understand the role of the nurse practitioner and the scope of your practice. Assess your comfort level and ease of conversation with them. And be sure that you understand their fee schedule and billing procedures so there are no unpleasant surprises down the road.

You may already have the connections—think about friends and family that you know. You may already be comfortable with an accountant you have met in another setting. Ask your friends and associates; people are usually happy to refer professionals to you. They can also warn you against professionals who do not do as they should. Some support business advisors that you should get to know include banker, insurance agent, financial advisor, lawyer, certified public accountant (CPA), and bookkeeper.

You can access free advice and counsel from various agencies; however, don't expect them to do your work for you. They will guide you along the way to success. Some organizations you may want to contact include the Small Business Administration (SBA), Service Corps of Retired Executives (SCORE), Small Business Institutes (SBI), and the Small Business Development Center (SBDC). Many states have small business support services to encourage economic development in the state and particular target areas.

Does the fear of being sued paralyze you? The thought of a lawsuit should keep you on your toes, but not paralyze you. You will not be able to provide good care if you don't have the confidence that your liability insurance company will support you. Be sure your insurance carrier will cover your independent practice. Select your insurance carrier carefully. Above all, even with good liability insurance, you will also want to do everything possible to prevent a lawsuit. Start building a policy and procedures manual for clinical practice and personnel management. This may sound like a cumbersome task, but there are a lot of resources and software available at minimum cost. Continuing education courses are available that feature liability reduction, record keeping, asset protection, and ethics. These courses may save you a lot of heartache and money down the road.

Your professional image is formed by every interaction you have with your patients, the community, and business associates. From your business cards, logo, store front, and personal appearance—all aspects of your practice reflect on you and your professional image.

You must convey confidence in both your clinical skills and in the business arena. Your confidence can be a motivating factor for your employees, referral providers, and patients.

Your "people skills" must be sharpened. As a good business coach, Susan Leventhal, of Susan Leventhall & Associates in Ft. Lauderdale, Florida, once told me "you have to get people to know you, to like you, to trust you, and then business is sure to follow."[2] This goes for business acquaintances, colleagues, potential patients, and current patients. Extending yourself to others in a networking situation may be awkward and a bit uncomfortable at first, but practice makes it easier.

DESIGNING YOUR PRACTICE

Over the years, as both a patient and a provider, you must have noticed details of the running of the practice that you think are either good or bad. When designing your practice, you can make it into what you feel is right. Such as no patient waits more than 15 minutes to see you, the cleanliness of the office is up to your standards, the receptionist greets every patient promptly and courteously, health education materials are available in the waiting area, to name a few examples.. Your employees' attitudes usually mirror your own—always be respectful of patients and employees. This is your practice and it reflects on you both personally and professionally. Make your practice into the practice you have been dreaming about.

CONCLUSION

In summary, independent practice may or may not be for you. Exploring your options is always a learning experience. Even if you decide not to launch an independent practice, your knowledge of the business of the practice will help you in your current work environment. You may be able to better understand why certain management decisions have been made. Also, you may want to keep notes, just in case you decide to venture into independent practice at another time.

Starting your own business is a huge undertaking. You will be working harder in more areas than ever before. So, why do it? Starting your own practice puts you in charge of your destiny. This is very appealing to many nurse practitioners.

Visiting other independent nurse practitioner's practices may give you more insight. You may be able to meet like-minded nurse practitioners at your local, regional, and state meetings. Ask whether you can come visit their practices. Prepare a list of questions so you can get the most out of your time together. This experience may help you decide whether or not you are ready to venture into independent practice.

If you do decide to launch the practice of your dreams, try to establish teamwork among your employees. But remember you are the captain of the team. Be determined and focused—and firm in a friendly but decisive way.

You may have some setbacks from time to time—that is to be expected. You must be resilient and keep moving forward towards your goals!

REFERENCES

1. Friedman C: *The girls guide to starting your own business,* New York, 2003, HarperCollins.
2. Leventhal, Susan: Personal communication, June 6, 2003.

HELPFUL RESOURCES

Aspatore J: *The Vault guide to starting your own business,* New York, 2002, Vault.

Lesonsky R: *Start your own business: the only start-up book you'll ever need,* Canada, 2001, Entrepreneur Media.

Letz K: *Business essentials for nurse practitioners,* Ft Wayne, IN, 2003, PreviCare.

Marciko D, editor: *The business of medical practice: advanced profit maximization, techniques for savvy doctors,* ed 2, New York, 2004, Springer.

Norman J: *What no one ever tells you about starting your own business,* Chicago, 1999, Upstart Publishing.

Paulson E: *The complete idiot's guide to starting your own business,* ed 4, Holiday, FL, 2003, Alpha.

Service Corps of Retired Executives (SCORE) (website): www.score.org.

Schine G: *How to succeed as a lifestyle entrepreneur: running a business without letting it run your life,* Chicago, 2003, Kaplan.

Small Business Administration (SBA) (website): www.sba.gov.

Small Business Development Center (SBDC) (website): www.sba.gov/SBDC/.

Small Business Institutes (SBI) (website): www.sbi.org.

Zaumeyer C: *How to start an independent practice: the nurse practitioner's guide to success,* 2003, Philadelphia, FA Davis.

THE BUSINESS PLAN

A Development and Management Tool

IVO L. ABRAHAM • KAREN M. MACDONALD • SALLY J. REEL

*T*he business plan is exactly what the name says it is: a plan to run your business, or in the context of this book, your nursing practice. Usually, people think of the business plan as part of starting a new business, launching a new service, or initiating a collaboration or joint venture—a focus on development. However, from the onset, we also want to underscore the importance of the business plan as a management tool through a cyclical process of planning, evaluating, and reevaluating, and replanning: a benchmark for gauging the business performance of your nursing practice.

In the enthusiasm of setting up a nursing practice or integrating a practice into a larger organization, we tend to focus in the first instance on the mission: the principles, models, and services we envision providing to patients, families, and communities. In the intensity of all this, we risk overlooking the pragmatic, often less exciting and sometimes even sobering, business realities that face us in the launch of a practice: operations, management, resources, finance, and marketing. This is where the business plan comes in.

This chapter is focused on the "money" side of things, specifically how to plan to provide the best clinical services within the inevitable financial constraints—from the long-term financing needs to the short-term cash flow crunches. The business plan, then, is your tool to plan and to manage your nursing practice. You will need it to get and manage money, and to survive in the periods when money may be short. Not that the business plan is just a financial plan; instead, it is the tool used to prepare for and deal with the various issues that impact on the money that comes into and flows out of your practice.

Developing a business plan is not an easy task, especially for nurses with the altruistic value set that characterizes them. It challenges you to think in a different framework and to adopt a new terminology—both of which are often seen as "hard core business," often with a tinge of reproach and resentment that you have to adopt such (seemingly) nonaltruistic perspectives. Bite the bullet, open your eyes, and be realistic. Otherwise you may fall prey to the (cruel) truism: "no money, no mission."

The business plan is integral to business communication. No doubt, you will need to raise money to launch your nursing service. You may need to convince yourself, family, friends, investors, bankers, leasers, and so on to finance such things as startup expenses, equipment, and initial personnel costs. They all are likely to ask for a business plan. They will review it thoroughly, and they will challenge assumptions and positions—all part of their due diligence as they consider supporting you new initiative. They will also hold you accountable to your business plan later on; or require a reevaluated business plan that responds to changing conditions or new opportunities. Just as it should be for you and your team internally, the business plan is also a development and management tool for the external world.

In this chapter, we provide a step-wise approach to the development of a business plan within the broader context of developing and managing a professional services firm[1] run by nurse practitioners. Though we realize that new nursing practices may emerge in many different settings, for the sake of clarity we chose the scenario of developing an independent nursing practice in the community (we will refer to it as the "practice"). With this focus in mind, we deviate here and there from traditional outlines of business plans because they may contain elements that are not relevant to the concept of an independent nursing practice. However, we encourage you to consult other resources to complement this chapter: books,[3,4] software programs (e.g. Business Plan Pro, Palo Alto Software; Business Writer, Nova Development), Internet resources, and especially, prior business plans (as to the latter, do ask permission!). Note that there exists a common platform for business plans and that some readers will prefer that format. More recently, especially with the "powerpointification" of business communications, narrative formats have been supplanted, in part or whole, by bulleted presentations, graphs, and tables.

We need to qualify our expertise in developing business plans. Admittedly, we have not developed business plans for independent nursing practices. However, we have authored business plans for our own independent ventures in health care consulting and research and have written a myriad of business plans for many of our clients (health care organizations; pharmaceutical, biotechnology, diagnostics, and medical device companies) as they moved from strategy development to new ventures.

GOAL AND OBJECTIVES OF THE BUSINESS PLAN

The business plan is the road map that outlines the different stages in the development of your practice. It assists you in shaping your thoughts, structuring the many aspects of a viable enterprise, anticipating opportunities and difficulties, providing a framework for your decision making, and structuring the outcomes of the many decisions that you need to make. The business plan is a tool, for development and for management, to assist you in such ventures as starting a new practice, launching a new service within an existing practice, positioning your practice within the local health care market, framing affiliations and joint ventures, and raising money.

Developing a business plan is not as much a writing exercise as it is a comprehensive exercise in strategic thinking and pragmatic operationalization. The goal of the business plan is to present to many stakeholders the "what," "why," and "how" of your new practice: how money well spent will enable you to achieve your mission. The business plan aims to make concrete (i.e., "to bring to pragmatic life") the strategy and operations of your practice in all its aspects: *services, market, marketing, development and setup, finance, organization,* and *key players*

A solid business plan is achieved through the following underlying objectives:

1. *To define the best strategy for your practice*—not *a* strategy, but the *best* strategy from all possible strategies that you have considered. The business plan is the culmination of your strategic thinking. If your strategic thinking is still unclear, your business plan will be unfocused. Don't start writing the business plan until you are absolutely clear about:

   - What services you will provide, to whom, how, when, where, with what resources, and why (services and market)

   - How you will make this known in your market (marketing)

   - What you need to do to get there (development and setup)

   - How much money will come in, how much money will flow out, and how much money you will need to get going (finance)

   - Who will be part of the clinical team, who will assure the business operations, and how these people are organized (organization)

   - What are the profiles of the leader(s) of the new enterprise (key players)

   A helpful test is what we call the "USA Today test" (as in: saying things simply and to the point): can you spec out in bullets, with a minimum of verbiage, all of the above? If yes, proceed with writing the business plan. If no, go back to the drawing table.

2. *To formulate realistic, pragmatic, and measurable objectives.* The business plan is about what objectives you want to achieve and how you will evaluate whether you have reached these objectives. This cuts across all areas of strategy outlined above: *services, market, marketing, development and setup, finance, organization,* and *key players.* State these objectives as clearly as possible, including the benchmarks that will tell you how much progress you have made. For instance:

   - Instead of stating that you want to get contracts with managed care organizations, specify how many contracts you want by a first milestone date, a second milestone date, and at the stage of business maturity of your practice

- Instead of stating that you want to be profitable, describe when your financial models predict break-even, how much margin you want by a first milestone date, a second milestone date, and at the stage of business maturity

- Instead of stating that you want to create a productive environment, specify the target number of visits and mix of services and procedures you want to reach under various staffing scenarios

Along with a clear description of your best strategy, the formulation of realistic, pragmatic, and measurable objectives will convey unambiguously your mastery over your concept and plans for a nursing practice. In turn, it prepares you well for considering the risks involved in your venture.

3. *To assess and preempt risks involved in your venture.* Invariably, with any new initiative, no matter how careful the planning, some things will not go as predicted. Some threats to the business may emerge and will require that you activate alternate plans or procedures. Likewise, some attractive opportunities may emerge, and you will need to be creative and responsive. Regardless of whether threat or opportunity, these events will require your practice to respond, reallocate resources, and proceed on uncharted paths. The business plan plays a critical role in reducing the likelihood that you will be unprepared for strategic and operational challenges and opportunities. Specifically, throughout the business plan's development, across all aspects of strategy (services, market, marketing, development and setup, finance, organization, and key players) you should consistently pose "what if?" questions? This is not always a fun exercise, for instance when you have to confront the possibility that you may not acquire the anticipated number of new patients in year one, or reach the targeted number of patient visits when your business should be at its peak. We recommend a very practical approach: take a sheet of paper (real or on your computer screen), turn it landscape-wise, and draw three columns (or use a spreadsheet formatted with three columns). In the first column ("Best Strategy Element"), state the actual element from your business plan (e.g., X new patients recruited in year 1). In the middle column ("What if?"), jot down any conceivable alternative, both positive and negative, that is halfway realistic (e.g., 10% less patients recruited, 20% less patients recruited, 10% more patients recruited, 20% more patients recruited). In the third column, state for each of these alternatives the actions you would need to take (e.g., reduce staffing by .5 FTE, increase staffing by .5 FTE, impact on infrastructure and equipment, etc.).

In summary, what you need to do is anticipate and hedge your risks, both the negative and the positive. You do so by constructing scenarios, from the best case to the worst case. Importantly, you show to future stakeholders that you are realistically aware of what may happen—to the good and to the bad—and that you are trying to be as well prepared as possible.

"What-if?" scenarios are seldom included in business plans with the attention and detail that is required for good management. People may want to avoid giving a "bad impression," but more likely they neglect this element because they have not been able to go through this difficult (and no doubt sobering) exercise. However, if you do not ask these hard questions, your stakeholders will—and you will need to be prepared to answer them. Consider adding your "what-if?" notes as an appendix to your business plan. It will impress any rational investor, lender, or leaser.

4. *To specify the action plan to achieve the strategic goals and objectives.* The next step is to specify how each element of the proposed strategy will be implemented. Be as concrete as possible because this section builds your operational profile as a leader and manager. It will contribute to a large extent to the confidence that external stakeholders will have in you. People don't invest, lend you money, or lease you equipment because they like your idea. They do so because they believe they will have a return on their investment, or that the loan or lease will be repaid. They will judge the likelihood of this happening from the confidence they gain in you and the key players on your team. They will put their money at risk only if they feel sufficiently assured that your practice will be successful. Here too, the best approach is to be as detailed as possible: specify for each element of your strategic and operational plan what will be done, by whom, when, and how. For instance, you propose to implement a quality management plan. In your business plan, state what this quality management plan will entail, how it will be rolled out, who will be responsible, and how results will be communicated and corrective action will be taken.

5. *To estimate the resources your practice will need.* As you develop your business plan, you will need to spend an extraordinary amount of time determining what human, physical, and other resources you will need. It is critical that your resource planning be as accurate as possible, because it will directly drive the expenditures included in your financial plan. If you underestimate your resources, your financial requirements will come out lower. You will find yourself in double jeopardy: insufficient resources and no financial means to make up the difference. We recommend the following approach. First, collect various budget planning templates for human services ventures—not only for clinical practices but also for other service companies where people serve other people (e.g., law firms, psychological counseling practices, accounting firms, etc.). Study these templates in great detail and identify every possible budget line item that may apply to you, from staffing down to waste management to insurance to legal and accounting support. This will provide you with a master list of budget items. Second, collect information about the cost of budget items. A very helpful strategy is to retain a colleague with an established practice as a consultant, and work with the practice's financial manager to link budget items with actual costs. This will give you the opportunity to compare a "budget-in-action" with the budget outline you developed earlier. It will help you put dollars to items. It will also help you identify budget items that did not make your original list. Important in this exercise is to adjust the dollar figures provided to you, which are based on that practice's patient and service volume, with the volume that you expect for your practice.

6. *To detail the financial implications under various scenarios.* The exercise of estimating resourcing and budgeting the appropriate expense items will help you in the final step of the business plan: the financial plan. However, the expenses are only part of the financial plan, because you will next need to estimate revenues from startup to maturity. Although underestimating expenditures is not uncommon in business plans, estimating revenues over time and through various growth stages is where most business plans fail. Too often, revenue projections are overly optimistic because the writer wants to cover expenses and become profitable soon; in part this also is a desire of wanting to present a positive picture to potential investors and lenders. Here too, working with real data from a parallel (noncompeting) practice might be helpful. As we specify later, your financial plan also will need to include various other calculations, some of which are quite complex and heavily dependent upon assumptions. Our recommendation is perhaps not cheap, but we believe essential: retain someone with expertise in business finance to assist you.

CORE QUESTIONS TO ANSWER IN A BUSINESS PLAN

Business plans come in various forms, from comprehensive narratives with supporting tables and graphs to structured sets of bulleted text outlines, tables, and graphs; and from long dossiers to focused briefs. Regardless of form (which is often a function of the target reviewer), the core content of a business plan is pretty much uniform.[3,4]

In essence, a business plan is an answer to anticipated questions. In other words, before anyone commits money to your venture, s/he will want to have answers to a set of core questions. These questions, which you will find below, should guide you in the development of your business plan in two ways: (1) developmentally, as you put the various parts of the business plan together and (2) evaluatively, especially when you are close to final draft, by using the questions to revisit various parts of the business plan and evaluate the extent to which the questions have been addressed.

Note that the questions below do not match up to the conventional sections of the business plan (see Boxes 7-1 and 7-2). Though some mapping of questions and corresponding sections of the business plan apply, it will be your challenge to weave the answers into and throughout the various sections of the business plan. This also will enable you to engender in your reviewer a sense of consistency and comprehensiveness and build your credibility in the eyes of the reviewer. Likely, then, the answers to your questions will be spread across sections, with perhaps one section providing the core answer and other sections adding to, reinforcing, or validating this information.

Let us now review the questions to which potential investors, lenders, leasers and other stakeholders will want detailed, informative, rational, and convincing answers.

1. **Who are the key players in this venture? How do they complement each other strategically and operationally? What are their professional and personal strengths? Do they form a qualified team?** Even before they consider operational and financial matters, potential stakeholders want a strong sense of assurance that the proposed venture is led by the right combination and integration of people. Do not focus only on describing individual strengths, but reflect in your business plan that it takes a team of people to bring together the right mix of knowledge, expertise, skill, and experience to fulfill the many clinical and managerial responsibilities that come with launching, building, and maintaining a new clinical venture. Avoid at all cost the "super-leader trap": the belief that the leader must have expertise in all areas. Instead, show how you have surrounded yourself with the expertise that you do not have, while also describing the areas where you will be the key expert.

2. **What is the history behind this venture? How did the initial idea evolve into a concept, and the concept into a business plan? What were the initial objectives and what are the objectives now?** Good initiatives do not emerge overnight. Rather, they evolve from prior experiences, passive and active incubation, "testing-the-waters," and sustained strategic and operational thinking about options and approaches, strengths and weaknesses, and opportunities and threats. Future stakeholders will want to understand how your practice venture gradually took shape. Describe with both enthusiasm and pragmatism your original thinking and how you translated this into your original objectives. Take your readers along on your planning journey—not sentimentally but pragmatically. Show them how you were able to gradually put your arms around the many elements of an enterprise, and specified these into a comprehensive set of strategic and operational objectives. Stakeholders want this information to (rationally) make decisions about potential support. At the same time, understanding the history adds to their confidence in you, your practice venture, and your team.

3. **What services will your practice offer?** Potential stakeholders reviewing your business plan may not have the depth of understanding that you assume they have. Granted, they may know what primary care is, but most likely they will define it in part by their own personal experiences. Though the role of nurse practitioners is evident to you, it may be novel or intriguing to your reviewers. Regardless of their level of understanding, you should provide, in excruciating detail, a listing of the services that your practice will provide—and the revenue sources associated with these services. Provide a context within which the reviewer can place your proposal and make clear what the boundaries of the context are. A bit of psychology plays here as well. A detailed yet conceptually organized listing and description of services and associated revenue sources will convey several different messages: "I know the operational parts of this business," "there is potential for volume in patient visits and thus revenue"; and "this venture is sufficiently mainstream and not a far-out idea."

4. **What is your market and what is it like?** A key challenge is convincing potential stakeholders that there is market need for what you propose. Just stating that people will need primary care will not cut it—nor will the argument that the population is aging. These arguments are givens, not market specifications. You need to demonstrate with statistics and argumentation that there is an unmet need; that you know exactly where it is; and, importantly, that the target market is responsive towards your practice and its service offerings. For instance, statistics about rural, medically underserved areas may highlight the need for a practice in a rural community, but do not assure that its residents will accept services provided by a nurse practitioner. The latter will require data from community assessments, resident surveys, and testimonials of need and support from individuals and community leaders. Importantly, give your reviewers a sense of the growth opportunities in your market. An unmet need today may indeed be met by your practice, but when will saturation of revenues occur?

5. **How will you promote your practice and its services?** Marketing is a reality of business life, even if for some people the term has negative connotations. A systematic, creative, responsive, and sustained effort to promote your practice and its services is critical to its success and survivability. Building a new practice is not enough: patients and families need to come to it and communities need to embrace it. Based on your assessment of the target market, what will your messaging say about your practice? How will this message be conveyed? You will need to be creative here and offer a number of strategies related to advertising, community participation and visibility, and networking with patient recruitment and referral channels.

6. **Where and how will you provide your services?** Your business plan needs to describe the physical setup of your practice and include a floor plan that identifies the functions of various spaces. Say also a few words about the interior and how it will be both a functional and welcoming place of care. Describe the location of your practice. Where in the community is it located? Is it accessible? Is there sufficient parking? Is it served by public transportation? Are there supporting service providers nearby (e.g., pharmacy)? Next, move into the pragmatics of service delivery. Describe who will do what; when your practice will be open; what after-hours backup it will have; what support services it can rely upon (clinical lab, imaging, specialty referrals, hospital alliances, etc.). Lastly, provide information about the quality management program that you will put in place.

7. **How will your practice's supply chain be organized?** Your practice will go through a lot of consumables such as clinical supplies and office items. Clinical supplies are important to address in the business plan because they will impact on your practice's ability to deliver care. Your business plan needs to document how you will assure that your practice will have the necessary inventory of supplies without the expense of overstock. Will you have one or a few distributors who will provide you with the full supply chain? Will it include support to monitor consumption and replenishment?

8. **How will your practice be managed?** Business plans for more conventional ventures typically describe the background and experience of the management team and board of directors. For clinical practice ventures, the needs may go a bit further. Your business plan will need to show that your practice has the managerial and clinical leadership to guide it through its startup and into its maturity. As to administrative functions, specify which services you may outsource, such as payroll, accounting and taxation, marketing, billing, and so forth.

9. **Which are the critical success factors for a venture like yours?** Your business plan will need to discuss these factors and demonstrate how they are present in your proposed plan. For instance, being part of managed care networks seems a logical critical success factor for a primary care venture. Do you have managed care contracts lined up? If not, can you show that you will be eligible for participation? Likewise, community visibility may be a critical success factor. Where do you stand in that regard? Do you have a referral network? A systematic review will be helpful in your efforts to benchmark your proposed venture to the critical success factors. In a table, list in a first column the critical success factors; in a second column, the extent to which they are present at this time; and in a third column, if not present, how you plan to develop this factor and, if present, how you will sustain it in the future.

10. **What are the financial requirements?** How do you propose to meet these requirements? No matter how you turn it, investors, lenders, and leasers are money people and their money is their primary concern. Your business plan will need to include several financial documents, including: revenue, expense, and profit/loss projections for several years; cash flow analysis; break-even analysis; and various returns on investment analyses. We recommend that you present at least two if not three scenarios: normal case and worst case scenario possibly complemented by a best case scenario. It will force you to formulate the different assumptions and to recognize that things could go various ways. It will also provide your stakeholders with perspective, not to mention an appreciation of your efforts to provide a balanced financial perspective. If you are seeking an equity investment, you will need to include a valuation of the proposed business: what will the business be worth on its first day of operations? This will enable you to determine the percentage of equity you can negotiate with investors. For this valuation, you will need to obtain external advice because it includes, among many things, an assessment of your potential value as a clinician and therefore your share of equity in the new venture.

TURNING CONTENT INTO BUSINESS PLAN: FIVE STEPS

Once you have defined the objectives and the core questions, then comes the challenge of turning all this content into a formal business plan. We propose a five-step approach. Four of these steps coincide with the major components of a typical business plan, whereas the fifth adds a quality management component to the whole exercise of business plan development. We suggest you read through these five steps first to get a sense of the challenge ahead of you. Next, use Table 7-1 as a checklist of key elements. Box 7-1 offers a typical business plan outline—regardless of its form. (See Appendix F for a sample business plan). Box 7-2 applies specifically to NPs.

Step 1: The venture and its context. It is critical that, from the very beginning, you delineate clearly what your practice venture is about. Set boundaries to your

TABLE 7-1	
Check List of Key Elements of a Business Plan	
Step 1. The venture and its context	Who are you?
	What is your history and trajectory?
	Within what context will you be working?
	What services do you offer?
	Who are the target recipients of your services?
	What is available on the market today?
Step 2. Developing the best strategy	What are your strengths?
	What are your weaknesses?
	What opportunities exist?
	Which threats are present?
	What is your core business?
	Who are your patients?
	How is your practice different from others?
	How do you see your practice evolving in the long term?
Step 3. Operationalizing strategy into an action plan	How will you deliver services?
	What is your supply chain?
	How will you price your services?
	How will you assure that your practice is known?
	How will you reach patients and families?
	How will you manage revenues and expenses?
	How will you innovate?
	Who will assume the administrative responsibilities?
	What is your quality management plan?
	What is the organizational structure?
Step 4. Financial plan	What revenues do you anticipate?
	What are your operating expenses?
	What are your investment requirements?
	What other financing mechanisms may you need?
	What are you cash flow projections?
	What does the total financial picture of your practice look like?

BOX 7-1	BUSINESS PLAN OUTLINE

1. Enterprise and management
    1.1 Mission
    1.2 Major objectives
    1.3 History
    1.4 Key players
    1.5 Legal organization
2. Services
    2.1 Service offerings
    2.2 Market analysis
    2.3 Competitive analysis
3. SWOT analysis
    3.1 Strengths
    3.2 Weaknesses
    3.3 Opportunities
    3.4 Threats
4. Strategic plan
    4.1 Core business
    4.2 Strategic goals and objectives
    4.3 Market positioning
5. Supply chain
    5.1 Sourcing
6. Commercial plan
    6.1 Pricing
    6.2 Promotion and marketing
7. Research and development
    7.1 Future growth opportunities
    7.2 Development plan
8. Organization and administration
    8.1 Governance
    8.2 Management
    8.3 Personnel and organizational structure
9. Financial plan
    9.1 Projected revenues
    9.2 Projected expenditures
    9.3 Required investments
    9.4 Company valuation
    9.5 Financing strategy
    9.6 Cash flow analysis
    9.7 Break-even analysis
    9.8 Profit and loss summary
    9.9 Balance sheet

BOX 7-2	SAMPLE OUTLINE OF A NURSE PRACTITIONER BUSINESS PLAN

Cover sheet
Table of contents
Executive summary
Detailed description of the business
Market analysis
Financial plan
Management or organizational plan
Financial documents
Supporting documents

From Reel S: Developing a business plan: getting down to specifics, Advance Nurs Prac 11(6):53, 2003.

ideas and concepts that are as clear and unambiguous as possible. What you want to avoid is that the reviewers of your business plan, as they set out to review (yet another) business plan, will try to set their own boundaries to the concept. In other words, you need to avoid having your reviewers conceive your proposed venture in their terms, not in yours. If your presentation at the onset of the business plan is not clear (let alone vague), even the best-intentioned reviewers will inadvertently begin to set their own boundaries. You may have "lost" your reviewer right then and there. Start with as crisp a description as possible of your proposed practice venture and how the team of key players will make it happen. Don't be modest when describing the team and be sure to project a sense of balance, competence, motivation, goal-directedness, focus, and enthusiasm that uniquely qualifies them to lead the proposed venture. Show that you and your team can shoulder the many responsibilities and challenges of a new venture. After describing the team, move into a review and discussion of the services you plan to offer. Refer your reviewers to tables and graphs that are part of your business plan—but don't repeat the details in the body of text. Instead, use text to tie things together to show that the total of your practice concept is more than the sum of its services. This is where you bring a sense of "holism" to your proposed enterprise. Include in this description the market in which you will be operating, the trends and dynamics in this market, and competition that currently exists or may emerge in the future. This first step ends with a synthesis exercise: you have described the services and the market, now you have to bring these together into a pairing of both (the "services/market" dyad). Show how your services will not only fill gaps in the market but also advance the market in terms of innovation, competitiveness, and eventual profitability. Too often, entrepreneurs naively assume that "if I build it, people will buy it."

Step 2: Developing the best strategy. After establishing what you want to do, design the best strategy for getting there. This step begins with an intensive and thorough analysis of the strengths and weaknesses of the enterprise coupled with the opportunities and threats that exist in the market. This is the so-called SWOT Analysis (Strengths, Weaknesses, Opportunities, and Threats). Most SWOT analyses limit themselves to a listing of elements under each of the headings. We suggest, however, that you add a column under each heading. As you identify a strength, describe briefly in the next column how you will apply this strength to the success of the enterprise. As you grapple with a weakness, specify what you will do to minimize its impact. For each opportunity, state how you will capitalize on it. Lastly, for each threat, explain how you will shield your practice from it. Once this SWOT analysis is developed, you will be in a position of strength to sketch out strategic options, to identify the best strategy, and to detail this strategy along the following dimensions:

a. Core business of your practice venture
b. Commercial objectives
c. Market positioning of the practice
d. Medium- and long-term objectives

Step 3: Operationalizing strategy into an action plan. This step in the process will take the longest to complete; your challenge is to explain *how* you plan to translate strategy into an operational plan. This plan is the nuts-and-bolts of your planned venture. The more detailed it is, the more likely you will receive the funding. In fact, in this step of the business plan, you need to describe each and every activity, clinical and administrative, as concretely as possible in terms of an action plan: objectives, resources, and target dates. In light of your financial plan, you may want to include the cost associated with each item of the action plan. The following are essential elements to be covered:

a. Delivery of services: how will you deliver your services?
b. Supply chain: how will you get the supplies necessary to deliver services?
c. Marketing: how will you promote your practice and attract patients?
d. Revenue management: how will you collect your money as fast as possible?
e. Expense management: how will you operate as "lean" as possible?
f. Development: how will you improve and expand initial services and what new services may you develop in the future?
g. Quality management: how will you monitor the quality of clinical and administrative services?
h. Administration: how will the clinical services be supported administratively?

Step 4: Financial plan. Present first the projected revenues for a given time period (typically 5 years for a small enterprise like a clinical practice) and, likewise, present the projected expenses. Analyze when you will achieve break-even, that is, the point at which revenues are sufficient to cover expenses and from whence one can assume a profitable enterprise. This will help you determine how much cash you will need to launch your practice and get through the stage where expenses exceed revenues. In turn, this will enable you to review options for getting this cash. Will you seek one or more investors: "angel" investors (individuals who invest limited amounts of their own money), FFFs (friends, families, and fools), or venture capital funds? How much equity will you give in return for certain levels of investment? Will you be borrowing money—and what collateral will you offer to guarantee this loan? Are there incentive programs for regional economic development that you can tap into, from low-cost loans to outright subsidies? Conduct a cash flow analysis in which you map expenses against the timing of revenue. For instance, it may take 45 days from the time a patient is seen until payment is received from the insurer. How will you bridge such time discrepancies and fund your operation before you have the cash in hand? Answering all these questions will enable you, preferably in collaboration with a finance person (accountant, consultant, banker...), to put together a solid, objective, and rational financial plan.

Step 5. Evaluation. This is not a part of the business plan, but rather part of the development of the business plan. Once you have developed particular sections of the business plan, revisit them to check on completeness, clarity, and objectivity. As you near the completion of the plan, revisit the plan as a whole. Be as critical of your own work as possible. Lastly, right before putting the business plan document into production, go through it again line by line to check for grammar and spelling—or better yet, have someone who is unfamiliar with your document do this for you.

THE EXECUTIVE SUMMARY

Realistically, investors, lenders, and leasers review many business plans as they seek synergies between their money, ventures, and returns. It is only in the later stages of due diligence that these people will read the entire business plan. We saved this perhaps discouraging information for the end of this chapter—mainly because you will not be able to write an executive summary until you have brought your business plan to near-final status. Reaching this near-final point is only possible if you have achieved such mastery over all the strategic and operational details of your venture that you know it inside out, can differentiate the major from the minor and the substantive from the substantiating, and can pitch your venture to prospective financiers in 10 minutes or less—including what is in it for them.

The executive summary is the text equivalent of your "10-minutes-or-less" pitch. Don't try to write it before you have finalized all other sections of the business plan and have answered all the questions and presented the major scenarios. The executive summary, which you should put at the front of your business plan, is the most critical section of your business plan. In it, you must be able to describe in a maximum of two pages the bare-bone essentials of your practice venture. You must convey to your reviewers an initial sense of why they should put some of their money at risk with you. Not to discount the enormous amount of work you have put into the development of the business plan, but the reality is that the first level of review by prospective financiers will be your executive summary and some of the summary financial tables. Only once their interest has spiked will they read the entire business plan (or at least the main sections).To summarize, your reviewers will (1) try to get an initial idea of the importance, relevance, and qualities of the document; (2) decide whether to read on; and (3) if so decided, dig into the details.

Think of your executive summary as the abstract with key tables and figures bunched together into two pages of narrative. To make the executive summary more digestible, use headings, bullets, and white space in a balanced fashion. Don't try to squeeze everything into the executive summary. Instead, think about the key messages you want to convey to (a) lay a foundation, and (b) pique the interest of your reviewers.

The executive summary is your gateway into your reviewers' attention sphere. By the time you have the business plan in near-final form, you will be tired and fed up with the exercise and will want to finish this "executive summary thing" as fast as possible. But do take your time—in two ways: (1) allow yourself some time to let the business plan settle before you write the executive summary and then (2) allow yourself the time to write the executive summary as if it were a different document, one to be developed, once again, from scratch.

Just as you may want to seek input from others in the development of various sections of your business plan, do the same with your executive summary. Ask some of your friends and colleagues to review it "cold" and without the backup of the entire business plan. Do they get it? Do they understand what you are proposing and why it makes sense? Does the executive summary pique their interest? Does it give them some initial assurances that it is worthwhile for them to read on and work through the entire business plan? In other words, does the executive summary "bait" them?

MANAGING YOUR BUSINESS (PLAN)

A variety of possible formats can be used for a business plan, but content-wise they are all the same. They all bring together critical information about a proposed business venture. They argue objectively and rationally that the venture is strategically relevant, operationally feasible, and financially realistic given the risk that may be involved.

However, as we argued early on in this chapter, the business plan is more than a development tool. For a moment, think ahead and imagine that you were successful in securing the money you need and are at the threshold of launching your new practice. Don't consider the business plan, which you developed so meticulously and with so much intellectual and physical effort, a document of the past in the evolving history of your practice. Instead, see it as a benchmark. What is it that we said we were going to do? Are we doing it? What were our objectives and targets? Did we meet them? What did we project in terms of revenues?

Are we at target, below, or above? In either case, what do we do next? What does our expense picture look like? Are we spending as projected, spending more, or less? Again, what do we do next?

Good businesses, from the very small to the mega-corporation, have adopted the business plan model as a management tool. Annually, and if necessary more frequently, they go through the most recent version of the business plan and compare it to reality. Next, they revise the business plan accordingly. If expenses need to be reduced, how will that be done? If new opportunities arise, how will we tap into them? If the market picture changes, how will we respond—not only to survive but also to take advantage of the new opportunities?

CONCLUSION

In European business circles, people often talk about a vademecum document—literally, "it travels with me"—in fact, the answer to the more widely known "Quo vadis?" (where are you going?). Your business plan should be your vademecum: the itinerary and roadmap and compass and co-traveler in your journey from conceptualizing to realizing your practice venture—not just launching your venture (i.e., securing the money)—but shaping it into a dynamic and innovative entity that provides good care to patients and families and thus strengthens communities.

Your challenge? Start by asking yourself, "Quo vadis?" Answer with a *vademecum*.

REFERENCES

1. Maister DH: *Managing the professional services firm*, New York, 1993, Simon and Schuster.
2. Reel S: Developing a business plan: setting down to specifics, *Adv Nurs Prac* 11(8): 53-54, 90, 2003.
3. De Thomas AR, Grensing- Pophal: *Writing a convincing business plan*, Hauppauge, New York, 2001, Barron's Educational Series, Inc.
4. Siegal ES, Ford BR, Bornstein JM: *The Ernst & Young business plan guide*, ed 2, New York, 1993, Wiley.

SOFTWARE RESOURCES

Business Plan Pro, Eugene, OR, Palo Alto Software.
Business Plan Writer, Calabasas, Calif, Nova Development.

Practice Management

SALLY J. REEL • IVO L. ABRAHAM

Managing day-to-day operations is the business plan in action and requires knowledge and skills to assure a successful practice. An independent NP practice is a business and in addition to the advanced practice skills needed to treat patients, an NP needs need to develop savvy business skills. A sound practice management plan should strike a balance between providing patients with high-quality care and making enough money to operate the practice and support one's lifestyle. Good businesses have a product, are profitable, respond well to market forces, and can weather changes in economic cycles.[1] An NP practice will be subject to sound business principles; thus an operational plan is an important tool for focusing the service mission of the practice and clear the books. Although it is beyond the scope of this book to describe in detail all the nuances of daily operations, this chapter discusses many operational issues that must be considered and managed within a successful NP practice.

LOCATION, BUSINESS HOURS, AND OFF-HOUR COVERAGE

Location is an important practice consideration. Location determines how easily patients can access the practice and can impact practice income—up or down—so determining the place of operations should not be taken lightly. Location should be carefully considered as the practice's business and marketing plans are developed. Although location is discussed more fully in Chapter 11, a few daily operational considerations are worth mentioning here.

Deciding where to locate often is about going where the patients are or where other providers are—and anticipating where patients and providers will be in the future. Location also may determine the mix of patients that will be seen by the practice. Be practical when considering practice location. Carefully look at and evaluate place and neighborhood. Who lives and/or comes and goes in the area? Is that the clientele the practice intends to target?[1]

Patients need to know when they can access services, including what to do during off-service hours. Business hours should be displayed and adhered to. Some practices use a voice-recorded answering message that includes office hours and what to do if care is needed when the practice is closed. There are advantages and disadvantages to using an on-call service, an answering service, or an answering machine, and what the practice can afford may determine the method used. Invest in a good sign that will be visible from the road. It assists patients in finding the practice and serves to market the practice as well. Include the name of the practice and the providers on the door.

An example of how location and patient-friendly services developed into a great business concept is MinuteClinic. MinuteClinic evolved from a business idea developed by Rick Kreiger and partners Douglas Smith, MD, and Steve Pontius, who first founded QuickMedx, a provider of retail health care centers that eventually became MinuteClinic. The first QuickMedx clinics opened in Cub Food stores in the Minneapolis-St. Paul area in 2000. Patients paid cash for services for the common conditions of strep throat, mono, flu, female bladder infections, ear infections, sinus infections, and pregnancy testing. As the company grew and insurance coverage grew as well, the company became known as MinuteClinic, and services were added to Target stores and corporate office locations in the Minneapolis-St. Paul area. MinuteClinic expanded to Target stores in the Baltimore area in 2004, followed by centers opening in CVS pharmacies in both Minneapolis and Baltimore and ultimately leading to national expansion.[2] Why does a concept such as MinuteClinic work? One answer is convenience and another is location. Patients can be seen quickly, at reasonable costs, and experience the convenience of shopping or getting prescriptions at the same time. For more about MinuteClinic go to http://www.minuteclinic.com/.

THE LEGAL BUSINESS STRUCTURE OF THE PRACTICE

The legal business structure of a practice has significant implications for operations. The most common legal business structures for practices include sole proprietorships, general partnerships, limited liability companies (LLC), limited liability partnerships (LLP), and professional corporations (PC), which may be either a 'C' corporation or an 'S' corporation. Sansweet[3] suggests that when choosing the legal business structure for the practice "... the two main factors to consider are liability protection and financial implications."

Business structures have different liability protections for malpractice or creditor problems that may occur. A business structure alone, for example, will not protect against personal professional negligence or malpractice, but certain types of business structures—PC, LLC, or LLP—may protect against personal liability for malpractice committed by another provider in the practice. General partnerships do not offer protection and sole proprietors do not need such protection.[3] Common business structures and potential tax liabilities for each are shown in Table 8-1.

Limited liability partnerships (LLPs) are developed to protect individual partners from personal liability for the negligent acts of other partners or employees not under their direct control, but LLPs are not recognized by every state. Some states recognize LLPs but limit LLPs to those organizations that provide professional services such as medicine or law, whereby each partner is licensed individually. Partners report profit and losses on personal tax returns. The Secretary of State's office in the state where the practice will be located may be contacted to determine whether the state recognizes LLPs and what occupations qualify for LLPs.[4]

Professional service corporations (PSs) are organized for the purpose of providing a professional service for which each shareholder is licensed. Professional service corporations have the advantage of limited personal liability for shareholders and are available to certain professionals such as physicians, attorneys, and accountants. Again, by contacting the Secretary of State's office one can find out whether PSs are recognized by the state and what occupations qualify for PSs.[4]

Limited partnerships (LPs) have complex formation requirements, require at least one general partner who is fully responsible for partnership obligations and normal business operations, and require at least one limited partner who may be an investor that is not involved in day-to-day operations and is shielded from liability for partnership obligations beyond the amount of their investment. Limited partnerships do not pay tax but file an informational return. LP partners report profit shares and losses on personal tax returns.[4]

One additional business structure to consider is a *nonprofit corporation*. Nonprofit corporations are formed for civic, educational, charitable, and religious purposes. These have tax-exempt status and limited personal liability and are managed by a board of directors or trustees. If the nonprofit corporation dissolves, any assets must be given to another nonprofit organization.[4]

Two examples of nonprofit organizations are federally qualified health centers (FQHCs) and rural health centers (RHCs) (NOTE: although FQHCs **must** be nonprofit, RHCs **may** be nonprofit). FQHCs are nonprofit organizations governed by a board of directors and also have potential to apply for and receive federal grants. An FQHC is a type of provider defined by the Medicare and Medicaid statutes and includes all organizations receiving grants under section 330 of the Public Health Service Act, certain tribal organizations, and FQHC look-alikes. Section 330 of the Public Health Service Act defines federal grant funding opportunities for certain types of organizations—for example, community health centers, migrant health centers, health care for the homeless programs and public housing programs—to provide care to underserved populations. FQHC look-alike organizations meet all of the eligibility requirements of an organization that receives a PHS Section 330 grant, but an FQHC look-alike organization does not receive grant funding.[5]

The benefits of an FQHC include enhanced Medicare and Medicaid reimbursement, malpractice coverage through the Federal Tort Claims Act, eligibility to purchase prescription and nonprescription medications for outpatients at reduced cost

TABLE 8-1		

Legal Business Structures and Tax Implications

TYPE OF BUSINESS	BASIC DEFINITION	POTENTIAL TAX LIABILITIES
Sole proprietorship	A simple, informal structure, usually inexpensive to form; is owned by a single person or marital community; owner operates the business and is personally liable for all business debts; owner can transfer all or part of the business usually without restraint; owner can report profit or loss on personal income taxes	*Income taxes Self-employment taxes* *Estimated taxes* *Employment taxes* (e.g., Social Security and Medicare taxes; income tax withholding; federal unemployment tax, depositing employment taxes) *Excise taxes*
Limited liability corporation (LLC)	Advantageous for a small business because an LLC combines the limited personal liability feature of a corporation with the tax advantages of a partnership and sole proprietorship; profit and losses can be passed through the company to company members or LLC can elect to be taxed like a corporation; LLCs do not have stock, do not have to observe corporate formalities, and owners are called *members* who manage the LLC	For information on the kinds of tax returns to file for LLCs, how to handle employment taxes, and possible pitfalls, refer to IRS Publication 3402, *Tax Issues for Limited Liability Companies.* Available online: http://www.irs.gov/pub/irs-pdf/p3402.pdf
General partnership	Are not expensive to form; require an agreement between two or more people or entities to mutually own and operate a business; profit, loss, and management is shared among partners; each partner is personally liable for partnership debts; partnerships do not pay taxes, but do file an informational return and each partner reports his/her share of profits and losses on personal tax return; joint ventures are short-term partnerships	Partnership: *Annual return of income* *Employment taxes* (e.g., Social Security and Medicare taxes; income tax withholding; federal unemployment tax, depositing employment taxes) Individual partner: *Income tax* *Self-employment tax* *Estimated tax*

TABLE 8-1

Legal Business Structures and Tax Implications—cont'd

Type of Business	Basic Definition	Potential Tax Liabilities
C Corporation	A complex business structure; startup costs can be expensive; is a legal entity separate from its owners who are company stock holders; may be profit or nonprofit organizations; may experience greater governmental regulation than other business structures; profits taxed at the business and shareholder levels; shareholders may not be personally liable for corporate debt unless corporate formalities are not observed; formalities include issuing stock certificates, holding annual meetings, recording minutes of the meetings, and electing directors	Corporation *Income taxes* *Estimated taxes* *Employment taxes* (e.g., Social Security and Medicare taxes; income tax withholding; federal unemployment tax, depositing employment taxes) *Excise taxes*
S Corporation	Very similar to the C Corporation but does not double tax; if corporation qualifies for S status with the IRS, then it is taxed like a partnership; income flow through the shareholders who report income on personal tax returns	S Corporation *Income taxes* *Estimated taxes* *Employment taxes* (e.g., Social Security and Medicare taxes; income tax withholding; federal unemployment tax, depositing employment taxes) *Excise taxes* S Corporation shareholder *Income tax* *Estimated tax*

Data from Business.gov, the official business link to the U.S. government: *Legal Structures* (website): http://www.business.gov/topics/business_laws/legal_structures/index.html. Accessed January 16, 2006; and Internal Revenue Service: *Business Structures* (website): http://www.irs.gov/businesses/small/article/0,,id=98359,00.html. Accessed January 16, 2006.

through the 340B Drug Pricing Program (see http://www.hrsa.gov/opa/introduction. htm), access to National Health Service Corps (see http://nhsc.bhpr.hrsa.gov/), access to the Vaccine for Children program (see http://www.cdc.gov/nip/vfc/ Default.htm), and eligibility for various other federal grants and programs. FQHC look-alikes receive many of the same benefits as FQHCs, such as enhanced Medicare and Medicaid reimbursement and eligibility to purchase prescription and nonprescription medications for outpatients at reduced cost through the 340B Drug Pricing Program.[5]

A rural health clinic (RHC) is a clinic certified to receive special Medicare and Medicaid reimbursement. The purpose of the rural health clinic program is to improve access to primary care in underserved rural areas. Rural health clinics are required to use a team approach of both physicians and midlevel practitioners—nurse practitioners, physician assistants, and certified nurse midwives— to provide primary care services. Rural health clinics can be a for-profit or not-for-profit, public, or private entity. One major benefit is that RHCs receive special Medicare and Medicaid reimbursement. RHCs must be located in a rural shortage area that has been named within the last 3 years as a federally designated health professional shortage area (HPSA), federally designated medically underserved area (MUA), or a state Governor–designated underserved area. How to form a RHC is discussed more fully in Chapter 17.[6]

COLLABORATIVE AGREEMENTS AND INDEPENDENT NP PRACTICE

Although this book deals with many of the nuances of advanced practice and considerations for opening an independent nurse practitioner practice, an NP, whether employed or in an independent practice, must be in compliance with state law as related to scope of practice and collaborative agreements. Klein[7] notes that:

> "Scope of practice determines who you can see, who you can treat, and under what circumstance or guidance you can provide this care. Scope of practice also determines the limits and privileges of your licensure and certification as an advanced practice nurse. In the United States, scope of practice determines your ability to bill and be paid for what you do, as well as your ability to be covered by malpractice insurance. Significant liability issues are created when NPs practice outside of their scope."

Most states have some type of physician and nurse practitioner collaboration (with some more formal or "stringent" than others) within an NP's scope of practice. When the NP is an employee of a practice, usually meeting the collaborative requirements is relatively easy because the employing physician serves as the collaborative physician. Meeting required collaboration laws can be more complex for the independent practitioner because issues such as increased liability risks for the physician and compensation for physician services arise.

Self-employed NPs often have to pay for collaborative services.[8] Practice management requires compliance with state law and business strategies that will mitigate some of the impact of these laws on an independent NP practice.

If the state where an NP is employed or intends to establish an independent practice requires that a collaborative physician review and sign charts, meeting this requirement must be managed in the practice's operational plan. Strategies to be in compliance include knowing what the law requires. This has legal implications for an NP's practice, including the ability to seek reimbursement. Buppert[9] notes that no state has laws that require physicians to sign every single NP's charts, and 35 states do not have any requirements for physician review of patient charts. However, some states have cosignature requirements. Tennessee, for example, requires a physician to sign 20% of an NP's charts every 30 days. Arkansas requires that physicians cosign NP orders, and practice protocols must specify when NP orders must be cosigned. Physicians must sign any prescription that an NP writes in the state of Georgia. Fifteen states also have some requirements for physician oversight in terms of collaboration, delegation, or supervision of an NP's practice—signing charts is one way to document this oversight. Chart review requirements vary greatly from state to state. Some states also have requirements for on-site physician consultation with an NP. Illinois, for example, requires a physician to consult on-site once per month, whereas Louisiana requires a physician to visit the NP practice site once per week.[9]

NPs also need a clear understanding of the practice laws that govern in the state where the NP intends to practice. From a business point of view, NPs cannot practice without being in compliance with the law. If a collaborative agreement is needed to practice as an NP, then an NP's business depends on having sound, collegial, legal agreements. NPs in business may need to be prepared to pay for a physician collaboration to meet collaborative requirements.[8] Costs for this service will vary depending on the complexity of collaboration mandated by law (e.g., will an NP need 24/7 access to a collaborative physician? Will an NP need weekly or monthly on-site collaborative visits? Will an NP need charts cosigned?).

One method of handling collaborative agreements is to enter into a professional services agreement. However, before entering such an agreement, an NP needs to know whether state law allows this type of agreement. For example, where prescribing laws call for "supervisory" contracts with physicians, a state may have rules that prohibit physicians from contracting with self-employed NPs—for example, one argument is can a physician that is employed by an NP remain objective when the possibility exists that the NP could fire the physician for an unpopular opinion or decision?[8] An attorney can provide assistance to develop a professional services agreement and review state laws. Depending on the nature of the collaboration, NPs operating independent practices may pay an hourly rate to the physician or may pay a flat rate monthly fee for this service based on an average time needed to complete collaborative actions. Past rates NPs have paid for such services ranged from $500 to $2500 per month.[8]

The good news is that NP scope of practice laws change. Many of the barriers that impact practice are addressed by professional stakeholder groups that help establish practice standards. Thus examples cited at the time of this writing may have changed, and the take home message is to know the governing scope of practice law and review the law at least annually for changes.

Practice Protocols

Many states also require that NPs have some kind of written description of practice guidelines, standardized procedures, or protocols that underpin the NP's practice. Protocols establish the NP's scope of practice and are generally used to meet state requirements, as a guide for practice excellence, and as a performance assessment [10] However, as providers move toward evidenced-based practice, best practice protocols need to be up-to-date, provide current best practice evidence-based on research, clinical expertise, and patient preference. Protocols also need to be modified to the population served by your practice and to the setting where the protocols will be used.[11]

Some states require that the protocols adopted for the NP practice be filed with the state board, such as being listed in the collaborative practice agreement. Arkansas, for example, requires that protocols be developed in collaboration with a licensed physician, and the requirements of protocols are described in the Nurse Practice Act and Rules. In the Arkansas example, protocols must (1) establish procedures for the management of common medical conditions in the practice, (2) describe the degree to which collaboration, independent action, and supervision are required, and (3) describe acts including, but not limited to, assessment, diagnosis, treatment, and evaluation.[12] Many protocols are already published that may serve as NP practice protocols, but the key is to make sure that the protocols adopted meet state approvals and requirements.

One additional word of advice regarding collaborative agreements and practice protocols is that if the state requires these, keep a copy of the signed collaborative agreement readily accessible. Hanson[13] suggests copying the collaborative agreement and taping the agreement inside the front cover of the practice protocol book or manual. Examples of various types of collaborative agreements are shown in Appendix B.

POLICIES AND PROCEDURE MANUALS

Several policy and procedure manuals should be developed for the practice. These include but are not limited to employment and office policies, bloodborne pathogen standards policies, hazardous materials handling policies manual, discrimination and sexual harassment policies, workplace violence prevention policies, Health Insurance Portability and Accountability (HIPAA) office policies, Medicare compliance, and individual managed care and third-party payer policies. Each type of policy manual is briefly described as follows.

Employment and Office Policy Manual

The employment and office policy manual details employment policies that provide a framework for operating the practice and managing the practice employees. The manual should describe in detail the various operational functions of the practice. This manual may be used to orient new employees and also to serve as a point of reference for the NP and other practice staff. A loose-leaf binder can be used to house the manual; this manual form easily accommodates additions, deletions, and periodic changes to policies. Use section dividers to separate the policy areas. These sections may include policies related to employees and employment benefits, office policy, correspondence forms, staff meeting policies, and office maintenance.[14] Policies for each section might include the following:

- *Employees and employment benefits*: Dress code, employment hours, staff meeting policies, smoking policies, job descriptions, employee benefits and procedures for enrolling or using benefits such as sick days, vacation time, holidays, personal leave days, salary, raises, productivity bonuses, health insurance, life insurance, pension plans, retirement, and profit sharing.[14]

- *Office policies*: Telephone priorities, fee schedules, third-party payers, vendor and supplier lists, names and contacts of who to call for office maintenance such as heating and ventilation repairs when the owner is away, standard office and practice supply list and approved vendors for stocking supplies, staff meeting policies.[14]

- *Correspondence forms*: Sample letters to be used by the practice, such as a request for records, request for consultation and referrals (patient and provider), patient information, collections, consent forms, assignment of benefit forms, insurance forms, medical-information release forms, patient instruction forms.[14]

Other Manuals

Other manuals that are necessary for a practice include a bloodborne pathogen standard manual, a hazardous communication standard manual, a material safety datasheet manual, a discrimination and sexual harassment policy manual, a workplace violence prevention manual or policy, a Medicare compliance manual, and a Health Insurance Portability and Accountability Act (HIPAA) manual.[14]

The practice also needs manuals for all individual managed care organizations and third-party payers with which the practice does business. These manuals help guide patient care and are a source of information if it becomes necessary to appeal denied claims or make other negative plan decisions. Finally, the practice needs an office emergency kit, and although not a manual or policy per se, equipment needed for emergencies should be readily available and organized for easy access.[14]

INSURANCE

Most health care providers understand the importance of having malpractice insurance to protect against liability costs associated with payment of defense and indemnity costs that are related to health service damage claims generally as a result of direct patient care.[15] When an NP opens an independent practice, other business insurances are needed. Business insurances are about preparing for the unexpected such as theft, embezzlement, a lawsuit, or a natural disaster.[4]

Unthinkable events do happen that disrupt business, and these can cause substantial loss. Many types of insurance are available to cover business risks and selecting what is needed for an NP practice reflects what is needed to protect the practice. A few types of business insurances are discussed here, but an NP needs to discuss with an insurance agent and an attorney what types of coverage are realistically needed for that particular practice.

Assets, including equipment and the buildings, money and securities, accounts-receivable records, inventory, and furniture can be protected by having *property insurance*. Property insurance provides coverage in the event of theft, fire damage, explosions, accidents, or acts of nature. Some insurers will provide policies to protect data and records in the event that records are destroyed and will take time to reproduce. Some insurers also provide computer virus protection for lost data and business related to computer viruses.[16]

Liability insurance protects business assets in the event a lawsuit occurs that is related to something the business did or did not do to cause an injury or property damage. With liability insurance, the insurer pays the legal costs of a business in a covered liability claim. Covered liability claims include things such as bodily injury, property damage, and personal injury. Insurers also cover compensatory and general damages but do not cover punitive damages because punitive damages are considered punishment for intentional acts. The amount of general liability insurance purchased for the practice depends on the perceived risks associated with the practice. Property and liability coverage may be purchased together under a general business owner's policy, but sometimes the coverage may be better if these are purchased separately.[17]

Worker's compensation insurance typically is mandated by state law for any business that has employees. Worker's compensation insurance covers loss of income, medical expenses, and rehabilitation and is designed to assure that injured or disabled employees hurt on the job are compensated whereas business liability is eliminated or reduced.[14,18]

Business interruption or *loss of income protection insurance* provides coverage for ongoing practice expenses and loss of income if the practice is forced to close because of fire or other disaster or another event such as a power failure or fire in a neighboring business. Business interruption insurance can save the practice in the event of unforeseen closure and loss of income.[14,19]

Fraud and abuse/billing errors and omissions insurance is an insurance that provides funding for unintentional billing errors and omissions when billing third parties. Coverage is also provided to cover the costs of governmental investigations that may result from Medicare and Medicaid billing investigations. Some policies provide coverage for the cost of audits, investigations, legal defense, judgments, settlements, civil fines, and penalties.[15]

As health information technologies become more embedded in health care, and because a practice is likely to do business that includes billing for patient services in an electronic environment, *cyber liability* insurance provides coverage against lawsuits for libel, invasion of privacy, inflictions of emotional distress, and copyright and trademark infringement. Cyber liability insurance also covers errors and omissions in content and errors and omissions in providing services for others.[15]

There are other insurances to consider as well, including employment practices liability insurance and dishonesty insurance. *Employment practices liability insurance* provides coverage for defense and indemnity costs incurred as a result of claims for damages brought by employees related to violation of employment practice laws and regulations such as sexual harassment, discrimination, and wrongful termination.[15] *Dishonesty insurance* protects against employee dishonesty and covers the loss of money, securities, or other properties resulting from acts by bonded persons.[14]

HIRING EMPLOYEES

According to the U.S. Small Business Administration (SBA), the following steps are important to filling a job position[20]:

- **Determine the need to hire a new employee.** Is the practice properly using the skills of current employees? Can the practice support a new employee?

- **Conduct a thorough job analysis.** What are the job's essential functions and key performance criteria?

- **Write a job description for the position based on the job analysis.**

- **Determine the salary for the position, based on internal and external equity.** Is the salary comparable and proportional with the salaries and responsibilities of other positions inside the practice and similar positions in the surrounding community?

- **Decide where and how to find qualified applicants.** What are the recruitment techniques to be used? What is the timeframe for conducting the job search? Advertising is not necessarily the best way to recruit.

- **Collect and review several applications, then select the most qualified candidates for further consideration.**

- Interview the most qualified candidates for the position.

- Check references.

- Hire the best person for the job.

If the applicant pool does not have a sufficient number of appropriately qualified applicants, consider expanding the timeframe for the search, rewrite any advertisements, and consider additional recruitment techniques.

How to Conduct an Employment Interview

Knowing what to do is an important part of conducting a successful job interview. The SBA suggests the following guidelines on how to conduct a successful interview.[20]

1. **Prepare in advance for the interview.**

   - Know what is desired in a candidate and review job specifications before conducting the interview.

   - Know the job and its responsibilities and review the job description before the interview.

   - Prepare a list of standard questions concerning the candidate's skills, abilities, and past work performance.

   - Prepare a list of prioritized and measurable criteria for analyzing and comparing the candidates.

   - Review the candidate's resume before the interview.

   - Set specific appointment times and reasonable time limits.

2. **Collect pertinent information during the interview.**

   - Past behavior is a predictor of future behavior, so try to get a sense of the candidate's behavior patterns as the interview is conducted. Often, by listening to how the candidate responds to interview questions about previous work, it is possible to get an idea of what the applicant's behavior will be like in the future.

   - Do not offer too much information up front during the interview to avoid coaching the candidate to formulate answers that fit the practice's needs. Do not put words into the candidate's mouth.

   - Ask questions that focus on the candidate's past performances. If, for example, the position, such as an office manager, demands an individual who is well organized and handles paperwork easily, ask how the candidate keeps track of schedules and workload in her/his current position.

- Ask specific questions about specific problems that the job holder may face. Focus on past behavior and the results of the candidate's actions in a particular situation. For example, "As the practice receptionist you may encounter a few unhappy patients who may yell at you over the telephone or in person. Have you had any experience dealing with difficult clients? What was the most difficult patient situation you have managed, and how did you resolve the problem?"

- Notice how well the candidate listens and responds to the questions asked.

- Note the candidate's choice of words and nonverbal behavior. Does the candidate answer the questions clearly?

- Listen to the questions the candidate asks and clarify why the questions are being asked. The questions a candidate asks first may be their primary concern.

- Take detailed notes about job-related topics that will help distinguish the candidates from one another

3. **Look and behave professionally during the interview.**

- Dress appropriately and set a businesslike atmosphere.

- Avoid appearing bored or tired.

- Structure the interview and inform the candidate of the structure. Let the candidate know that the interview will be focusing on past results and that interviewers will take notes.

- Provide information on the practice and the job position to each candidate.

- Record information about the job position's criteria that will help evaluate the candidates.

- Organize and analyze the candidate's information immediately after the interview when memory is fresh. Consider rating each candidate on each of the job criteria immediately after the interview.

4. **Treat candidates fairly.**

- Use the list of standard questions during each interview so that all candidates are treated the same.

- Refer to the job criteria to analyze the candidates. Keep all questions job-related.

- Do not ask any discriminating questions.

- If possible, have at least one other person meet and/or interview and rate candidates who are "finalists." Compare ratings among interviewers to help control for personal biases.

5. **Be courteous and respectful.**

- Begin on time and conduct the interview in a private place away from distractions and without interruptions.

- Allow enough time for the interview.

- Appreciate the candidate's accomplishments.

- Do not patronize or argue with the candidate.

- Thank the candidate for his/her time and interest in the position.

6. **Facilitate open communication.**

- At the onset of the interview, attempt to establish a rapport with the candidate by breaking the ice; look for something on the resume such as experiences in a particular practice or geographical location.

- Promote a relaxed environment with free-flowing conversation, and do not dominate the discussion. Many experts recommend an 80/20 rule, meaning that the interviewer talks 20% of the time and the candidate talks 80% of the time.

- Politely query the candidate for information by asking open-ended questions that will provide insight into the candidate's values and traits.

- Ask structured questions that require some thought on the part of the candidate and listen carefully to the candidate's answers. If the person does not provide you with specific results, ask questions until you do get detailed answers.

- Explain the selection process to the candidate. Offer realistic timeframes for the selection process and adhere to these.[20]

What Not to Ask During an Employment Interview

There are several areas that should not be asked about during an employment interview because these subjects relate directly to federal and state employment laws. Equal Opportunity legislation is complex and individual state laws vary as well.

In an interview, or on an employment application, do not ask questions about the following[14,20]:

- **Age or birth date.** Asking about high school graduation date may be interpreted as age discrimination in some states. It is also a good idea not to use words like "overqualified" when interviewing older candidates.

- **Arrest record.** Although it is discriminatory to ask about an arrest record in most states, it is permissible to ask whether the candidate has ever been convicted of a crime. If the candidate is asked whether he or she has ever been convicted of a crime, follow the question with a statement that a conviction is not necessarily a bar against employment.

- **Race or ethnicity**. Do not ask questions about the candidate's ancestry, where the candidate was born, or what the candidate's native language is because this could be perceived as discrimination based on national origin. It is permissible to ask about the person's ability to speak English or a foreign language if required for the job.

- **The candidate's citizenship or immigration status in the United States before hiring.** It is permitted to ask whether the candidate will be able to provide proof of eligibility to work in the United States if hired—but do not ask to see proof before hiring the candidate.

- **Religion or religious customs or holidays.** If the practice is open on both Saturdays and Sundays, it is permissible to state that the office is open on Saturdays and Sundays and then ask whether the candidate can work on these days and satisfy this requirement. This question is allowable only if working weekends is a central job expectation. If the practice is closed, it is not permissible to ask this question.

- **Candidate's height and weight if it does not affect ability to perform the job**.

- **Names and addresses of relatives.** Candidates may be asked only about those relatives employed by the organization.

- **Whether or not candidates own or rent their homes or who lives with them.** Because minorities may have a lower rate of home ownership, asking this question may be discriminatory. It is permissible to ask for the candidate's address for future contact.

- **Candidate's credit history or financial situation**. Although in some situations credit history may be considered job-related, it is wise to proceed with great caution.

- **Education or training not required to perform the job**.

- **Sex or gender.** Avoid any language that may be found inappropriate by the candidate because it is the candidate's standard of conduct that must be met.

- **Pregnancy (actual or planned) or medical history**.

- **Family or marital status or child-care arrangements**. It is permissible, though, to ask whether the candidate will be able to work the required hours for the job.

- **Membership in a nonprofessional organization or club that is not related to the job**.

- **Physical or mental disabilities.** A candidate may be asked whether he or she can perform the essential duties of the job. Under the American Disabilities Act of 1990 candidates may be asked questions about disability accommodations if the disability is overt or voluntarily disclosed.

- *The key point*—if in doubt, think carefully about whether the question is job-related. If not, do not ask and keep it out of the conversation.[14,20]

As a final point, how might the dishonest applicant who lies or embellishes a resume be spotted during the interview? It may not be possible to determine dishonesty from a review of the resume. However, some steps to gain more information may be taken. Specifically, have applicants complete a job application even if a copy of the resume has been provided. Make sure the job application has a statement on it that indicates giving false information on the application is grounds for termination. Always ask for and check references. Contact previous employers listed in the application or resume. Have more than one person interview the candidate, and ask the candidate questions that directly relate to the job.[21]

MANAGING PRACTICE FINANCE AND DAILY OPERATIONS

Few NPs hold MBAs or are certified public accountants, and unless an NP has a solid business background, having an accountant and an attorney for the practice is simply good business sense; their fees are worth the advice and protection they can provide as the practice is operated. Accountants provide bookkeeping and tax services, but more importantly, a good accountant can help with financial planning necessary for the health and growth of the practice.

It is important here to distinguish between accounting and day-to-day bookkeeping. Bookkeeping is the recording of every financial transaction, both on the revenue and the expense side. It is a trail of every dollar received and every dollar spent. Bookkeeping can be outsourced, or bookkeeping may be performed as an internal function within the business—however, bookkeeping does require some specific skills and expertise. The practice's accountant, on the other hand, is the business finance and taxation expert. He or she may help you set up the practice's accounting system of accounts, revenue, and expense codes, cash management procedures, and financial reports. Just as much, he or she is your financial planning adviser, who brings both analytical and planning skills. He or she can help an NP understand the practice's patterns related to cash flow, revenue and expenditures; perform future projections, and advise the NP as to growth management and decision making; estimate needed resources; identify crunch periods; and set realistic goals.

The practice's attorney ideally will understand business and employment laws plus have a background in health care. The attorney can provide valuable guidance on health care transactions, contracts and litigation, credentialing and peer review, federal and state fraud and abuse, elder care law, professional liability and malpractice defense, third-party payers and managed care contracts, and advise on investments, retirement, and estate planning. A reputable attorney may be found by obtaining a referral from a colleague or contacting the state bar association and getting a list of qualified names. Confine the search to attorneys specializing in the area of law an NP needs counsel about. NPs also can consult the *Martindale-Hubbell Law Dictionary*, which provides a complete listing of domestic and international lawyers by state and specialty. Hetico and Pentin-Maki[22] describe the ideal attorney as "… one that is pleasant to be around, though not a 'yes' man, and who will also serve as a relentless advocate for you and your practice."

Payroll Taxes

Once an NP becomes a business owner, a new partner is acquired—tax agencies. There are several business taxes that an NP business owner should become familiar with to ensure meeting all tax obligations. Major payroll taxes include federal and state taxes and FICA. Employers are responsible for withholding taxes from employees' paychecks, sending these withholdings to the right government agencies, as well as other tax obligations.

• FICA is the Federal Insurance Contributions Act and provides for a federal system of old-age, survivors, disability, and hospital insurance. Old-age, survivors, and disability are financed by the social security tax and hospital insurance is financed by Medicare taxes.[23]

• Federal unemployment taxes and state unemployment taxes provide for payments of unemployment compensation to workers who have lost their jobs. Most employers will have to pay both a federal and state unemployment tax. Only the employer pays the federal unemployment tax, and this is not deducted from the employee's salary. Each state has a different unemployment tax rate and different wage limits from which the taxes are calculated, and state unemployment taxes are also paid by the employer.[23]

Some business owners may use a professional payroll service to manage payroll, especially if payroll varies from pay period to pay period. A benefit to using a payroll service is avoiding costly mistakes during payroll processing such as failing to send payroll taxes on time. If a professional payroll service is used, one should expect a payroll service to determine the amount of each paycheck and the tax obligations for each employee as well as print the checks and provide the business with payroll reports.[23]

Revenue collections are part of the everyday life of any NP practice. Although billing and coding are discussed in Chapter 9, successful revenue collections are a daily affair. As an NP business owner, the NP and the practice's providers have ultimate responsibility for coding clinical encounters, which means that providers and billers need to be up-to-date on coding practices. Some practices outsource billing and other daily operations because there are many firms that will provide billing and other practice management services. Billing firms may charge a percentage of income for each billed encounter or take a set fee.

Outsourcing is a viable alternative if an NP lacks the knowledge or skills necessary to manage all aspects of the practice but wants to maintain general management or ownership of the practice. Outsourcing is about using services outside the practice to handle activities traditionally managed by the NP or the practice staff. Outsourcing can enhance business profits if the practice does not have in-house expertise to manage areas such as accounting and bookkeeping, quality assurance, fee schedule review, marketing, legal contracting, budgeting, negotiating, formulation of scheduling systems, evaluation of staffing needs, and billing and reimbursement analysis. Other areas where the practice may benefit from external support include business planning, health information technology, laboratory and radiology services, credentialing, staffing and managed care/third-party payer contracting.[24]

How to Avoid Revenue Loss

Inefficiency and waste can wreck havoc on a practice's financial health. Borglum[25] identified 10 areas of revenue loss that affect practice revenue. These include (1) lack of a budget, (2) lost productivity, (3) inadequate and inaccurate coding, (4) poor billing practices, (5) poorly reimbursing insurance plans, (6) infrequently and improperly updated fee schedules, (7) excessive overtime and staffing, (8) inefficient supply purchasing, (9) petty theft and embezzlement, and (10) unmanaged risk. An NP needs to understand potential sources of revenue loss and manage appropriately.

To illustrate, one caveat with outsourcing practice billings is that the practice owner must be certain the billing company will investigate unpaid claims by third-party payers; otherwise the practice may lose potential income. For this reason, some recommend in-house billing.[1] Billing is only one part of practice revenue generation. Practices need a collections policy to ensure payments are received. Billing and collections begin when a patient makes an appointment. At the time of appointment scheduling, tell the patient that the office policy is to collect all deductibles and co-payments and fees at the time of service. Verify insurance and have patients bring their insurance cards to the appointment.[26]

Educate staff to expect payments at the time of service as well. Third-party billing also begins when the appointment is made and at the time of service when patient demographic data is gathered and insurance verified. Third-party billing is finalized during the visit when appropriate codes are known. It is advisable to verify insurance and what is covered before the patient's actual visit. Staff can call the insurance carrier before or at the time of service and determine eligibility for benefits, whether the plan covers services for NPs or other practice providers, whether the service or procedures are covered, and how much the plan will pay for services and procedures. These questions are the same questions the staff should ask before the patient's appointment. Bill daily and use electronic billing whenever possible because bills are paid more quickly. Have a mechanism for follow up on all claims not paid within 45 days. Follow the rules of third-party payers to receive the maximum reimbursement allowed for services in the shortest timeframe.[26]

The Practice Budget

An operational budget is essential for a practice. Without one the practice is subject to many things including embezzlement, over- or understaffing, supply waste, inappropriate purchasing, inadequate savings for practice improvements and higher-than-necessary income taxes—hence profit loss for the practice. Developing a practice budget is challenging but can be learned. Three strategies can be used to get started: tracking expenses, using published benchmarks, and regularly comparing the practice's actual financial status with its budget. Start tracking practice expenses by recording what the practice spends money on. Create a practice-specific list of expense categories. This is the "general ledger" and should be as detailed as possible because this allows for ready extraction of information. A sample chart of accounts is shown in Figure 8-1. These account categories should be modified to reflect the expenses of a particular practice. It may be necessary to document an expense in more than one place on the ledger. Avoid combining categories such as accounting for clinical and administrative supplies in the same category. Combining accounts may make it difficult to identify theft, determine appropriate staffing ratios, or conduct appropriate cost analyses.[27]

Benchmarks for physician practices are also available to provide some idea about medical practice expenses. Although the author does not endorse any particular benchmark, one benchmark to look at can be obtained from the Medical Group Management Association's (MGMA) *Cost Survey* ($255 for members, $465 for nonmembers; http://www.mgma.com) and the *Statistics Report on Medical and Dental Income and Expense Averages* (for a specialty report: $99 for members, $249 for nonmembers; for the full report: $495 for members, $795 for nonmembers; http://www.healthcon.org). Both reports include information on staffing counts, accounts-receivable levels, and contractual disallowance percentages, and both present data as a percentage of collections (revenue).[27]

By regularly comparing a practice's actual finances with its budget, it is possible to see how the numbers in the actual practice finances vary from the expected norm, how much these numbers vary, and why they vary. This is known as a *variance analysis* and should be done quarterly.[27]

Lost Productivity

Lost productivity is a significant source of practice revenue loss. Lost productivity occurs when providers see fewer patients than optimum, provide fewer services per visit, or have visits that have less than optimum complexity. Several thousand dollars can be lost annually simply by missing one fee-for-service patient visit per day. Productivity also can be lost by scheduling too many unnecessary visits, because these types of encounters are usually less complex and require minimal services. Failure to offer services patients want also is a productivity risk because patients may go elsewhere as a result.[25]

Improving productivity and preventing revenue loss involves setting and achieving daily productivity goals such as maximizing complexity and services per visit and providing alternatives to unnecessary patient visits.[25] Practice revenues fluctuate and offering diverse services helps mitigate lean revenue periods.

	Budget	This month	Last month	This month last year	This year to date	Last year to date
ALL EXPENSES	100%					
Capital (IRS section 179) purchases						
Donations and contributions						
Dues						
Fees: Lab						
Fees: Retirement plan						
Insurance: Business						
Insurance: Malpractice						
Janitorial/maintenance						
Journals						
Lease payments: Equipment						
Legal, accounting and consultants						
Loan payments: Principal						
Loan payments: Interest						
Marketing: Ads, promotion and yellow pages						
Marketing: Meals and entertainment						
Meals: Business/staff meetings						
Miscellaneous						
Outside services						
Postage						
Rent and utilities						
Repairs and maintenance: Building						
Repairs and maintenance: Contracts						
Repairs and maintenance: Equipment						
Staff wages						
Staff benefits						
Staff retirement plan						
Staff continuing education						
Supplies: Clinical						
Supplies: Office						
Taxes and licenses						
Telephone/answering service/pager						
Travel and professional meetings						
Uniforms and laundry						
Provider associate wages						
Provider associate benefits						
Provider associate retirement plan						
Provider associate continuing education						
Ancillary provider wages						
Ancillary provider benefits						
Ancillary provider retirement plan						
Ancillary provider continuing education						
Owner's wages/draws						
Owner's benefits						
Owner's retirement plan						
Owner's auto						
Owner's dues						
Owner's individual and student loans						
Owner's insurances						
Owner's journals						
Owner's marketing: Meals and entertainment						
Owner's other						
Doctor-owner net income (practice profit)						

Figure 8-1

Chart of accounts. Variance analysis template. *Adapted with permission from Medical Practice Forms: Every Form You Need to Succeed. Copyright © 2004 PMIC. Physicians may adapt for use in their own practices; all other rights reserved. Borglum K: Three Steps to an Effective Practice Budget: Family Practice Management 11(1):46-50, 2004 (serial online): http://www.aafp.org/fpm/20040100/46thre.html.*

For example, avoid relying on one major payer by contracting with many third-party payers. If not prohibited by state scope-of-practice laws, offer services such as wellness evaluations or home visits for cash payments. Negotiate with hotel managers or large resorts and have them place the practice's business card in the guest rooms; when these patients are seen charge cash. The key to diversifying services is to maximize profitability by choosing services wisely and not being afraid to think in terms of maximizing profitability.[1]

Understanding Cost Per Unit as Related to Practice

Understanding the costs per patient visit in the practice is good business. Kullgren and Sibella (2004) provide several steps to understanding cost unit analyses within a practice and several of their suggestions are included in this section. A unit cost analysis examines all the resources associated with providing a particular service and calculates just what it costs to deliver that service to the smallest unit—for example, a well woman exam, an adult physical or procedure. Costs per unit information helps with budget preparation, setting service fees, and negotiating rates with third-party payers. The goals of a unit costs analysis is to understand accurate practice cost information because this informs making good practice management decisions. One starting point for a unit cost analysis is to identify the type of service for which costs will be determined; this might be a particular type of patient care or perhaps an evaluation of what all comprises the costs of a 15-minute patient encounter. Once a service for analysis is identified, a time period for conducting the analysis is established. Many computerized practice management systems have tracking functions that support analyzing the number of units of a particular service during a specified timeframe. A chart audit can be done to estimate the units of service when a computerized practice management system is not used.[28]

Part of unit analysis includes calculating direct costs related to the service. Direct costs include provider and support staff salaries and benefits, medical supplies, laboratory tests and any other resources used at the time of the service. The largest direct cost is usually the amount of time the provider spends on one unit of service. Provider time may be determined by direct observation of the provider's activities, time sheets completed by the provider, time sheets completed by the patient, or patient cycle time from check-in to check-out. Support staff time can be calculated in a similar manner. An average time per type of patient visit can be determined and salary associated with that time prorated to determine what the provider for the service is. Supply costs can be analyzed by comparing a list of items used against the practice supply catalog.[28]

In addition to determining direct costs, indirect costs should be analyzed too. Indirect costs are those costs that are shared by more than one area of the practice. Indirect costs involve resources that are not directly used when a particular service is provided but without which providing the service would not be possible. Typical indirect costs are administrative staff salaries and benefits, facility costs, insurances premiums, and other office equipment and supplies. Indirect costs can be determined by listing and totaling all the indirect costs of the practice such as rent and utilities per year, administrative salaries and benefits per year, and malpractice and general liability insurances per year. Once indirect costs are known a decision should be made about how much of the practice's indirect costs should be allocated to the particular service. Several methods can be used to determine the percent of indirect costs and a couple methods include determining the ratio of the particular service to all the services provided in the practice or determining the percentage of the practice's total direct costs that are generated by the particular service. To illustrate, if 15% of the practice visits are pediatric well child visits, this percentage may be used as a rationale to determine that 15% of the practice's indirect costs are attributable to well child visits.[28]

Depreciation costs are also factored into the cost analysis of a particular service, and if not considered, may result in an underestimation of expenses and long-term planning. A straightforward way to determine depreciation is to take the initial cost of the equipment and subtract the estimated resale value and the end of the equipment's useful life. Divide this figure by the number of years the particular equipment will be used by the practice. Using a cost allocation similar to determining direct costs, calculate the amount of depreciation attributable to the service, then divide this number by the number of units of service during the analysis time period.[28]

Last, to determine full cost per unit of service add direct, indirect, and depreciation costs to arrive at the final cost per unit of service. One note—if donated goods or services are part of practice operations, the market value of these services should be added into practice cost calculations, particularly if resources to purchase these are not available to the practice. This is especially relevant if the practice relies on fundraising.[28]

Conclusion

As discussed in this chapter, many considerations go into a sound practice management plan. A few final points about daily operations are also worth mentioning. A practice requires establishing efficient daily operations to track and purchase supplies, purchase equipment, repair equipment, deposit cash at the end of the business day, and dispose of hazardous waste. A system also must be established to protect the confidentiality and storage of patient records no matter what the format of those records (e.g., paper versus electronic). An NP owner also must comply with fire marshall inspections and building codes and must also comply with maintaining any laboratory facilities in accordance with federal and state laws.[9]

A call system should be established so that patients know how to access providers 24-hours per day. The practice manager should keep a copy of all providers current state licenses, national certification, malpractice history, the practice agreement for all NPs and collaborative physicians, and prescriptive authority numbers.[9]

Housekeeping, laundry, snow removal, Occupational Safety and Health Administration (OSHA) and Clinical Laboratory Improvement Amendements

(CLIA) compliance, proper storage and dispensing of pharmaceutical samples if allowed by state law are areas of consideration too. A security plan may be necessary, and drafting a policy about how the physical facilities may be used by staff members during after-hours should be considered as well. Avoid keeping narcotics or large sums of case on site.[9]

Finally, develop a practice organization chart. An organizational chart is needed when the business plan is written and the practice management structure is outlined for daily operations. An organizational chart should demonstrate the practice's decision-making chain of command; and if used as part of the business plan and fund-raising efforts for the practice, append written job descriptions for each position and biosketches of key personnel. The business plan is discussed more fully in Chapter 7.

REFERENCES

1. Ranier, C: *Practice management: a practical guide to starting and running a medical office,* Lima, Ohio, 2004, Wyndham Hall Press.
2. About MinuteClinic (website):http://www.minuteclinic.com/Home/About/tabid/55/Default. aspx. Accessed January 10, 2006.
3. Sansweet JB: Choosing the right practice entity, *Family Practice Management* 12(10):42-44, 2005 (serial online):http://www.aafp.org/fpm/20051100/42choo.html. Accessed January 17, 2006.
4. Business.gov, the official business link to the U.S. government: *Special Structures* (website): http://www.business.gov/phases/launching/choose_structure/special_structures.html. Accessed January 17, 2006.
5. Rural Assistance Center: *What is a Federally Qualified Health Center (FQHC)?* (website): http://www.raconline.org/info_guides/clinics/fqhcfaq.php#whatis. Accessed January 17, 2006.
6. Rural Assistance Center: *What is a Rural Health Clinic?*(website): http://www.raconline.org/ info_guides/clinics/rhcfaq.php#whatis. Accessed January 17, 2006.
7. Klein T: Nurse practitioners: defining scope of practice, *Topics in Advanced Practice Nursing* eJournal 5(2), 2005 (serial online): http://www.medscape.com/viewarticle/506277_1; quote: section 3 of 10. Accessed January 2, 2006.
8. Tumulo J: Paying for collaboration. *Advance Newsmagazines, Advance for Nurse Practitioners,* June 2002 (serial online): http://nurse-practitioners.advanceweb.com/Common/editorial/ editorial.aspx?CC=35731. Accessed January 2, 2006.
9. Buppert C: Does a Physician Need to Sign All NP Charts? *Medscape Nurse* 7(2), Dec 20, 2005 (serial online): http://www.medscape.com/viewarticle/518049?src=search. Accessed January 2, 2006.
10. LeMaire B: *Winifred Star, on nurse practitioner protocols, Nurseweek.com,* January 23, 2004 (serial online): http://www.nurseweek.com/5min/wstar.asp. Accessed January 9, 2006.
11. Lucas J, Fulmer T: Evaluating clinical practice guidelines: a best practice. In Mezey M, Fulmer T, Abraham I, editors: *Geriatric nursing protocols for best practice,* ed 2, New York, 2003, Springer, pp 1-14.
12. Arkansas State Board of Nursing: *Nurse Practice Act/SubChapter 3/Section 17-87-303, Registered nurse practitioner* (website): http://www.arsbn.org/pdfs/practice_act/chap3.pdf.
13. Personal communication between Charlene Hanson and Sally Reel, March 23, 2006.
14. Marcinko D, Hetico H, Pentin-Maki R: Medical practice strategic operating plan. In Marcinko D, editor: *The business of medical practice: advanced profit maximization techniques for savvy doctors,* ed 2, New York, 2004, Springer, pp 49-66.

15. Brown and Brown Insurance (website): http://www.ephysiciansinsurance.com/policydetail. html#medmal. Accessed April 13, 2006.
16. AllBusiness: *Property Insurance Basics* (website): http://www.allbusiness.com/articles/ Insurance/1248-30-1831.html. Accessed January 10, 2006.
17. AllBusiness: *Understanding General Liability Insurance* (website): http://www.allbusiness.com/ articles/Insurance/389-30-1801.html. Accessed January 10, 2006.
18. AllBusiness: *Does Every Business Have to Have Workers' Compensation Insurance?* (website): http://www.allbusiness.com/articles/Insurance/1662-30-1862.html. Accessed January 12, 2006.
19. AllBusiness: *Interruption Insurance for Your Small Business* (website): http://www.allbusiness. com/articles/Insurance/2603-30-1801.html. Accessed January12,2006.
20. U.S. Small Business Administration: *The Interview Process—How to Select the "Right" Person* (website): http://www.sba.gov/managing/growth/interview.html. Accessed January 14, 2006.
21. Strada H: *How to Spot a Lie on a Resume or Application* (website): http://www.sba.gov/ managing/growth/employeelie.html. Accessed January 14, 2006.
22. Hetico H, Pentin-Maki R: Selecting practice management advisors wisely. In Marcinko D, editor: *The business of medical practice: advanced profit maximization techniques for savvy doctors,* ed 2, New York, 2004, Springer, pp 443-460, quote: p 453.
23. United States Small Business Administration: *Payroll Taxes* (website): http://www.sba.gov/ managing/taxes/payroll.html. Accessed January 14,2006.
24. Mackey T, McNiel N, Klingensmith K: Outsourcing issues for nurse practitioner practices, *Nursing Economics* 22(1): 21-26, 2004.
25. Borglum K: 10 ways family practices lose money, *Family Practice Management* 10(6):51-56, 2003 (serial online): http://www.medscape.com/viewarticle/457397_print. Accessed January 4, 2006.
26. Cascardo D: Overlooked factor in successful practice collections, *Medscape Money and Medicine,* 2001 (serial online): http://www.medscape.com/viewarticle/403796_print. Accessed January 12, 2006.
27. Borglum K: Three steps to an effective practice budget, *Family Practice Management* 11(1): 46-50, 2004 (serial online): http://www.aafp.org/fpm/20040100/46thre.html. Accessed January 5, 2006.
28. Kullgren J, Sibella M: Calculating your cost per visit, *Family Practice Management* 11(4):41-45, 2004.

REIMBURSEMENT

GAIL P. BARKER • VALERIE LIGHT

*B*illing for clinical services in the health care industry is unlike that of any other business in the country. In this chapter we explore this unique practice and learn not only how to bill for professional clinical services but also what to expect in terms of reimbursement and how to determine whether a billing operation is performing well.

THE PATIENT ENCOUNTER

Understanding how to code patient encounters is discussed in this section using evaluation and management (E/M) service information that comes directly from the Centers for Medicare and Medicaid Services—*Evaluation and Management Services Guide.*[1]

Each clinical encounter begins when the patient calls to make an appointment with a provider. To assist with all aspects of the visit, several pieces of information must be collected including the patient's name, address, date of birth, phone number, insurance information, and reason for visit. Another source for retrieving this information may be a hospital or other clinic/provider's office. If the service requested for the patient requires an authorization or referral for the visit, one must be obtained by calling the patient's insurance company and/or the referring provider. Insurance dates of eligibility also must be obtained to determine whether the visit and services will be covered or payment from the patient will be required.

When the patient arrives for the visit, it is recommended that a copy of the patient's insurance card be made for the patient chart. The next step in the patient encounter is to determine what type of visit will be established. Has the patient been seen in the clinic within the last 3 years? If yes, this is an established patient in the practice. If no, this is a new patient visit.

It is important to understand and record why the patient has come in for services.

Every visit requires a documented chief complaint regardless of the level of service performed. A chief complaint is "a concise statement describing the symptom, problem, condition, diagnosis, or other factor describing the reason for the encounter—in the patient's words. This may be recorded by the nurse, but the provider must refer to the nurse's documentation if it is separate from his/her note.

Once the patient has been escorted to the exam room, the patient encounter begins with a history of present illness (HPI). The HPI is a chronological description of the development of the patient's present illness from the first sign and/or symptom or from the previous encounter to the present. The elements to be included are listed in Table 9-1. All of these elements should be documented in the patient's chart. They are considered pertinent facts, findings, and observations about the patient's health history. This communication also allows for continuity of care among providers.

The provider will next explore the past, family and/or social history (PFSH) of the patient. This is where the provider is able to identify any hereditary information pertinent to the patient's medical evaluation.

- *Past history:* Patient's past experience with illness, operations, injuries, and treatment

TABLE 9-1

Elements of the HPI

ELEMENT	DESCRIPTION	EXAMPLE
Location	Place, whereabouts	Groin area
Quality	Characteristics, grade	Burning in groin
Severity	How hard to endure	Mild burning has become more intense
Duration	Length of time	Pain for last 2 wk
Timing	Regulation of occurrence	Intermittent becoming more intense/frequent
Context	Circumstances of event	Activity that caused the pain such as bending/picking up
Modifying factors	Altering elements, conditions	Is patient taking medication for pain?
Associated signs/ symptoms	Other related complaint(s) to presenting problem	Pain in other related areas such as bladder urgency

- *Family history*: Review of medical events in the patient's family, including diseases that may be hereditary or place the patient at risk

- *Social history*: An age-appropriate review of past and current activities

After the chief complaint has been obtained, with the elements of HPI and PFSH being noted, the review of systems (ROS) may begin. The ROS is an inventory of body systems obtained through a series of questions seeking to identify signs and/or symptoms that the patient may be experiencing or has experienced. The following systems are recognized:

- Constitutional symptoms (fever, weight loss)

- Eyes

- Ears, nose, mouth, throat (ENT)

- Cardiovascular

- Respiratory

- Gastrointestinal (GI)

- Genitourinary (GU)

- Musculoskeletal

- Integumentary

- Neurologic

- Psychiatric

- Endocrine

- Hematologic/Lymphatic

- Allergic/Immunologic

The last part of the patient visit is the physical exam. Upon listening to the patient's description of symptoms, the provider then physically examines the patient, performing skills such as listening to the patient's heart and lungs. The provider might also palpate the abdomen or touch the skin. The following areas may be examined:

- Constitution/general appearance

- Skin

- Eyes

- ENT

- Neck

- Respiratory

- Cardiovascular

- Chest/Breasts

- GI/GU

- Lymphatic

- Musculoskeletal

- Neurologic

- Psychiatric

Patient Encounter Documentation

Each patient encounter must be documented. If documentation does not exist, there is no proof that the encounter took place, and the rationale for ordering diagnostic tests or medications cannot be substantiated. The documentation should be complete and easily interpreted. Documentation is also required to bill a patient encounter.

Third-party payers require documentation that services are consistent with level of service billed (using Current Procedural Terminology [CPT]). A payer may request information to substantiate the appropriateness of diagnostic and/or therapeutic services provided and that the services provided have been appropriately reported and documented.

Seven components are recognized when documenting E/M services:

- History

- Examination

- Medical decision making

- Counseling

- Coordination of care

- Nature of presenting problem

- Time

History, examination, and *medical decision making* are the key components in selecting the level of E/M services to bill. Whereas, if a visit is predominantly counseling or coordination of care (more than 50%), then *time* may be considered the key or controlling factor to qualify for a particular level of E/M services.

The levels of E/M services are based on four types of examination:

- *Problem focused:* Limited exam of the affected body area or organ. Documentation requirements: (1) Chief complaint, (1) ROS, (1-5) Physical exam elements

- *Expanded problem focused*: Limited exam of affected body area or organ system and any other symptomatic or related associated signs and symptoms.
  Documentation requirements: (1) Chief complaint, (1-2) PFSH, (2-9) ROS, (6-11) Physical exam elements

- *Detailed*: Extended exam of the affected body area, organ and any other symptomatic or related body area or organ system.
  Documentation requirements: Documents (1-3) Chief complaints, (2-3) PFSH, (12-14) ROS, (12) Physical exam elements

- *Comprehensive*: a general multisystem exam or complete exam of a single organ system and other symptomatic or related body area or organ system.
  Documentation requirements: Documents (1-3) Chief complaint, (2-3) PFSH, (12-14) ROS, and *all* (14) Physical elements

An example of documenting a patient exam, using all of the information provided above, is given in Box 9-1.

BILLING FOR CLINICAL SERVICES

There are usually three separate clinical encounter billing scenarios:

- Patient or self-pay billing (a patient pays for services directly)

- Third-party payer billing (a claim is submitted to an insurance company for payment)

- Sponsoring organization billing (a claim is sent to a sponsoring organization)

Patient or Self-Pay

If a patient has no insurance, services must be paid for directly. If there is a hardship circumstance, a patient's bill can be discounted, particularly for prompt pay (paying at the time of the service). However, charges must remain at the same level regardless of the pay source. A discount is applied to the full charge, rather than reducing an individual charge itself.

A patient with insurance might also want to obtain services that are not covered by his or her insurance. A cosmetic procedure is a common example of this type of self-pay patient.

Billing a Third Party

Most clinical service billing is adjudicated through third-party payers, or insurance companies. Although every third-party payer has it own billing regulations and reimbursement policies, almost without exception, third-party payers

BOX 9-1	DOCUMENTATION OF A PATIENT EXAM

Chief Complaint
A 49-year-old female presented to the office with symptoms of dizziness and difficulty maintaining her balance. Thus patient had two chief complaints, dizziness and unstable balance.

History of Present Illness (HPI)
The nurse performed an initial evaluation that consisted of taking the patient's blood pressure, weight, height, and pulse. The patient was asked if she was allergic to any medications. The patient responded that she had no adverse reactions to any medications. The patient stated that she could not walk a straight line. When asked, the patient also denied use of any alcohol or drugs. She also reported that she was unable to sleep well and was having a hard time hearing.

Past, Family, Social History (PFSH)
The patient described the following conditions in her *medical history:*
- Broken femur 1985
- Seasonal allergies, currently taking no medications
- Did not drink alcohol
- Smoked ½ pack of cigarettes per day

The patient described the following conditions in her *family history:*
- Mother still living
- Father died of cardiovascular disease

The patient described the following conditions in her *social history:*
- Married, stable environment
- 2 grown children

Review of Systems (ROS)
The provider began the patient exam by asking about the patient's constitution; the patient reported she was fatigued. The provider then examined the patient's skin, eyes, ears/nose/throat, listened to the heart, listened to and examined patient's stomach, GI tract, and GU tract. Finally the provider reviewed the patient's musculoskeletal system.

Physical Exam
The patient appeared tired and had an unbalanced gait. The patient was borderline obese. She had a 3-mm skin tag on her neck, and her eyes appeared normal. The ear, nose, and throat (ENT) exam showed the patient's right ear was inflamed with drainage. The lymph glands in the neck were also swollen. The respiratory area was clear and the cardiovascular exam indicated a heart rate of 54 beats per minute.

Assessment
The provider suspected severe otitis media, so the plan was to check blood sugar; check urine for ketones, and order an EGK with interpretation. The procedures performed included a fingerstick blood, EKG, and urinalysis.

Diagnosis
Vertigo, severe otitis media, and fatigue. The patient was put on 50 mg erythromycin for 10 days and told to return if the symptoms persisted.

BOX 9-1	DOCUMENTATION OF A PATIENT EXAM—cont'd

The provider spent approximately 30 minutes face-to-face with the patient.

Summary of Patient Exam Documentation for Selecting an E/M Service Category

Chief complaint/HPI = 3
PSFH = 3
ROS = 9
Physical exam = 7
Time = 30 minutes

The above scoring pointed to a detailed, extended exam. This translates to CPT 99203, an Office or Other Outpatient Visit, Level 3.

require both a CPT and ICD-9 (International Classification of Diseases, ninth edition) code for payment. These payers can be clustered into three particular groups:

1. Centers for Medicare and Medicaid (CMS)

2. Commercial managed care organizations

3. Commercial indemnity insurance companies

Centers for Medicare and Medicaid (CMS)

Although Medicare and Medicaid are both regulated by the CMS, they are very different programs. Medicare is a federal program administered through subcontracted regional carriers. Medicaid is a federal program administered by the individual states.

Medicare

Medicare is considered the gold standard for third-party billing and reimbursement. The Medicare program covers enrolled patients 65 years of age and older, and the long-term disabled who qualify for social security benefits. Medicare offers different types of programs to its beneficiaries, including both discounted fee-for-service and HMO (health maintenance organization) products. Advanced practice nurses are recognized as billable providers in the Medicare program; however, fees are reimbursed at 85% of the approved Medicare physician's fee schedule, unless the incident-to method is used. *Incident-to billing* can be reimbursed at 100% of the Medicare physician fee schedule if the supervising provider is a physician. Incident-to billing is described later in the chapter.

- *Medicare discounted fee-for-service (FFS)*. The Medicare discounted FFS service program is based on the resource-based relative value scale (RBRVS) schedule, wherein each CPT-coded service performed (e.g., outpatient visit, clinical procedure) has a value assigned. The value is multiplied by a conversion factor resulting in a standard payment. The payment schedule is established nationally (but varies based on geographic region) and is not negotiable.

- *Medicare health maintenance organization (HMO).* Medicare also offers an HMO plan in which a flat per member per month (PMPM) amount is paid to a provider and is calculated based on criteria such as age and gender.

- It is through *CMS,* and in particular the Medicare program, that the importance of billing and coding compliance evolved. Billing and coding compliance was first addressed in the 1996 Health Insurance Portability and Accountability Act (HIPAA). Embedded in the legislation was a provision for the investigation of billing fraud and abuse. The responsibility for enforcement of appropriate billing activities became the responsibility of the Office of the Inspector General (OIG) and the Department of Justice (DOJ). An entire book could be written about billing and coding compliance, however, for this chapter the important thing to remember is you must follow the published billing and coding guidelines, such as those described above. This will ensure accurate claims are submitted to CMS.

- *Incident-to services.* The incident-to service billing method is unique to Medicare. The term *incident-to* is short for *incident to an approved provider's professional service.* Services are furnished as an integral yet incidental part of an approved provider's professional services as part of the course for diagnosis and treatment of injury or illness.[2] The top eight rules for billing incident-to services are as follows:

1. Outpatient services that must be billed under the direct supervision of an approved provider:
   Physician
   Clinical psychologist
   Nurse practitioner
   Nurse midwife
   Clinical nurse specialist
   Physician assistant (in a physician-directed clinic)

2. Services are furnished as an integral but incidental part of the approved provider's services in the course of diagnosis and treatment of an injury/illness.

3. The approved provider must initiate treatment and see the patient frequently enough to illustrate active involvement in the care.

4. Advanced practice nurses may bill incident-to under a physician or have incident-to billed under herself/himself. The supervising provider's fee schedule is billed.

5. Both providers' names go on the claim form.

6. The typical incident-to code is an office or other outpatient visit for an established patient (CPT codes used are 99211-99213.)

7. Incident-to does not require all the E/M components for billing. Only a brief description of the minimal services provided during the course of treatment is needed (e.g., follow-up or reevaluation).

8. An incident-to code cannot be billed on the same day as a therapeutic diagnosis (which has its own Health Care Financing Administration Common Procedure Coding System [HCPCS] code.). However, it can be billed on the same day with some other services (i.e., a vaccine) IF a separately identifiable E/M service is also performed and documented.

Medicaid

Medicaid, a federal program administered through each state, is adjudicated based on a patient's proximity to the poverty level. The patient base consists primarily of mothers and children, and short-term (less than 1 year) disabled individuals. Unlike the Medicare program, there is some variance in programs from state to state. In addition, a "waiver" program can be granted to states. This allows states to offer managed care plans to Medicaid beneficiaries. With the waiver, Medicaid, like Medicare, can offer patients a variety of programs including both FFS and HMO products. Advanced practice nurses are recognized as billable providers in state Medicaid programs and can even have their own panels. Reimbursement can average between 70% and 100% of the approved physician Medicaid fee schedule, depending on the state and services approved.

Commercial Managed Care Organizations (MCO)

Almost all third-party payers now offer managed care products to their constituents, which include both employer groups and individuals. The most popular include discounted FFS, HMO, and provider of services (POS) options. In the past two decades, HMOs were on the rise, but as the new century emerged, discounted FFS and POS plans started to erode the HMO market share. Patients wanted more influence in regard to their health care decisions and appeared to be willing to pay for it. Rates paid to providers for commercial MCOs are negotiated between the practitioner (or provider group) and the MCO. Today, most advanced practice nurses are recognized as billable providers, and reimbursement usually varies between 80% and 100% of the approved physician fee schedule.

Commercial Indemnity Insurance Companies

Today commercial indemnity insurance is a small percentage of the health care market, and most commercial payers have migrated to managed care product offerings. Indemnity insurance is reimbursed on a per service (CPT) basis, and claims are paid as a percentage of billable charge. Any amount not reimbursed by the indemnity insurance company is balance billed to the patient. Contributing to the decline of the indemnity insurance model was the incentive driver, which encouraged the provider to increase charges, and thus increase health care costs. As costs continued to increase, the commercial indemnity model started to fall out of favor. With the introduction of managed care, indemnity insurance offerings declined dramatically, and now indemnity plans represent only a small percentage of health care plans.

Billing a Sponsoring Organization for Services

In some instances a claim is sent to a sponsoring organization for payment, particularly when a patient is unable to pay at the time of service. For example, an inmate patient does not maintain eligibility during the period of incarceration. Therefore, the correctional facility is billed for an inmate patient's services. There may also be an instance wherein an institution requests services be billed back to them, and they in turn bill a third party. This is not uncommon with bundled services billing because a "package price" has been agreed upon and only one bill is sent for all services included in the package.

REIMBURSEMENT METHODOLOGIES

With the introduction of managed care, the health care industry's method for reimbursing clinical services differentiated dramatically from traditional payment for services. There are no other industry markets in which fees are set with the express expectation they will be methodically negotiated down by a factor of 50% or less. Yet in today's managed health care market, this is the prevailing circumstance. The notable exceptions include some self-pay services and indemnity insurance (where it is expected full payment from a combination of the third-party payment and balance billing to the patient will be forthcoming.)

Managed care insurers (including Medicare and Medicaid) reimburse services based on a FFS schedule or on a PMPM basis regardless of the charges. Let's look at a FFS example (numbers are estimated.) A clinical encounter charge, identified as an outpatient visit for a new patient, Level 3 (CPT 99203) has a set charge of $173.00. Medicare, based on a relative value unit (RVU) of 2.55 and a conversion factor amount of $37.8863, would pay $96.61 (2.55 × $37.8863.) Medicaid might pay $95.36, commercial payer #1 might pay $125.88, commercial payer #2 might pay $117.86, and so on. The balance between what is charged and what is paid is written off as a contractual adjustment (also called *disallowance*.) In managed care, the patient is not billed for the balance owed, and the amount is not considered an account receivable. When a provider (or provider group) enters into a managed care agreement, and the deductible and co-pay are met, the provider (group) agrees not to balance bill the patient.

Why wouldn't a provider then just reduce fees to the negotiated payment rate?

1. Regulatory compliance guidelines require practitioners to bill the same fee to all patients regardless of their respective funding sources.

2. There are a small number of indemnity insurance payers that still pay as a percentage of charge. If the charge is lower, the reimbursement will be less.

3. As charges are decreased, managed care organizations might also continue to reduce reimbursement. They might see it as a signal that the cost to deliver health care has declined. This becomes a spiral of reduced charges and reimbursement.

Important management tools are available, however, to determine whether the fees charged are at an appropriate level and to check that all fees legitimately owed to you are being collected.

- *Gross collection rate (GCR).* The gross collection rate, or GCR, helps you set charges at an appropriate level, stay competitive, and yet not fall behind the prevailing market. A simple calculation can be performed to determine the GCR: (gross charges ÷ average reimbursement.) This calculation is generally performed in aggregate and is weighted based on payer mix. But to illustrate, using the example above, the charge for CPT 99203 is $173.00. The average reimbursement based on the payers above is $108.93 (average of $96.61, $95.36, $125.88, $117.86). The GCR = ($108.93 ÷ $173.00) or 63%. Academic practices generally have a GCR of approximately 45% to 65%; private practices are generally higher. Some practices set fees as a percentage of the highest payer. For example, 137% of $125.88 = $173.00. Regardless of how fees are determined, it is important to perform an annual review of fees to ensure they are higher than any payer reimbursement, yet are not so high that collection rates fall too low.

- *Net collection rate (NCR).* This calculation provides a very quick view of how the biller is performing in regard to collecting the allowable reimbursement. Again, this calculation is generally performed in aggregate, but for our example, we will again use the figures above. The formula is actual collections ÷ expected collections.) For CPT 99203, let's say the average collection is $105.00. From the payer table you know the expected collection should average $108.93, thus $105.00 ÷ $108.93 = 96%. Collection rates should be in the 90th percentile, so this is a very good collection rate.

HMO reimbursements are based entirely on a formula that calculates reimbursement on a PMPM monthly flat amount regardless of the services rendered. Factors such as age, gender, geographic area, and sometimes lifestyle (e.g., smoker versus nonsmoker) are considered. Generally ancillary services (e.g., labs, radiology) are calculated separately and can be included either in the PMPM total reimbursement or negotiated separately. It is the responsibility of the provider group to manage care within the PMPM amount. Certain specialty services are sometimes 'carved out" of the PMPM amount and paid separately.

Denied Claims

Not all claims are paid upon submission. There are four scenarios for a submitted claim.

1. The claim is paid in full.
2. The claim is partially paid.
3. The claim in pended.
4. The claim is denied.

When the claim is *paid in full*, the provider [group] accepts payment and writes off the balance (if any) as a noncontracted or disallowed adjustment. When the claim is *partially paid*, the reason must be researched. Possibly the patient owes a balance due for the deductible or copayment. It is also possible to balance bill a secondary insurance if one is available. When the claim is *pended*, more information is generally required. This could include additional demographic information required on the patient or additional documentation for the services being billed, such as chart notes.

When the claim is *denied*, the insurance company does not feel they have an obligation to pay for the service. A reason is almost always stated for the denial; some of the most frequent are (a) because the service is not covered, (b) the insurance company thinks it is a duplicate bill, or (c) because the patient's eligibility is questioned. A provider [group] can choose to write off the claim to bad debt, appeal the claim, or bill the patient directly as a noncovered service (if the contract allows it).

CREDENTIALING

Credentialing is the collection and review of professional qualifications for practicing providers.[3] Almost all third-party payers require credentialing and generally have their own individual guideline requirements making this a time-consuming, labor-intensive activity. This is not to suggest credentialing is not an important element to ensure health care is delivered by qualified individuals. However, a one-size-fits-all credentialing process could significantly reduce time and cost. Some payers are moving in that direction. Recredentialing is usually done every 2 to 3 years.

Some of the components of credentialing include, but are not limited to, verification of training, board certification, current medical license, Drug Enforcement Agency (DEA) certificate, hospital privileges, malpractice insurance and history, national practitioner databank status, and clinical competence. This information is generally stored in a database, and through the recredentialing process, information is updated and reverified.

Conclusion

Health care billing and reimbursement can be a complex process. However, it is the accepted method for payment of health care services in the United States. Therefore it is imperative for practitioners to understand the process not only for purposes of reimbursement but also in order to comply with the requirements of a highly regulated industry.

REFERENCES

1. U.S. Department of Health & Human Services, Centers for Medicare and Medicaid Services: *Evaluation and Management Services Guide*, 2004, revised April 2006, (website): http://www.cms.hhs.gov/medlearn/emdoc.asp. Accessed August 1, 2005.
2. *Incident-To Service: the University Physicians Documentation and Coding Policy Procedure*, revised July 29, 2004.
3. Wolper LF: *Health care administration*, Miami, FL, 1999, Warner Brother Publications.
4. Bench S, Magnani R, Parkinson J, editors: *2006 Professional: HCPCS Level II*, Salt Lake City, 2005, Ingenix.

MARKETING

Understanding Strategies to Build an NP Practice

SALLY J. REEL • IVO L. ABRAHAM

*F*or any business to succeed, including an NP practice, customers must be attracted and retained. Marketing strategies are about convincing people to use a product or service and to make them into loyal customers who are convinced of the value provided. A successful NP practice will need good, well-planned marketing strategies to attract and keep satisfied patients.[1]

MARKETING DEFINED

Marketing is about the importance of attracting customers to a business and keeping them as customers as long as possible. According to the U.S. Small Business Administration,[1] marketing has two important principles:

1. All company policies and activities should be directed toward satisfying customer needs.

2. Profitable sales volume is more important than maximum sales volume.

To best utilize these principles, a small business such as an NP practice must learn the needs of their customers (patients) by doing *market research*; analyzing competitive advantages to develop *market strategies*; selecting specific markets to attract patients through target marketing; and determining how to satisfy patient needs by identifying a *market mix*.[1]

Market research is about systematically gathering, recording, and analyzing data about challenges relating to the marketing and delivery of products and services. Market research can help pinpoint new markets and customers, track customer (dis-) satisfaction, analyze trends that affect sales and profits, and

137

identify competitors' market strategies. By conducting market research, it is possible to find out what customers want, not just what a business wants to sell.[1]

Market research is what a business owner does when the owner comes up with a new idea but is not sure whether or not to run with that new idea. Market research is about determining characteristics of current customers so that new ones can be found. There are several techniques for conducting market research that fall basically into qualitative and quantitative strategies. *Qualitative strategies* are about what questions to ask and *quantitative strategies* are about what to do with the answers. In other words, qualitative strategies provide meaning and are open-ended in nature. Quantitative strategies provide measurable data suitable for statistical analysis.[2]

Market research strategies may be direct or indirect. Direct means the information is gathered by the owner or the owner's marketer, such as by way of surveys and questionnaires. Indirect means the information is found in existing sources such as government reports, industry data, financial institutions, or other media. Significant information also may be found online. Table 10-1 describes techniques for market research and the relationship between qualitative and quantitative and direct and indirect methods.[2]

Marketing strategy is about identifying customer groups—or target markets—that a business can serve better than its competitors. Marketing strategy customizes product offerings, prices, promotional efforts and services toward the target market. A well-planned marketing strategy helps a business focus on the customers it can serve best.[1] Market segments exist as well. Market segments are groups of people who have identifiable similarities—a niche. Target marketing is deciding which segment to market to.[2]

Marketing mix—or the combination of activities that comprise a marketing approach—is usually a blend of four P's: products, places, prices, and promotions. Good marketing strategy is about understanding people too—why people do what they do and why they buy what they buy. Thus "people" is the new target behind current marketing strategies as marketers use psychology to induce desired behavior in people. People, from a marketing perspective, include staff, suppliers, customers, and competitors.[2]

TABLE 10-1

Techniques for Market Research

	QUANTITATIVE	QUALITATIVE
Direct	Example: Questionnaires	Example: Focus groups
Indirect	Example: Research reports	Example: Case studies in textbooks

From White S: *A complete idiot's guide to marketing,* ed 2, New York, 2003, Alpha Books, p 72.

"Why" people buy is often that they have hopes that the product or service will solve problems and/or fill needs. The "what" is often the solution to a problem; in other words, people buy the benefits they expect to derive from a product or service. When a business does not focus on the benefit a customer expects to receive from the product or service, the business is left open to challenge from others who have not forgotten this. Customers and competitors are people and people change. In a good business, products and services evolve to meet the changing needs of customers.[2]

A good business strategy includes understanding competitors. Competitors, while being those businesses that can provide the same or better services, are also mentors. It is also wise to research competitors—a practice that is fair and necessary.[2] Beckwith[3] suggests asking this question: "If I ran a competing firm, how would I beat ours?" Once the weakness is determined, eliminate the weakness.

Marketing is also about value and understanding what customers are really looking for in terms of value. "When" customers buy they often look for the following qualities in a product or service:[2]

- Something that performs as expected
- Something that is offered in a convenient manner
- Something that is readily available in a timely manner
- Something that can be obtained easily and at a fair price

Value, the relationship of quality and price, is defined by the market, and a satisfied customer will usually pay for good value.[4] Figure 10-1 shows a Customer Value Pyramid. Customer value theory contends that customers hope to find an

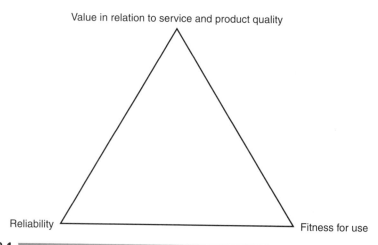

Value in relation to service and product quality

Reliability

Fitness for use

Figure 10-1

Customer value pyramid. *From White S: A complete idiot's guide to marketing, ed 2, New York, 2003, Alpha Books.*

appropriate mix of product quality (fitness for use), service reliability (service quality) and reasonable price (value in relation to service and product quality). The objective is to blend these three items in such a way that customers are attracted and the business profits. Customers perceive value when each element meets or exceeds their expectations.[2]

A much used term in the business literature is *branding*—the creation and management of brands. A brand is a unique and identifiable symbol, association, name, or trademark that serves to differentiate competing products or services. A brand is both a physical and emotional trigger for creating a relationship between consumers and the product/service. Inherent to branding is the development of an identity or profile that customers associate with the triggering of a brand. Does branding apply to nursing practices? Maybe not at first sight, although the MinuteClinic concept in the Practice Management chapter (see Chapter 8) has a clear branding component: customers know what they can get and what they can't, they associate it with quality, and they discern the value it provides. Though an independent nursing practice is unlikely to become a brand (even on a small community scale), its success will be determined by the extent to which current and potential customers understand the profile or identity of the practice and how this differentiates the practice from other health care providers.

Today's marketing concepts also integrate ideas from the field of strategic planning with commitment to quality management and customer (both discussed later in this chapter and also in Chapter 19). Warshaw[5] suggests that "... every small business owner... must ask the following questions to come up with effective marketing strategies:

- Who are the potential customers?

- What kind of people are the potential customers?

- Where do potential customers live?

- Can and will potential customers buy?

- Is the business offering the kind of goods or services that customers want at the best price, best time, and in the right amount?

- Are prices consistent with what customers view as the product's or service's value?

- How does the business compare with competitors?

- Are promotional programs working?"

Beckwith[3] also suggests that successful businesses ask "What would people love?" But as Warshaw[5] notes, market research is not a perfect science. It is about people and their constantly changing feelings and behaviors that are influenced by a multitude of factors; thus to do marketing research, facts and opinions need to be collected in an orderly, objective way to find out what people want.

The "take home" is that it is impossible to sell a product or service that customers do not want.

Last, a word about customer relations: ... It is among the best persistent marketing activities in which a business can engage—especially in the professional services sector.

What Does All This Mean for Effective NP Practice Marketing?

An NP practice is subject to the same marketing needs as other small businesses and needs an effective marketing strategy for long-term success. Start with good patient relations in all aspects of practice operations. It is the cheapest marketing activity, the return is significant, and it assists with profile and identity development.

Marketing resources may be limited for many small businesses including NP practices; therefore target marketing may promote the best marketing "bang for the buck." Target marketing, for example, focuses on a few key market segments such as geographic segmentation and customer segmentation. Using geographic segmentation, NP practice marketing would focus on serving the needs of patients in a specific geographic area; thus marketing strategies would focus on advertising to and attracting patients from within a defined geographic radius. Customer segmentation, on the other hand, is about identifying those patients most likely to use the NP services and targeting marketing efforts to those patients.[1]

Providing quality services is a key marketing strategy. Baum and Henkel[6] describe a number of strategies for promoting quality services, and several of those strategies are discussed here. Specifically, a successful practice requires going the extra mile for patients, referral sources, and third-party payers—knowing what they want and do not want—and designing practice services around this knowledge. It is important to exceed expectations of patients as well. Current patients are the foundation for a successful practice because it costs more to attract a new patient than to retain a current patient. Good market strategy for the NP practice is about attracting and retaining patients and continuously improving that practice for those served by it. Market strategy is about avoiding complacency and keeping the appointment book filled during natural peaks and ebbs throughout the year.[6]

There are external and internal marketing strategies to attract and retain patients. External sources include referrals, word of mouth, and public appearances such as writing newspaper columns or fulfilling community speaking engagements. Advertisements might take the form of formal newspaper announcements, newspaper columns (that are written by the provider), websites, newsletters, direct mailings, brochures, and business cards. A well-designed ad in the yellow pages should be considered because this is a major marketing tool that has been identified as being how most patients locate a physician. It is worth investing in a good display ad, and it is important to track the impact of this ad, which can be done when the patient registers for an appointment by asking how they heard about the practice.[6]

Internal marketing strategies go back to quality management and value. Good service is about making people feel special—it is personalizing the service and going that extra mile. Market strategy takes this into account. For example, Baum and Henkel[6] explain that personalizing an encounter can be as simple as creating a mechanism that shows you care about patients and their families—for example, remembering a birthday or acknowledging an achievement of a family member. Great first impressions begin the minute the patient walks through the door— for example, a reception process and waiting area that lacks appeal will do little to give the impression that great service can be expected. Think also about what patients will benefit most from your effort to go that extra mile—for example, someone new to the practice, someone having outpatient procedures and/or diagnostic studies, someone on a new medication, or someone that had an insurance claim denied[6]—in other words, people who may be feeling an extra measure of stress.

There are strategies to evaluate quality service. Some reasonably straightforward strategies include developing sound market research surveys (including patient satisfaction surveys) or putting a suggestion box in the waiting area. Surveys should be kept simple and easy to take. A professional approach to collecting and analyzing the information also should be taken. People collecting the information need to be trained on what and how to collect the data because lack of training and supervision may lead to incorrect information. Pretest the survey by having various people take it—including regular patients, staff, and colleagues; get feedback on the survey's style, simplicity, and their perception of the survey's purpose. Analyze the data for patterns, common opinions, and relevant information that focuses on the practice's marketing needs so that evolving market trends can be identified. Keep the marketing plan up-to-date because markets are ever changing[5] and failure to meet patients' needs may result in losing patients to competitors.

Evaluating quality services also requires paying attention to how patients are treated. A poorly motivated staff can hinder a practice, particularly if patients perceive rude or negative treatment—this begins with first contact and is an ongoing process. For example, telephone etiquette can go a long way in establishing a positive (or negative) rapport with patients. Although it may be obvious that connecting with the patient in a personal and professional way is important, you should recognize this begins with instructing staff on how to screen calls and provide information and also on how they should present themselves and interact with callers. Evaluate what the patient hears when he or she calls, which should include the name of the practice, the name of the person answering the call, how the person answering the call may be of assistance, and referring to the caller by name throughout the encounter. It is also a good idea to have a general information "cue card" about the specifics of the practice and general services, as well as the credentials and professional background of the providers. Include written guidelines for telephone technique in the employee policy manual and train employees on how to manage practice calls consistently and positively—negative impressions could cost the practice patients.[6]

Hiring a "mystery shopper" is another way to evaluate how patients are treated in the practice. A mystery shopper is a marketing professional trained to evaluate how a business serves their customers. These people are usually hired through a marketing or public relations firm. If a mystery shopper is hired, evaluate and modify, if necessary, all questionnaires that will be used prior to their assessment of the practice. Have the shopper go through the scheduling process by calling for an appointment, then asking for one earlier than the date given, asking for directions, asking how fees are handled at the initial visit, and asking about provider credentials. When the shopper arrives, instruct her (him) to not identify herself (himself) until after she (he) is in the exam room and with the provider (stop short of asking the shopper to disrobe or go through the exam). Finally, have the shopper go through the exit process. Avoid telling staff about the shopper until after the encounter. Get a written summary of the report.[6]

Quality service includes positively managing difficult patients. Difficult patients can be challenging—not to mention the negative impact they can have on marketing through word of mouth with family and friends about their perceptions of poor service. These patients take extra attention and may be managed best when the provider or staff is not tired or preoccupied and sufficient time is allocated for the patient to air their complaints. Another challenge is the patient who requests a record transfer. When this happens, consider promptly calling the patient but do not take it personally when a request for transfer happens. Send the record and follow up a few weeks later by phone to inquire about the patient's health.[6]

Understanding how providers and staff relate to colleagues is an important marketing strategy as well. Referrals can be a major source of patients to the practice. Networking and collaborating with colleagues foster several things, including getting to know other providers in the community, getting to know the nature of other practices in the community, and sending a message to other providers in the community about how easy the practice is to work with, and it gets the practice's name out to referring colleagues. Take colleagues to breakfast or coffee and make a point to get to know them.[6] This practice also provides an opportunity to assess competitors as well. When building a referral network, emphasize as appropriate the concept of reciprocity and the NP practice's commitment to refer patients to other members of the network.

Specialty markets are business opportunities too. If attracting and serving ethnic groups is a potential specialized market, doing homework about these groups is essential because it is important to know where the ethnic groups in the practice's community originally come from to avoid treating all people with an ethnic designation the same. Foreign-born groups, for example, may present with health care needs that are not common among Americans, and they may take medications that are not common as well (e.g., folk treatments). Belief systems also may vary significantly. Good service depends on knowing community demographics and being linguistically and culturally competent.[6]

Other specialty markets include "boomers, seniors, and/or generation X'ers" because these groups represent population trends. Boomers are members of the generation born after WWII, between 1946 and 1964 and are the most populous group in the United States. When marketing to boomers, it is a good idea to keep in mind that they like to choose their own providers, want control of decision-making processes, and spend money on health care that helps them feel and look better, as well as live longer. It is important to see them on time, make one-stop shopping a regular experience, and exceed their expectations.[6]

Seniors, on the other hand, require some unique marketing strategies. The physiologic and mental changes that occur with aging impact how well patients can see, hear, walk, and move, and maintain their attention span. Marketing to seniors includes proper lighting in the practice, limiting sounds (piped music, for example, can interfere with the ability to hear), and adequate space to negotiate chairs, corridors, and exam rooms, as well as providing furniture that also facilitates "navigating" through the practice. Seniors also may need transportation (is public transportation readily available?), good signs and directions, safety rails and door levers, nearby parking, and printed materials they can read. Avoid calling them elderly and/or reminding them of their age and infirmities. Instead, preserve their independence and provide sufficient time for socialization during the encounter—especially for the isolated senior.[6]

Summarized, a successful NP practice needs to develop a quantitative and qualitative system to (analogy intended) keep a finger on the pulse. A good marketing strategy should enable this; in other words, not just promote the practice but first of all understand the market and its customers. In turn, this finger-on-pulse system will enable the practice to monitor its performance, assess what is working well and not working well, and identify the need for tuning up or changes.

A Word About HIPAA and Marketing

HIPAA (Health Insurance Portability and Accountability Act of 1996) is a new set of federal regulations that set national standards for the privacy of health information, the activities of institutional review boards, and informed consent for the use of health information.[7] HIPAA privacy rules must be followed when marketing a health care practice because the privacy rule gives individuals significant controls over whether and how their protected health information is used and disclosed for marketing purposes. Although there are a few exceptions, the privacy rule requires an individual's written authorization before the use or disclosure of any personal protected health information for marketing purposes. Under HIPAA's privacy rule, marketing is defined as making "a communication about a product or service that encourages recipients of the communication to purchase or use the product or service." In terms of marketing, the communication can occur only if the covered entity first obtains an individual's consent.[8]

Basically, under the HIPAA privacy rule, covered entities may not sell protected health information to any business associate or any other third party for that party's own purposes. Furthermore, if a covered entity wants to sell lists of patients or enrollees to third parties, then the covered entity must obtain authorization from each person on the list. HIPAA describes the following examples of when marketing occurs:

- A managed care plan sells a list of its members to a company that sells glucometers, and the company intends to send the plan's members brochures on the benefits of purchasing and using that monitor

- A pharmaceutical company receives a list of patients from a covered health care provider and provides remuneration, then uses that patient list to send discount coupons for a new antidepressant directly to those patients[8]

Exceptions to the HIPAA privacy rule fall into three categories. Basically, a communication is not marketing if:

- The communication is made to describe a health-related product or service (or payment for such product or service) that is provided by, or included in a plan of benefits of, the covered entity making the communication

- The communication is made for treatment of the individual (e.g., a primary care provider refers a patient to a specialist for a follow-up test or provides free samples of a prescription medication)

- The communication is made for case management or care coordination for the patient, or to direct or recommend alternative treatments, treatments, health care providers, or settings of care to the patient[8]

The take-home message for practice marketing is that any consultant or company associated with the practice will be held to the same HIPAA privacy compliance standards as the practice itself. Under the HIPAA rules, any communication that encourages recipients to purchase or use a product or service would be defined as marketing; thus an entity that sends such communications must get the recipient's individual permission if any protected health information will be used in that communication, even if clinical information is not used. Individual authorization is usually not required to provide certain types of marketing such as distributing marketing materials for products and services within the practice's facility; to run television or radio ads; to use a practice website as a health education or marketing vehicle; and to send e-mail newsletters to patients and the public who request these.[6] HIPAA is discussed more fully in Chapter 12.

CONCLUSION

Several books are available from which you can learn more about marketing, and how to write ads, design websites, newsletters, brochures, and flyers; a walk through the business section of the local library or bookstore will usually reveal a wealth of resources. Ultimately, marketing is about attracting and keeping patients. Stout and Grand[9] summarize a number of strategies for accomplishing this:

- *Stay humble:* come across as competent, professional, and confident but avoid being perceived as a know-it-all.

- *Respect the right to charge money for services provided:* avoid undercutting the practice's services and value the right to set reasonable, competitive fees.

- *Speak with confidence:* hesitating, mumbling, and fidgeting during conversation with patients and colleagues creates an impression of weakness, not confidence.

- *Ask the right questions:* inquire about what goals patients have and how they would like their lives to be different because this is why they come to the practice and spend money.

- *Explain how the patient will be helped:* most patients want to know the plan.

- *Follow up:* call back when a patient has been told to expect the call.

- *Take responsibility for how the practice is doing:* do not blame managed care or short-change the knowledge needed for success. Make a running list of things that can be done right away to build the business.

- *State the bottom line:* communicate to people why they should utilize the practice rather than some else's.

- *Make the practice services easy to buy:* look for ways to make obtaining services easy and convenient for patients to obtain.

- *Focus on the positive:* eliminate anything in the marketing plan that does not focus on a positive result.

Building a successful NP practice will take work, and as Stout and Grand[9] noted "... there are no overnight successes. But being successful is quite doable."

REFERENCES

1. U.S. Small Business Administration: *Marketing Basics: What is Marketing?* (website): http://www.sba.gov/starting_business/marketing/basics.html. Accessed January 20, 2006.
2. White S: *A complete idiot's guide to marketing,* ed 2, New York, 2003, Alpha Books.
3. Beckwith H: *What clients love: a field guide to growing your business,* New York, 2003, Warner Business Books, p 4.
4. Webster F: *Market driven management: how to define, deliver, and deliver customer value,* Hoboken, NJ, 2002, John Wiley.
5. Warshaw A: Rule no. 1 in doing market research: keep it simple, February 6, 2006, *Tucson Citizen,* p 1D.
6. Baum N, Henkel G: *Marketing your clinical practice ethically, effectively, economically,* ed 3, Boston, 2004, Jones & Bartlett

7. Clause S, Triller D, Bornhorst C, Hamilton R, Cosler L: Conforming to HIPAA regulations and compilation of research data, *Am J Health-Sys Pharm* 61(10):1025-1031, 2004 (serial online): http://www.medscape.com/viewarticle/478848_print
8. Office of Civil Rights (OCR): OCR HIPPA Privacy, December 3, 2002; revised April 3, 2003, *Marketing* [45 CFR 164.501, 164.508(a)(3)] (website): http://www.hhs.gov/ocr/hipaa/guidelines/marketing.pdf. Accessed February 15, 2006.
9. Stout C, Grand L: *Getting started in private practice: the complete guide to building your mental health practice*, Hoboken, NJ, 2005, Wiley.

PHYSICAL PRACTICE SPACE CONSIDERATIONS

SALLY J. REEL

*T*he physical nature and location of a health care practice is a significant factor in the success of a practice. Location determines how easy or difficult it will be for patients to access care. Location can impact income—up or down—so careful planning is essential. Although it may not appear challenging on the surface of practice planning, location planning includes reviewing multiple issues related to space, aesthetics, disability access, fire, laboratory, building vs. leasing or renovating, and convenience and parking.

Location and space are components of a practice's marketing plan; marketing is discussed in Chapter 10. From a building or renovation perspective, consider consulting with an architect experienced with health facilities design to assure an aesthetically pleasing, functional practice space that meets all required codes and regulations. This is especially important if using or renovating an existing space. An experienced architect can determine "hidden" challenges such as asbestos in older buildings and can determine what is necessary to meet local, state, and federal building codes. Consulting an attorney is also recommended during practice space planning because many legal issues relate to building, renovations, or leasing. This chapter briefly discusses some key space planning questions and issues.

HEALTH CARE CONSUMERS

Health care design today includes both the needs of the health care provider and the patient. A visit to a health care facility is traumatic for many patients. Patients may feel vulnerable during a health examination and may feel that personal space is being invaded. Patient satisfaction is part of the current health care market as well and is "… the difference between providing what a patient needs and what a patient wants."[1]

Research demonstrates that ambulatory health care consumers want a physical environment that:

- Facilitates connection to staff
- Is conducive to well-being, including room temperature, color, lighting, and avoidance of stressors
- Is convenient and accessible
- Is confidential and private both in the waiting room and the exam room
- Is caring for the family
- Is considerate of patient impairments, which includes appropriate seating and signage to accommodate the elderly
- Is close to nature, with views of gardens, sky, natural lighting, and indoor plants, aquariums, and water elements[2]

Health care consumers also share four basic design-related needs: physical comfort, social contact, symbolic meaning, and wayfinding. Physical comfort includes such things as appropriate room temperature, lighting, comfortable furniture, freedom from such things as unpleasant odors or noise. Social contact includes personal privacy and limiting what others see and hear about self and others. Symbolic meaning consists of the nonverbal messages embodied in the design. An uncomfortable waiting area, for example, can be physically offensive. Large facilities also have the challenge of wayfinding, and strategies to promote ease with finding one's way through the facility is important.[3]

First impressions count, and once the patient walks into the practice, the environment needs to immediately establish rapport and ease. Outdated furniture, worn upholstery, and grimy spots on walls may send a message that the patient's comfort is not important or that the health care provider is outdated on health matters too. Seating arrangements also enhance or detract from a patient's experience. To illustrate, Americans generally do not like to sit in close proximity to strangers, whereas Middle Eastern and Latin cultures encourage closeness. Seating arrangements in a waiting room for Americans should not force strangers to sit close together, but considering the cultural diversity of American people, flexibility should be built into seating arrangements to allow families, for example, to wait in groups. However, if the practice will serve a particular ethnic group, using research about how that ethnic group uses space is an important planning consideration.[1]

General Thoughts about Practice Space Planning

Good practice space planning involves knowing something about the health care consumers the practice will target because the facility design must be responsive to that market. Design planning ideally needs to consider the current market as well and be flexible enough to serve future markets. This includes designing for future technologies also. Flexible design means creating a facility that can be quickly and economically modified to accommodate health service change.[3]

For some primary practices a modular design concept is one design strategy that adapts well to rapid changes. The modular approach allows decisions to be postponed about what service or specialty will occupy a specific space. Modular designs also allow practices to expand and contract as demands for services change. Modular designs also allow smaller practices with different peak usage periods to share examination rooms and other spaces. These designs result in predictable practice layouts that foster locating equipment and instruments easier, as well as assisting patients to find their way through the practice more easily.[4]

The medical office building is a traditional facility that many practices relied upon for years. Traditional health facilities included the hospital and doctors' offices. For convenience, many offices were located in a medical office building attached to or adjacent to a hospital.[3] The medical office building is one of the most familiar designs, but changes in services from hospital to outpatient-based care is also fostering changes in the types of practice facilities. Free-standing ambulatory care and outpatient surgery centers are becoming more common, as are other atypical facilities such as workplace-based facilities and those designed for patient convenience such as urgent care facilities or those located in shopping malls.[3]

FUNCTIONS OF A PRACTICE SPACE

The functions of the practice space usually include administrative, patient care, and support services.[1] Administrative functions include waiting and reception, appointments, insurance, and clerical. Patient care functions include examination, treatment, and consultation. Support services include laboratory, storage, staff offices and lounge, and any technologies such as x-ray machines. Layout of these functions impacts flow and efficiency. For example, grouping exam rooms and consultation space together enables more than one provider to practice simultaneously. Arranging toilets close to lab stations facilitates obtaining urine specimens. Another consideration is where the lab is located. If patients obtain lab work after seeing the provider or come to the clinic for lab work only, having the lab located near an exterior exit allows patients to enter or leave the clinic without going through the waiting room. The circulation path for staff should enable them to move quickly across all parts of the suite. Medical records and business functions are usually centrally located.[1]

SPECIFIC FUNCTIONAL ELEMENTS OF PRACTICE SPACE

Toilets

The nature of patients served and practicality generally determines whether or not to locate a toilet in the practice waiting room area. Although a toilet in the waiting area saves staff the trouble of directing patients to the toilet in the exam area, a waiting room toilet has the disadvantage of patients being able to empty their bladders before a urine sample can be requested. However, in practices where children are patients, a toilet in the exam area facilitates a parent's ability to change an infant's diaper. From a practical standpoint, ceramic tile floors provide long-term finishes for toilets. Dark grout conceals stains. Americans with Disabilities Act (ADA) requirements are also important toilet design considerations for persons with disabilities; ADA issues are discussed later in this chapter.[1]

Reception Area

The receptionist often schedules appointments and maintains the day's schedule and sees the patient on arrival and just before leaving. The receptionist needs a good view of the waiting area and adequate counter space. Space for computers, fax machines, printers, and copiers needs to be included in the reception area. It is also convenient if the receptionist can easily serve patients on entry and exit of the clinic, such as with an L-shaped area that has a receiving and exit window.[1]

Patient Education

Patient education is an essential component of health services. If possible, creating a small room or alcove for educational purposes may facilitate education. Education space may include written materials and handouts such as brochures, a small television monitor, and a recording device such as a video or DVD recorder. Privacy also should be taken into consideration when education is provided.[1]

Business Office

This business office sometimes is referred to as the "front office" because appointments are scheduled there, patients are billed, medical records are stored, patients are greeted, and routine insurance and bookkeeping functions occur there. If the practice is small, two people may perform all of these tasks, but in a large practice, it may take more people to manage these duties. One consideration when space planning is the ratio of one administrative assistant for every two providers in a low-volume practice and one administrative assistant per provider in a high-volume practice. If the provider is seeing four to six patients per hour, the administrative assistant may actually spend more time with patients than the provider. A gated door in the receptionist's area allows the patient to talk to the office staff without blocking corridor traffic, but for longer or more private encounters, the gated door would also permit the patient to enter the business office.[1]

Although some practices use an outside agency for bookkeeping and/or billing services, a review of how these services will be managed within the practice has space implications. If, for example, on-site bookkeeping and insurance billing is anticipated, operational space separate from the front office should be considered.

The front office is a busy place with ringing phones and patient traffic that may not promote a conducive work environment for people such as billers, who need to concentrate. Modular workstations are an alternative possibility when a separate room is not available. However, if a large practice is anticipated, one employee may be needed to handle insurance billing alone, and adequate workspace will be needed, such as an L- or U-shaped desk and space for office machines and computers, especially because many insurance claims are now processed electronically.[1]

Medical records must be accurate and easily retrievable to provide continuity of health care and protect against legal complications. Storage should consider the nature of recordkeeping. Lateral file cabinets have been a preferred method of storage and remain so for paper records. Color-coded file jackets are convenient and are a common way to organize files. Record storage planning also should consider the future needs of the practice and be projected for 3 to 5 years to accommodate the numbers of new patients added each month. Location of these records may be the business office or another area, but location should provide ready access to staff. Also, some practices are integrating patient records into electronic records that also have implications for storage.[1] Electronic health records are discussed more fully in Chapter 12.

Exam Rooms

Several things influence the location of exam rooms. If a nurse controls traffic to and from the exam rooms, clustering a nurses' station and exam rooms together enables the nurse to prepare patients quickly while also traveling back and forth to obtain equipment or other items needed for the examination. Consultation rooms also should be close to the exam area for provider convenience. An alternative design plan is to combine the exam room and the consultation room for some practices, but many consultation rooms also function as private offices for the providers. Routine consultation may occur in a well-designed exam room. Arranging the exam room corridor so that patients must pass through the business office on the way out is another functional consideration.[1]

The exam room, as the place for diagnosis, needs to be designed for functionality, including an understanding of equipment that needs to be available for the provider and the psychological well-being of the patient. When planning the exam room, design space to facilitate patient/provider rapport and provide space where interviews can occur eye-to-eye. Technology is such that integrating a computer into the room enables the provider and patient to review digital x-rays, lab reports, and video images of procedures, and to retrieve electronic patient records.[1]

The exam room layout should also enhance the examination process. The provider needs to be able to readily wash his or her hands, pivot to face the patient on the exam table, reach for routinely used instruments with the left hand, and examine the patient on the right. The room layout puts the provider on the patient's right side, which is standard, even for most left-handed providers. If during the building/design phase, plumbing is placed back to back for economic reasons, this will result in right- and left-handed exam rooms. It is better to lay out every exam room in the same way for efficiency and same degree of comfort for the provider in each room.[1]

For functionality, 8×12 feet is identified as an ideal size for exam rooms because this size accommodates a full-size exam table, a sink cabinet with storage, a dressing area, small writing desk, an exam stool, and a guest chair for the patient, as well as a treatment stand and portable equipment. Room size may vary depending on provider preference and the nature of the examination and testing that may occur in the room. The functionality of the exam room also should accommodate positioning of the exam table in such a way as to angle the foot or stirrup end of the table away from the door to allow the provider access to all sides of the patient and assure that the patient is out of the view of passersby when the door is opened. Further, the door should be hinged so that it opens away from the wall because this shields patients from corridor traffic and gives the patient more privacy when dressing because one has to walk around the open door to enter the room. ADA door requirements must also be accommodated.[1]

Exam room functionality also includes easy access to equipment, including those pieces mounted on the wall by exam tables and biohazardous waste disposal. These waste disposal units and other needed items such as glove dispensers, paper towel dispensers, and liquid soap may be wall mounted but done so with regard for the aesthetics and functionality of the room, usually close to the sink area. Sufficient electrical outlets also need to be available to accommodate equipment and extra light sources.[1]

A dictation space with little distraction should be considered if providers are likely to dictate records. A dictation niche may be no more than a countertop work surface adjacent to or located within the exam rooms so that dictation may occur throughout the day. A dictation niche might include a phone, an x-ray film viewing box, a storage area for routinely used forms and diagnostic instruments, and a computer terminal if electronic health records are part of the practice.[1] Avoid placing a dictation niche in a corridor or space that does not protect patient's private information.

Treatment Room

A treatment room serves a variety of purposes and may be valuable for the practice, particularly if minor surgeries or procedures such as casting or splinting will be performed. Treatment rooms are also useful when electrocardiograms are performed, minor procedures such as wound closures are done, or emergencies are managed. Good lighting such as a ceiling-mounted surgical light over the treatment table in addition to standard lighting is needed in treatment rooms.[1]

Nurses Station and Laboratory Space

Many primary care practices have a dedicated nurses' station. If a registered nurse or other assistant for the practice will be hired, a nurses' station should be considered. A nurses' station is an area where the nurse or medical assistant performs a variety of assessments and duties such as taking vital signs and weighing patients, sterilizing equipment, dispensing drug samples, performing lab tests, communicating with patients, or handling paperwork. The size of the space depends on the number of persons that will use it and the functions to be performed in the space. Locating this space close to the front office has the advantage of allowing the nurse or assistant easy access to patients as they are led from the waiting area to the exam area. Some practices combine this space with laboratory, and whether combining space works for the practice is determined by the nature of the practice because some practices have greater laboratory needs than others.[1]

When planning a laboratory space for the practice, include a double sink, microscope, and full-size refrigerator (depending on what is stored), a blood drawing station and chair, a centrifuge, and sufficient countertop space for it. A toilet room with a pass through window located adjacent to the lab allows personnel access to the specimen without having to leave the lab. Lab space planning is impacted by the CLIA (Clinical Laboratory Improvement Act discussed later in this chapter). Although providers may do some tests without CLIA compliance (tests known as "CLIA waived'), the practice's lab must still register with CLIA. Examples of CLIA waived include tests that could be purchased over the counter at a pharmacy, such pregnancy tests and dipstick urine tests. Common nonwaived CLIA tests, or tests that do fall under CLIA regulation, are blood counts, kidney and liver function tests, cholesterol testing, or a full lipid panel. For these tests, the lab would need benchtop hematology equipment and chemistry analyzers.[1]

Workroom and Storage Space

There are several things to consider when planning practice storage space, including how to manage the flow of paper and communication and how to prevent repetitive strain injuries among staff. Ergonomic considerations are essential in today's work space designs. HIPAA regulations will impact the need for confidential storage and handling of patient data. Storage also is about having enough storage where it is needed so that people do not have to keep getting up to get forms that are frequently used and so that countertops are not cluttered with so many machines or manuals that there is no work space left. Cabinet height impacts storage too because the height of the staff may not facilitate storage on high shelves.[1]

CODES AND SAFETY REGULATIONS

The practice space design team needs to understand the codes and safety regulations under which the practice will be reviewed and licensed. This includes applicable codes related to building, fire, plumbing, mechanical, electrical, and accessibility codes.[5] Health-related codes and regulatory issues also impact space planning. All of these codes are important reasons why working with architects and designers is needed during the planning phase for practice space.

Specific codes that most likely will impact space planning include fire protection, the Americans With Disabilities Act, sanitation, minimum construction requirements, energy conservation and environmental impact, Certificate of Need, and other codes relating to medical office buildings, including OSHA and CLIA. Fire protection includes flammability of materials such as carpet, wall-coverings, and upholstery fillings and fabrics, exit requirements, storage of combustible solids or medical gases, fire-fighting equipment and where these are located, electrical systems, and fire detection devices.[1]

The Americans with Disabilities Act

Complying with the accessibility guidelines of the Americans with Disabilities Act (ADA) became law in 1990. ADA is civil rights legislation, enforced through the U.S. Department of Justice in accordance with complaints of private citizens and other organizations; it was enacted to assure equal access in public accommodations. Both federal and state codes provide for creating accessible public places. The ADA defines disability broadly to include the visually or hearing impaired, those with motor or neurologic disorders, and individuals with arthritis, asthma, and cardiac insufficiency. Space planning in terms of complying with ADA is about creating spaces that are universally accessible to persons of different stature, age, and abilities.[1,5,6]

ADA affects many public facilities including health care facilities. ADA requirements need to be considered when planning the location of ramps, curb cuts, parking stalls, placement of exits, dimensions of elevators and restrooms, door width, restroom fixtures, countertop heights, and elimination of protruding objects in corridors and lobbies.[5] ADA requirements have specific toilet guidelines too. Toilets must be able to accommodate wheelchairs or those with disabilities that may need additional space to transfer onto the toilet or use the sink. In a single-use toilet, for example, the door may not swing into the clear floor space required for either the toilet or sink, but it can swing into the required 5-foot turning radius. Height issues for service countertops and dressing rooms also have ADA requirements. It is important to note that required accessibility guidelines vary from state to state, and it is important to follow the most stringent guidelines.[5] The take home message for practice space planning is that although most health care providers are aware of ADA requirements, an architect familiar with health facility design is able to review space to assure code compliance.

Employee Safety and OSHA

Employee safety also must be addressed in space planning. The Occupational Safety and Health Administration (OSHA) of the U.S. Department of Labor publishes guidelines, standards, and regulations governing many settings, products, and situations to protect workers from occupational risks. These do not come under the domain of the architect or designer.[1,5]

OSHA periodically visits worksites including health care offices. Employee safety issues to consider include personal use and food storage, emergency eyewash station, places where lab coats can be removed before leaving a space where staff are exposed to bloodborne pathogens, and placement of sharps and hazardous waste disposal equipment. These are just a few of the things that must be considered during space planning. Examples of how OSHA compliance can be violated include the following:

- Personal-use and food items cannot be stored in the same refrigerator as blood or tissue samples.

- An eyewash diverter valve device mounted to a faucet is required in any workplace where the employee's eyes may be exposed to injurious materials.

- In offices where staff are exposed to bloodborne pathogens, staff should remove their lab coats before leaving the suite, so a place to change clothes may be of value

- Selection and placement of sharps containers should be carefully considered because inappropriate placement of the sharps container can lead to needlestick injury.

The last example is especially important because research demonstrates that nurses sustain the most needlestick injuries and that as many as one third of all sharps injuries occur during disposal.[7] Because bloodborne pathogen exposure was the most significant standard cited and penalized in offices and clinics of physicians by OSHA between October 2003 and September 2004,[8] adherence to OSHA safety standards during space planning is essential.

Certificate of Need

In the early planning stages of the practice, it is important to determine whether a certificate of need is necessary. A certificate of need (CON) is established by state law and may be required when a provider begins, upgrades, expands, relocates, or acquires a covered health service or entity. CON legislation began in New York in 1966. Thirty-six states and the District of Columbia currently require CON. States vary in how CON is implemented, and it is difficult to compare across states. Although attention under a CON is often given to the construction and related costs of capital expansion and improvements, the focus in many states is on the increase in health care costs that can arise from the availability of unneeded service capacity and total operating expenses that are more costly than necessary. CON is directed at constraining excess capacity by requiring health care service providers to demonstrate the need for the initiation, upgrading, expansion, relocation, and acquisition of services. CON also addresses the potential impact of excess capacity or inefficient design on the higher total operating costs that are the concern for those who make payments for care—particularly employers, health insurers, and the state and federal governments.[9]

WHAT TO CONSIDER IF PRACTICE SPACE WILL BE LEASED

Whether or not to buy, build, or lease space is something that will at some point be part of space planning. There are some issues to consider before leasing space, and it is beyond the scope of this chapter to discuss all the nuances of leasing. Key questions related to leasing space are presented here to help with the issue of getting a clearly written lease.

From a business perspective, if space is leased, it is important to evaluate and know how many offices will be in the practice and how many patients the waiting room will accommodate, how late the building will be open and whether there will be evening or weekend access, what charges will be incurred for putting names on the door or in the building directory, and whether there will be support services such as secretarial, fax, or answering services available. When leasing, it is better not to make assumptions, and it is important to learn the language needed to be informed when you enter a lease arrangement. Common lease terms are listed in Table 11-1 and common business terms for leases are shown in Table 11-2.

In addition to becoming familiar with leasing terminology, common business questions to bring up about the lease include the following:

- Does the lease specifically state the square footage of the premises and the total rentable square footage of the building?

- As a tenant, is your share of expenses based on total square footage of the building or the square footage leased by the landlord? If the lease is based on the total square footage, your share may be lower.

- Do the base year expenses in the lease reflect full occupancy or are these expenses adjusted to full occupancy (e.g., base year real estate taxes that are based on an unfinished building may be lower than in subsequent years)?

- When increases occur, must the landlord provide a detailed list of expenses, prepared by a CPA, to support increases?

- As a tenant, does the lease clearly give you the right to audit the landlord's books or records?

- If use of the building is interrupted, does the lease define the remedies available to you, such as rent abatement or lease cancellation?

- If the landlord does not meet repair responsibilities, can you as the tenant make the repairs, after giving notice to the landlord, and deduct the cost from the rent?

- Is the landlord required to obtain nondisturbance agreements from current and future lenders (if not, you may be forced to move or sign a new lease if the building is sold or undergoes foreclosure)?

- Does the lease clearly define how any disputes will be decided?[10]

TABLE 11-1

Common Lease Terms

TERM	DEFINITION
Lessee	Tenant
Lessor	Landlord
Right of first refusal	Before vacant space is rented to someone else, landlord must offer it to the current tenant with the same terms that will be offered to the public.
Gross lease	Tenant pays flat monthly amount; landlord pays all operating costs, including property taxes, insurance, and utilities.
Triple net lease	Tenant pays base rent, taxes, insurance, repairs, and maintenance.
Percentage lease	Base rent, operating expenses, common area maintenance, plus percentage of tenant's gross income (most common for retailers in shopping malls).
Sublet	Tenant rents all or part of space to another business; tenant is still responsible for paying all costs to landlord.
Assign lease	Tenant turns lease over to another business, which assumes payments and obligations under the lease.
Anchor tenant	Major store or supermarket that attracts customers to a shopping center.
Exclusivity provision	Shopping center cannot lease to another who provides the same product or service that existing tenant does.
CAM	Common area maintenance charges including property taxes, security, parking lot lighting, and maintenance; may not apply to anchor tenants in retail leases.
Nondisturbance clause	Tenant cannot be forced to move or sign a new lease if building or shopping center is sold or undergoes foreclosure.

From U.S. Small Business Administration: *Getting Started: How to Start a Small Business* (website): http://www.sba.gov/starting_business/startup/guide2.html#lease. Accessed July 16, 2005.

Also, is the space code compliant or will there be any problems associated with making renovations or changes to bring the space up to code? It is worth having an architect review the space to assure code compliance. It is also worth consulting with an attorney and having your attorney review any business lease agreement before you sign it.

TABLE 11-2

Common Business Terms for Leases

Term	Definition
Escalation clause	Defines how much the rent will escalate with inflation; lessee should ask for documentation on what the percentage has been over the past 5 years
Heating and air conditioning (HVAC)	The lease should describe the hours of operation for the HVAC system, especially if you plan business hours that are not within the usual time frame; the lease should also clearly describe your responsibility for heating and air conditioning; questions to ask and be clear about include whether HVAC is a percentage based on square footage and whether costs in the common areas are included
Improvements	Any improvements that are negotiated should be reflected in the lease; ownership of all improvements also should be reflected in the lease and what happens to improvements when the lease is terminated should be clearly described; the lease should describe the lessees rights and the extent to which change within the space may be done; this may be as simple as putting in a security system to more complex renovations such as wall removal/relocation
Insurance	Lessor may ask for proof of insurance coverage before lessee moves in; minimum coverage the lessor expects needs to be detailed in the lease
Maintenance	The lease should clearly describe what repairs or maintenance you are responsible for; as examples, who provides cleaning services? Who repairs a door lock if it jams?
Move-in and delivery regulations	When moving into a multioccupancy building, the management company may have designated rules about hours you may move in and specific doors and elevators that must be used to do so; there may also be restrictions on times and types of deliveries once you have moved in; the lease should describe these rules
Renewal option	This clause provides the option of renewal under the original base rent
Renovations and repairs	Any repairs that are negotiated before or after move in should be described in the lease
Restrictions on use	Any restrictions for use of the leased space should be described in the lease
Storage space	If storage space is needed, the lease should describe what space is available and the costs to lease storage space; the lease should also clearly describe whether storage space can be built in the leased space
Sublease	The lease should describe whether a sublease is permissible and the specific terms for a sublease
Termination	The terms by which either the lessee or lessor may terminate the lease should be clearly described

From U.S. Small Business Administration: *Online Women's Business Center: Business Terms for Leases* (website): http://www.onlinewbc.gov/docs/finance/lease_terms.html. Accessed July 21, 2005.

CONCLUSION

Practice space planning is important from a location and marketing perspective; planning also assures compliance with the multiple codes that govern practices. Although it may seem costly to consult architects and attorneys during planning phases, the long-term payoff may be designs that foster patient satisfaction, enhance practice functionality for providers and staff, and aid in the avoidance of code violations. Space planning also anticipates change and future markets and technologies.

REFERENCES

1. Malkin J: *Medical and dental space planning: a comprehensive guide to design, equipment, and clinical procedures*, New York, 2002, John Wiley, p 1.
2. A report by the Center for Health Design and the Picker Institute: *Consumer perceptions of the healthcare environment: an investigation to determine what matters*, Lafayette, CA, 1998, Author; cited in Malkin J: *Medical and dental space planning: a comprehensive guide to design, equipment, and clinical procedures*, New York, 2002, John Wiley, pp. 1-6.
3. Miller RL, Swensson ES: *Hospital and healthcare facility design*, ed 2, New York, 2002, W.W. Norton.
4. Arsenault B: Adapting to change: the advantage of modular clinic design, *J Ambul Care Manage* 27(3):237-241, 2004.
5. Bell K: Planning ahead: practical hints for designing ambulatory care facilities, *J Ambul Care Manage* 22(1), 74-88, 1999.
6. Department of Justice: *Codes of Federal Regulations, ADA Standards for Accessible Design, 28 CFR Part 36* (website): http://www.ada.gov/adastd94.pdf. Accessed June 26, 2005
7. U.S. Department of Labor, Occupational Safety and Health Administration: *Bloodborne Pathogens and Needlestick Prevention: Possible Solutions* (website): http://www.osha.gov/SLTC/bloodbornepathogens/solutions.html. Accessed July 1, 2005.
8. U.S. Department of Labor, Occupational Safety and Health Administration: *Standards Cited for SIC 8010; All Sizes; Federal* (website): http://www.osha.gov/pls/imis/citedstandard.sic?p_esize=&p_state=FEFederal&p_sic=801. Accessed June 28, 2005.
9. Citizens Research Council of Michigan: *The Michigan Certificate of Need Program, February 2005, Report 38* (website): http://crcmich.org/PUBLICAT/2000s/2005/rpt338.pdf. Accessed June 22, 2005.
10. United States Small Business Administration: *Getting Started: How to Start a Small Business* (website): http://www.sba.gov/starting_business/startup/guide2.html#lease. Accessed July 16, 2005.

THE ELECTRONIC PRACTICE

Electronic Health Records, Health Information Technologies, and HIPAA Considerations

SALLY J. REEL

*M*any experts, including the Institute of Medicine (IOM) Committee on Quality of Health Care in America, recognize that information technology (IT) systems have profound potential to improve practice efficiency and the overall quality of health care.[1,2]

The automation of patient-specific clinical information is central to many IT applications, and efforts to automate clinical data date back several decades. Although the IOM called for the implementation of computer-based patient records in 1991, progress toward implementation has been slow.[1] However, legislation through the "Wired for Health Care Quality Act"[3] may promote the use of IT in health care if approved by Congress, so understanding the implications of an electronic practice is essential for nurse practitioners.

THE MOVE TOWARD ELECTRONIC HEALTH RECORDS IN THE U.S.

Despite calls for widely implementing electronic health records, most patient health records are stored on paper. Paper records mean that health records cannot be used to coordinate care, routinely measure quality, or reduce medical errors, and consumers generally lack the information they need about costs or quality to make informed decisions about their care. Research shows that moving the U.S. health care system to broad adoption of standards-based electronic health record systems could also reduce national health care spending.[4]

Challenges exist in the United States (U.S.) related to applying IT to health care. The U.S. lacks national standards for protecting health data and capture, storage, communication, processing, and presentation of health care information, and the costs of implementing IT systems can be prohibitive for some practices.[1] Miller, West and Brown, et al, found that for small group practices with electronic health records (EHR) initial costs to implement per provider averaged $44,000 with ongoing costs per provider per year averaging $8,400. This study also found that the average practice would cover costs of EHR implementation within 3 years and profit afterward. However, despite potential profitability, the study also found that providers spent more time at work initially when EHRs were implemented with revenue losses during training and implementation averaging $7,473 per FTE provider. Some practices also faced substantial financial risks including long payback periods, billing problems, disrupted revenue streams, and data losses.[2]

The U.S. Office of the National Coordinator for Health Information Technology (ONC) estimates that health information technologies (HIT) may reduce national health care costs by up to 20% per year through time savings and reduced duplication and waste. The ONC also estimates that HIT could reduce medical errors by providing complete patient histories, computerized ordering, and electronic reminders. Computer order entry, for example, may reduce errors associated with poor handwriting or when the wrong drug is ordered by prescribers such as NPs and physicians. HIT may save time simply because patients do not have to routinely give over and over again their address, insurance information, or other basic information. HIT also may alert providers when tests or treatments may be unnecessary. HIT improves portability of patient records as consumers get care from different providers by making sure that health information follows the patient throughout the healthcare system.[5]

The ONC identifies several barriers to widespread adoption of HIT. First, payers generally reimburse based on volume not efficiency or quality. Second, there are adoption issues that include a negative business case for a typical HIT adopter and significant electronic health record adoption gap based on organization size. Third, there is a high failure rate for EHR implementation, often because there is variable availability of HIT expertise in provider offices and limited implementation support for small practices. Finally, HIT has limited interoperability capacity issues because there are few rigorous HIT product standards and a limited health information exchange infrastructure.[6]

Implications for Nurse Practitioner Practices

So what is the take home message for nurse practitioners who are establishing independent practices and thinking about implementing EHRs and other electronic devices? HIT is coming, and it is anticipated that EHRs will have a pivotal impact on health care transformation.[7] As noted, it is suggested that HIT will improve safety, quality, and health care spending, and some advocate "... for government policy to facilitate widespread diffusion of interoperable HIT."[4] Nationally, President Bush called for the adoption and widespread use of HIT within 10 years starting in 2004.[8] Congress will consider the "Wired for

Health Care Quality Act" that would require the U.S. Department of Health and Human Services to disseminate HIT standards and require that all federal HIT purchases conform to those standards (as of this writing the Senate approved this bill). This bill would (1) authorize grants and loans to health care providers to support adoption of HIT, (2) require privacy protection for online health information and notification of patients if health information about them is wrongly disclosed, and (3) call for the development of health care quality measures and then reporting the quality scores of providers who receive federal funds.[3]

Although currently the widespread use of HIT among hospitals and providers in the U.S. is low, there is a rapidly growing consensus in the policy community that HIT is essential for improved patient safety and health quality and pending legislation recognizes this. Some of the potential drivers of HIT change include Congress, as noted, and Medicare, which as the single largest purchaser of health care services in the county could over time influence the adoption of HIT if Medicare adopts some type of HIT incentive or financing program that could influence provider use of HIT.[9]

Other possible drivers include quality incentives to promote provider adoption of HIT. It is known that costs, complexity of implementation, and uncertain financial returns are barriers to HIT adoption. Some advocate for incentive payments based on quality performance as an incentive for providers to adopt HIT systems and suggest that Medicare might reward providers "... who perform quality-increasing activities associated with IT use."[10]

For NPs considering HIT adoption, the costs and overall utility of EHR software and systems varies widely. Although there are many commercial vendors, the Veterans Administration (VA)—a leader in EHR development—in collaboration with the U.S. Department of Health and Human Services is presently developing a public domain EHR based on its present core VistA technology. It is anticipated that the technology product will be developed and released to the public in the near future and will be suitable for use in office-based practices and clinics. As public domain software, this VistA-based tool will provide an affordable option for HIT acquisition by decreasing resources necessary for installation and maintenance. It is expected that such a tool may be adopted directly by physicians and clinics, or acquired by private sector entities that support them.[11]

NPs should plan carefully how HIT will be integrated into the practice. Walker notes that implementation of an EHR requires an analysis of how work is conducted in the practice because work will also need to be redesigned with the implementation of an EHR.[7] In addition, effective implementation of an EHR needs commitment and capability to transform the ways the practice provides patient care. Walker also suggests that few health care organizations will be able to recruit, train, and retain information technology personnel with the necessary skills to implement an effective EHR, and that "Scarcities of both the passion and the capability are probably reflected in the low rate of EMR project failures."[7]

NPs also need to understand what features of an EHR are necessary for the type of practice use the system will serve when moving toward purchasing an EHR.

Consultation is probably needed for NPs without significant IT knowledge because a current caveat with EHR systems is that there are several hundred vendors nationally, and multiple vendors compound clinical data exchange. A starting place to gather information is to find out whether there are "preferred" vendors for the geographic region of the NP practice. As HIT is implemented, one trend in other countries and within some regions of the United States is that "preferred" vendors are identified for regions because this approach facilitates clinical data exchange regionally. Specifically, a few vendors are identified for a region, and these vendors are required to adhere to certain standards to facilitate clinical data exchange between different health care facilities. Massachusetts is an example of a state that has identified preferred vendors.[12]

One source of information is the Health Information and Management Systems Society (HIMSS) Ambulatory EHR Selector. This tool is an online database of EHR products and vendors that compares multiple characteristics including practice size, specialties that use the product, software pricing, product features and functions, regulatory compliance, contract details, and training and support. The HIMSS Ambulatory EHR Selector is available online at http://www.solutions-toolkit.com/EMRtoolkit/ASP/default.asp and currently is offered to individual physician practices for an annual subscription fee of $149.

Another source of information is the American Academy of Family Physicians (AAFP) Center for Health Information Technology available online at http://www.centerforhit.org/x11.xml. This center is about increasing the availability and use of low-cost, standards-based information technology among family physicians, and the center collaborates with government, industry, and other professional organizations to apply HIT to improve patient care and safety, and to increase the efficiency of health care delivery. Several tools/tutorials are available through this site including "Introduction to Electronic Health Records" at http://www.centerforhit.org/x1072.xml or "EHR 120—Understanding Features & Functions" available at http://www.centerforhit.org/x1070.xml.

PDAs, cell phones, tablet PCs, and other wireless devices are revolutionizing mobility and information exchange within many practices too. Knowing how these devices work, particularly in relation to assuring privacy of patient information is another important electronic practice consideration. For example; there are two types of major networks: a wide area network (WAN) and a local area network (LAN). An example of a WAN is the internet, which is open to users. A LAN is a closed, private network of computers such as is found in an office that has one large server and many computers and printers. A LAN may be connected to a WAN, and a firewall may be used to prevent outsiders from accessing the LAN. Hardwired networks rely on Ethernet wiring to physically connect computers. Wireless networks (WLANs) transmit data over radio waves and are comparable in speed to Ethernet. Several versions (protocols) of WLANs allow wireless transmission of data at varying speeds and distances. These WLAN protocols are commonly known as "Wi-Fi."[13] Wi-Fi's allow laptop portability (without all the Ethernet cords) between examining rooms and other physical areas and can provide great support in clinical decision-making.

Under HIPAA the Wi-Fi system must be secure and data encryption must meet HIPAA standards.[14]

Although it is relatively easy to set up a wireless network in an office setting, wireless networks are susceptible to security breeches, and seeking a consultant or networking expert for initial setup may help maximize functionality and security—which is essential in the HIPAA era. Hackers can access unprotected wireless networks and access private files. Routers, wired equivalent privacy (WEP), and virtual private network (VPN) are methods to protect systems from hackers.[13] The convenience of mobility and portability is a practice revolution, and taking steps to ensure privacy and security is essential.

There are considerations for devices such as personal digital assistants (PDAs), BlackBerries, and other electronic devices that allow managing patients on the go and away from the office too. Sharing patient data is an infrared "beam" away from one PDA to the next.[14] Lab data may be available wirelessly through the touch of a screen, however carrying around patient data on a PDA or other portable devices is now a potential HIPAA compliance concern because HIPAA's privacy rule (discussed later in this chapter) applies to all media of a patient's protected health information. A login and auto logout feature reduces the risk of someone seeing patient data they should not see, but as Bergeron[14] points out, "Consider the liability issues if you forgot your PDA at a coffee shop and someone picked it up and scanned through your list of patients. But with a login screen, one of the major benefits of a PDA—instant access to data—is lost." But it does not end here. Wireless PDAs, such as BlackBerry, have additional HIPAA-related issues, and it is essential to know whether these devices support encryption of e-mail and patient data they send over the Internet and whether the encryption is enabled—and is the level of encryption at HIPAA compliance levels?[14]

AAFP's Center for Health Information Technology also has information about the various electronic devices used in practice such as PDAs and tablet PCs on their website under "Hardware 101—The Basics" at http://www.centerforhit.org/x1067.xml.

HIPAA AND ELECTRONIC DATA

HIPAA (Health Insurance Portability and Accountability Act of 1996) is a new set of federal regulations that set national standards for the privacy of health information, the activities of institutional review boards, and informed consent for the use of health information.[15] Although HIPAA was passed in 1996, the privacy rule did not become effective until April 14, 2001, and April 14, 2003, was the compliance date for health care organizations. HIPAA has many parts including insurance portability and administration simplification (e.g., privacy, security, and electronic data interchange). HIPAA began as a means to allow employees to maintain their health insurance coverage when changing jobs. HIPAA also increases the federal government's authority over fraud and abuse in the health care industry.[16]

The Standards for Privacy of Individually Identifiable Health Information establishes, for the first time, a set of national standards for the protection of certain health information. The U.S. Department of Health and Human Services (USDHHS) issued the Privacy Rule to implement the requirement of HIPAA. Within USDHHS, the Office for Civil Rights (OCR) is responsible for implementing and enforcing the Privacy Rule. A major goal of the Privacy Rule is to assure that patients' health information is protected yet allows for the flow of health information needed to provide high quality health care and protect the public's health and well being. The Privacy Rule is about permitting important uses of information while protecting the privacy of people who seek health care. The Privacy Rule applies to health plans, health care clearinghouses, and to any health care provider who transmits health information in an electronic form in relation to transactions that are regulated under HIPAA.[17]

The development of EHRs was part of the impetus for HIPAA. The Constitution provides a fundamental right to privacy, and although the moral and ethical obligation to protect patient health information is not a new concept, the electronic environment provides significant challenges to protecting patient information. HIPAA was designed to assure that information transferred between facilities is protected. HIPAA also protects individuals from losing their health insurance when leaving or changing jobs by providing insurance continuity (Portability), and HIPAA increases the federal government's role and authority over health care fraud and abuse.[16]

With respect to EHRs, the HIPAA privacy rule does not single out an EHR for special treatment, and HIPAA does not establish special requirements that apply exclusively to patient information contained in an EHR. HIPAA regulations relate to the use and disclosure of a patient's protected health information regardless of the format that is used to maintain or transmit the patient information. Maintaining patient records in an EHR may affect the way a health care organization ensures compliance with HIPAA regulations. The HIPAA privacy rule, for example, applies to protected health information stored in or transmitted through electronic information systems, and security rules for protecting confidentiality, integrity, and availability of protected health information applies directly to the EHR.[18]

Three new terms that are related to HIPAA must be understood to comply with the new rules and regulations: covered entities (CE), protected health information (PHI) and designated record sets (DRS). *Covered entities* include health care providers, health plans, and health care clearing houses that must protect individual information. Some responsibilities of CEs include establishing oversight committees, clarifying exemption status, validating research practices, conducting risk analyses, developing polices and procedures for the disclosure of information, monitoring access, and handling privacy complaints.[16]

Protected health information refers to all "individually identifiable health information" held or transmitted by a covered entity or its business associated in any form or media, including electronic, paper, or oral. This information may include identifying information such as name, address, social security number, birth date, medical record number, telephone number, and patient account number. Any information that can be used to discover a patient's identify or leads to the access of the patient's medical information is protected health information. PHI also refers to any information about the patient's past, present, or future health conditions and treatment as well as billing and payment records related to the provision of health care services.[17]

Designated record set refers to that group of records maintained by or for a covered entity that is used to make decisions about individuals, or that is a health provider's medical and billing records about individuals or a health plan's enrollment, payment, claims adjudication, and case and medical management record systems.[17]

DRS includes health and billing records, but usually not peer review documents, appointment and surgery schedules, or employer records.[16] Patients do have the right to see and obtain a copy of their health records, and patients may amend protected health information in their DRS when that information is inaccurate. However, the privacy rule excepts the following from patient right of access: psychotherapy notes, information compiled for legal proceedings, lab results to which the Clinical Laboratory Improvement Act (CLIA) prohibits access, and information held by certain research laboratories.[17]

In terms of an NP practice, there are some key points to know about HIPAA and the workplace. First, it is essential to be in compliance with HIPAA rules and regulations. HIPAA privacy rules apply sophisticated technologies for controlling access to health information. Failure to maintain compliance with HIPAA privacy regulations can result in significant penalties including either civil or criminal penalties that can be as high as $250,000 and/or a prison terms of 10 years for anyone who sells, transfers, or uses individually identifiable health information for commercial advantage, personal gain, or malicious harm. The penalties may increase if the patient suffers serious injury from the violation.[16]

Technologies used in practice need to be reviewed in terms of HIPAA compliance. Today's technologies such as wireless devices and PDAs, as noted, offer added practice functionality and workflow efficiencies—as well as new HIPAA security compliance issues. How a practice conducts business with vendors also has HIPAA compliance issues. If as part of practice management, for example, digital audio files are sent overseas for transcription, it is crucial to know how patient data is handled on the other end (and if confidential patient files become public, would the practice be covered for a HIPAA violation lawsuit under its insurance coverage?).[14]

These are not unrealistic HIPAA compliance situations. The notion of the examining room computer is a reality of current practice.[19] Providers use personal computers and handheld electronic devices for many aspects of patient care. As noted, the Institute of Medicine and the U.S. Department of Health and Human Services advocate the use of computerized patient records and interoperable EHRs within the next decade. Providers are using computer physician order entry (CPOE) systems to order medications and lab studies. PDAs are used to gain access to drug information, clinical guidelines, decision aids, retrieval of patient test results, electronic prescribing and data collection in research. E-mail and the Internet are also used in many practices.[20]

Assuring HIPAA compliance is crucial because patient information is stored and exchanged electronically through these various technologies. There are steps that can be taken to meet HIPAA security compliance. First, avoid complacency. Security breeches do happen—computer viruses, eavesdropping on wireless communications, unintentional pharmaceutical company distribution of e-mail addresses of hundreds of patients taking an antidepressant are examples of such breaches. Second, take steps to prevent patient health information from falling into the wrong hands or being inadvertently altered or destroyed.[21] Kibbe[21] describes some practice steps to improve security and meet HIPAA compliance standards as follows:

1. Install appropriate computer security to protect patient and practice information.

2. Implement written security policies and procedures including those that cover personnel training and sanctions for security policy violations, and appoint a practice HIPAA security manager (written policies and a security/compliance manager is required under HIPAA).

3. Limit physical access to computers, printers, faxes, monitors, and other display devices.

   a. Avoid busy corridors and placement of display devices where someone without appropriate access can walk up to the display and see what it on it.

   b. Make sure the display access has a 30-second time out feature.

   c. Implement password management to control access to personal health information based on a person's role, authority, or need to know.

4. Know the capabilities and weaknesses of information systems used in the practice and how these are HIPAA compliant.

   a. Hardware: computers, laptops, tablet PCs, PDA, printers, servers, scanning devices, and modems/Internet connections

   b. Software: operating systems, billing software, practice management software, e-mail software, database and office productivity software

   c. Network components: routers, dedicated phone and cable lines, Wi-Fi systems, firewall software and hardware

5. Take steps to protect electronic data from loss or corruption by having a backup system that will allow retrieval of critical data needed to run the practice in the event of a disaster.

6. Secure any network and communications used by the practice through firewalls and up-to-date antivirus software

7. Consider whether any of the practice's electronic data transfers should be encrypted such as patient billing and administrative information exchanged with payers, utilization and case management data, lab and other clinical data electronically sent to and received from outside labs, word processing files used in transcription or other patient reports that are transferred electronically, and e-mails between providers and patients and between referring providers.

8. Evaluate chains of trust with business vendors such as insurance companies and transcription and billing services because each entity that shares information with the practice is an extension of that practice. HIPAA requires that a practice obtain assurances from business associates that they will implement necessary safeguards to protect the confidentiality, integrity, and availability of electronic health information they create, maintain, or transmit on behalf of the practice

9. Insist that vendors fully understand HIPAA security standards, including any local contractors used for installation or maintenance of hardware and networking components.

10. Evaluate the current computer security of the practice for HIPAA compliance gaps.

    a. One tool to start with is the AAFP's Center for Health Information Technology "Needs Assessment 101" available at http://www.centerforhit.org/x74.xml.[21]

CONCLUSION

David Bates notes that the current level of adoption of EHRs in the United States is low, with the major barriers to EHR adoption being related to reimbursement because providers pay for EHR systems, yet many of the benefits go to payers and purchasers.[12] Successful, widespread EHR adoption may require some financial incentives for providers as well as greater EHR interoperability (the ability of EHRs to operate well with other applications). Agencies such as the Centers for Medicare and Medicaid Services may play key roles as the Nation transitions to EHRs by providing financial incentives to providers who use EHRs, measure quality data, or achieve quality benchmarks. States may help in the transition too by creating mechanisms for small provider practices to form virtual groups to leverage a better financial advantage with EHR vendors.[12]

Meanwhile, the current governmental climate has embraced the adoption of EHRs, but strategies toward widespread EHR implementation appears to embrace market-based strategies.[22] Although providers may initially bear substantial startup costs, this does not mean that an NP should take a wait-and-see approach toward adopting an EHR because the future broad adoption of EHRs in the

United States is likely, particularly as issues of quality are addressed. Instead, before adopting any EHR system, investigate options for the practice by doing a careful practice risk and benefit appraisal and analyze how an EHR would enhance the work within the practice. It is equally important to review current knowledge about the quality of any EHR systems including HIPAA compliance before adopting any product as and finding out whether there are any regional preferred vendors; a consultant may help alleviate some of the confusion surrounding this.

REFERENCES

1. Committee on Quality of Health Care in America, Institute of Medicine: *Crossing the quality chasm: a new health system for the 21st century*, Washington, DC, 2001, National Academies Press.
2. Miller RH, West C, Brown TM, Sim I,. Ganchoff C: The Value of electronic health records in solo or small group practices, *Health Aff (Millwood)* 24(5):1127-1137, 2005.
3. Ferris N: Senate passes health IT bill: bipartisan 'wired for health care quality act' now goes to House for action, *Government Health IT*, November 18, 2005 (serial online): http://govhealthit.com/article91485-11-18-05-Web&RSS=yes. Accessed November 21, 2005.
4. Hillestad R, Bigelow J, Bower A, Girosi F, Meili R, Scoville R, Taylor R: Can electronic medical record systems transform health care? Potential health benefits, savings, and costs, *Health Aff* 24(5):1234-1245, 2005.
5. U.S. Office of the National Coordinator for Health Information Technology (ONC): *Value of HIT* (website): http://www.hhs.gov/healthit/valueHIT.html. Accessed November 1, 2005.
6. U.S. Office of the National Coordinator for Health Information Technology (ONC):*Barriers to adoption* (website): http://www.hhs.gov/healthit/barrierAdpt.html. Accessed November 1, 2005.
7. Walker JM: Electronic medical records and health care transformation, *Health Aff (Millwood)* 24(5):1118-1120, 2005.
8. U.S. Office of the National Coordinator for Health Information Technology (ONC): *Health IT (HIT) Adoption Initiative*, October 12, 2005 (website): http://www.hhs.gov/healthit/measuring.html. Accessed November 6, 2005.
9. Rosenfeld S, Bernasek C, Mendelson D: (2005). Medicare's next voyage: encouraging physicians to adopt health information technology, *Health Aff (Millwood)* 24(5):1138-1146, 2005.
10. Hackbarth G, Milgate K: Using quality incentives to drive physician adoption of health information technology, *Health Aff (Millwood)* 24 (5):1147-1149, 2005.
11. U.S. Department of Health and Human Services: *Health IT Strategic Framework. Attachment 2. V. Other VA Approaches—Knowledge and Technology Transfers to Benefit Target Populations* (website): http://www.hhs.gov/healthit/attachment_2/v.html. Accessed: November 9, 2005.
12. Bates D: Physicians and ambulatory electronic health records, *Health Aff (Millwood)* 24(5):1180-1189, 2005.
13. Lewis M: A primer on wireless networks, *Fam Prac Manag* 11(2):69-70, 2004.
14. Bergeron B: Where is HIPAA taking physician practices? *Medscape General Medicine* 7(2), 2005 (serial online): http://www.medscape.com/viewarticle/497977_print. Accessed November 18, 2005.
15. Clause S, Triller D, Bornhorst C, Hamilton R, Cosler L: Conforming to HIPAA regulations and compilation of research data, *Am J Health-Sys Pharm* 61(10):1025-1031, 2004 (serial online): http://www.medscape.com/viewarticle/478848_print. Accessed November 1, 2005.
16. Harmon L: HIPAA: a few years later, *Online J Issues Nursing* 10(2), 2005 (serial online): http://www.medscape.com/viewarticle/506841_print. Accessed November 21, 2005.
17. U.S.Department. of Health & Human Services, Office of Civil Rights Privacy Brief: *Summary of HIPAA Privacy Rule*, May 2003 (website): http://www.hhs.gov/ocr/privacysummary.pdf. Accessed October 20, 2005.

18. Hatton M: Medical privacy and electronic medical records, *Medscape Business of Medicine* 5(2), 2004 (serial online): http://www.medscape.com/viewarticle/492785_print. Accessed October 11, 2005.
19. Ventres W, Kooienga S, Marlin R, Vuckovic N, Steward V: Clinician style and examination room computers: a video ethnography, *Fam Med* 37(4):276-281 2005.
20. Mosley-Williams A, Williams C: Computer applications in clinical practice, *Curr Opin Rheumatol* 17(2(:124-128, 2005.
21. Kibbe D: Ten steps to HIPAA security compliance, *FamPract Manag* 12(4):43-49, 2005 (serial online): http://www.medscape.com/viewarticle/502875. Accessed November 18, 2005.
22. Iglehart JK: Pursuing health IT: the delicate dance of government and the market, *Health Aff* 24(5):1100-1101, 2005.

CHAPTER *13*

MANAGING GROWTH, THINKING BEYOND THE BOX

The (Not-So-Obvious) Opportunities and the (Not-So-Hidden) Dangers

IVO L. ABRAHAM • KAREN M. MACDONALD

*T*hink a few years ahead. You have your practice up and running. Things are going well, in fact better than expected. With great skill, you have circumnavigated some obstacles. You are generating good revenue, you are managing your expenses well, and you are turning a profit. You have paid off your personal credit cards, which you used to finance some of your practice. You have secured a line of credit from the bank to weather potential rainy days. Your investors have been offered an attractive exit package. Yet, notwithstanding all these indicators of success, you feel a bit antsy, perhaps ill at ease. You see further growth on the horizon and this prospect, exciting as it may be, is pulling you out of your comfort zone in ways you have not felt before in the years of building your practice. Welcome to managing growth! Welcome to being pulled out of the box! Welcome to new business opportunities and challenges! This chapter aims to help you stay in your current box (the practice you built) and think, not outside of the box, but beyond the box. Building on our experience, launching various health care businesses and consulting with numerous others, we too have been confronted with the opportunities and challenges of managing (fast) growth.

Business growth is usually measured in increased revenues and sustained profitability. However, these are proxy measures of much deeper processes. Mostly, young businesses grow (fast) because they have been building expertise, are maturing in their processes, and do not stray from their core competencies (yet grow as these core competencies expand). Young businesses grow successfully because they emphasize in the first place "growth-in-depth" (getting better

175

at what we do) rather than just "growth-in-breadth" (simply doing more of what we do).

THE BENEFITS OF FAST GROWTH

Fast growth is seldom a deliberate marketing strategy. Your patients may be asking you for more services and referring family and friends because they realize the value you provide. Also, you may have been anticipating what your patient population might need, you have consulted with them on those needs, and you have resourced accordingly. In other words, you are fueling your growth by way of requests for more and increasingly diversified clinical services.

This is good news! More services and new kinds of services provide you and your staff with more learning opportunities. Certainly, it keeps you on our toes ... There's no room for complacency or hesitation. It all fosters organizational and staff maturation and leads to faster innovation cycles. It supports growth-in-depth and positions you for growth-in-breadth. All along, growth produces more revenue, which in turn allows you to invest in the design of new services, support new initiatives, and fund additional marketing activities.

If managed well, fast growth can fuel staff enthusiasm and generate a "can-do" attitude. It engenders in staff both pride and satisfaction by being an active part in the intense process of creating something new. Fast growth stimulates the design and implementation of services that are direct derivatives of what you currently deliver. Thus it enables short-term strategic development. Fast growth enables you to keep pace with, and benefit from, economic trends. At the risk of using a corny metaphor, think about the growth of your practice in anatomical terms: fast growth enables your practice to build its muscle system (getting the work done); nervous system (central and peripheral); sensory and motor systems (to get things organized and processed); the gas-exchange part of the pulmonary system; the endocrine and the upper GI systems (to get energy sources in, processed, coordinated, and available); and the cardiac and central vascular systems (to get energy distributed).

THE RISKS OF FAST GROWTH

Unfortunately, growth can get out of hand. Too much growth in absolute terms produces too many commitments for the resources you have or can marshal. Too much growth in relative terms makes it difficult or impossible for you to deliver the quality and value you are committed to providing.

Growth rates often run faster than revenue flow. For instance, cash flow problems may occur when many services are delivered in a short period, but payment for those services is lagging. True, fast growth generally attracts greater access to capital. But if you are not careful, your practice could develop a "live it up" attitude. You can never afford to ignore sound (conservative) financial management.

Success due to fast growth may cause people to believe they can run a business enterprise "by-the-seat-of-their-pants-with-only-an-occasional-burning-feeling-due-to-excessive-seat-to-surface-friction". Occasional or not, burning the unmentionable anatomical region is painful. Fast growth may make you forget that a growing company requires more structure, formalized processes, and outcome parameters than a small company. Fast growth and early success may make you forget to keep your eyes on the business development radar screen and forget to populate the radar screen with new targets. To return to the (corny) metaphor... Because of the demands of fast growth, you may forget to build a healthy corporate body: the skeletal system (to keep you standing up); the integumentary system (to set your boundaries); the immunologic system (your resistance to noxious external influences); oxygen delivery pathways such as the peripheral vascular system (to enable creativity and productivity); nephrologic system (cleansing your blood); and the urological and lower GI systems (to get rid of excess and waste).

WHAT CAN YOU DO TO PROTECT YOURSELF?

Never cease to invest in people (both in numbers and in mix of expertise) and in enabling technologies, even if you need to put off other (needed) investments for the time being. This growth-in-depth will soon translate into growth-in-breadth, giving you additional stability.

Move from a focused leadership model (you) to a more generalized leadership model (you and your core team), because this will allow your practice to grow more naturally. Your strategic priority should be to shift the identity of your practice away from being mainly associated with you and your talents—superstar leaders who can do it all just do not exist.

As your current employees grow in knowledge, experience, and maturity, emphasize the recruitment of "entry-level" staff and empower more experienced employees to share their knowledge, expertise, and skills within a learning context. Keep on creating a "great place to work hard," building resilience into your team and giving it the strength to "go the distance." Institutionalize training and career development opportunities, and try to build informal learning experiences into the life of your enterprise.

Harness fast growth by investing even more in a quality management program. It signifies your commitment to doing things right the first time ... every time. In turn, this will build internal confidence among your employees but also expand patients' confidence in your services.

Harness fast growth by improving in your financial operation: accuracy of coding of patients, procedures, and services; optimizing the revenue-generating potential of staff; and shortening collection cycles. Still, conservative financial management should always be a way of life in your enterprise.

Challenge the thinking of your senior staff and build their business skills:

- Expect beyond-the-box thinking (but still within the gravity sphere!).

- Coach them to question themselves.

- Help them listen to patients, families, community leaders, other employees, and external advisors.

- Together, actively seek and use the individual and collective wisdom of your auditors, bankers, and legal advisors.

- Teach them to follow intuition but not to succumb to "gut" feelings ("[right] brain over stomach").

Fast growth requires you to take good care of your employees. Provide them with generous benefits, from the persistent to the occasional. Sharing benefits this way helps to balance short-term success with long-term rewards and recognition (Remember how long it took Eric Clapton to win a Grammy?)

SOME UNDENIABLE REALITIES

Regardless of the benefits and risks of fast growth, and what you may do to buffer your enterprise against the risks, there are some undeniable realities. Young companies are volatile companies, no matter how careful and strategic they are. In fact, you will always have to be volatile (that is, creative and responsive) to be successful, regardless of how old and experienced you and your colleagues become.

Your fast growth probably happened because you carved out a niche and created a new market. This gives you a window of opportunity within which to further define that market and assume a competitive and leadership "first-to-new-market" position—before the (much more capitalized) competition catches on. To grow, you will need to keep on redefining this market, expanding it so that you can graft new services onto it, and stay ahead of the dangers of both external competition and internal stagnation.

Your employees need to understand what it means to work for a young enterprise. They should understand that your practice is not a place for them to work if they can't stomach the volatility, the relative unpredictability, and the required individual and collective flexibility. It is not the place to work if they cannot assume the responsibility of individually and collectively creating new services through increasingly improved processes. If they are looking for stability, predictability, and rigidity, they may be on the wrong bus.

PART III

ACADEMIC PRACTICES AND ALTERNATE BUSINESS FORMS

ACADEMIC PRACTICE AND ACADEMIC NURSING CENTERS

DONNA BEHLER MCARTHUR

he relationship of faculty practice to professionalism and scholarship is inherent in the definitions of both *faculty practice* and *academic nursing practice* offered across the past decade. Early (1993) definitions of faculty practice were forwarded by the National Organization of Nurse Practitioner Faculties (NONPF) Faculty Practice Committee: *Faculty practice includes all aspects of delivery of nursing service through the roles of clinician, educator, researcher, consultant and administrator.*[1] In 1996, a more comprehensive definition included direct nursing services to individuals and groups as well as technical assistance and consultation to individuals, families, groups, and communities. While providing opportunities for promotion, tenure, merit, and revenue generation, the distinguishing characteristic of faculty practice within a school of nursing was the integration of teaching, research, practice, and service to achieve excellence.[1]

The succinct definition by Saxe et al.[2] captures the essence of faculty practice. "Faculty practice is a formal arrangement between a school of nursing/academic health center and a clinical facility/enterprise/entity that simultaneously meets the service needs of clients, while meeting the teaching, practice, service and research needs of the faculty and students (p 166)."

Academic nursing practice is described as "the intentional integration of education, research and clinical care in an academic setting for the purpose of advancing science and shaping the structure and quality of health care"[3, p. 63]. Key concepts include deliberate integration, providing evidence-based care and educating health care professionals, and contributing to the development of nursing knowledge and improvement of health care delivery.[4]

ACADEMIC PRACTICE

Reflecting on the above definitions, it is evident that academic practice is often synonymous with faculty practice. There is little doubt that the core foundation of professionalism is nursing practice. As such, faculty/academic practice is a venue for initiating, sustaining, and enhancing direct and indirect services to clients, students, and the community. Academic nursing practice enhances opportunities for role modeling service as well as autonomy and self-regulation.[5] Clearly, each school of nursing should have its own definition of faculty practice—capturing their roles, settings, and structural and economic models.

History of Academic Nursing Practice

The trajectory of academic nursing practice should be viewed within the context of nursing education. It is well known that early nursing education took place in hospital schools of nursing. Nurse historian Dr. Joan Lynaugh[6] clearly describes the shift in focus from educating those who cared for the sick to those preparing to be administrators or educators at the college level, thus weakening the relationship between education and practice. The historical record supports that academic nurses' experience with clinical practice is a recent event occurring within the past five decades.

The Division of Nursing of the Public Health Service was founded in 1946 and was a major force for improving nursing education. Throughout the 1960s, federal support increased after the Surgeon General's initiative to address the nursing shortage. During this time the practice-education gap, as defined by Lynaugh,[6] began to close. This was facilitated in part by the growth of advanced practice nursing, representing a new independence within the profession. On a practical note, faculty teaching clinical components of nurse practitioner programs must maintain current licensure and certification. Certification from both the American Nurses Credentialing Center (ANCC) and the American Academy of Nurse Practitioners (AANP) require a minimum of 1000 hours of nursing practice every 5 years.

An ambitious effort, beginning in 1999 the Penn-Macy Initiative to Advance Academic Nursing Practice assisted 21 schools of nursing in the development of their academic practices through an intensive 1-week institute with consultation and follow-up over a 2-year period.[7] The majority of the schools were from large public universities. Practice history varied widely to include several schools reporting evolution of practices in the 1970s. Each school identified an academic practice resource team representing three perspectives essential for academic practice success: research/practice nursing faculty, health care business manager, and/or academic financial administrator. As a member of the team from Vanderbilt University School of Nursing, this author participated in the intensive summer institute. Follow-up consultation and support, a senior fellows exchange, and participation in evaluation were part of the process. Key indicators for success of the individual programs included having a place for practice on the school's organizational chart, having a critical mass of faculty in practice, and having clear and achievable goals. It appeared that the importance of each characteristic was dependent on the history of the individual school, its location in the university and health environment, the commitment and vision of the dean and administration, the composition and mission of the faculty, strategic plans for the school, and access to external and internal resources. Individual successes were independent of the length of practice history in the school. A school's understanding of its own history, mission, and environment was essential. Research integration continued to remain the biggest challenge; the necessity for collaboration between clinical and research faculty was highlighted in their evaluation. Perhaps the addition of nurses prepared at the Doctorate of Nursing Practice level will facilitate this collaboration.

Recurring themes related to academic nursing practice include the following: (1) clinical expertise is a prerequisite for most nursing faculty in higher education; (2) to implement a tripartite mission, schools must find ways to link revenues from teaching, practice, and research to build viable and balanced budgets; (3) many schools of nursing are still tuition-driven; and (4) faculties of the future will continue to maintain their flexibility, recognizing and responding to environmental changes.[6]

Models

The model selected for an academic nursing practice lays the foundation for the types of risk and benefits the nurse practitioner and school will face, and influences the schools' ability to meet its strategic goals.[8] Practice models may be conceptualized based on sites of practice (e.g., community centers, hospitals) or form of service such as case management. Conceptual dimensions used to evaluate models of nursing practice include structure, function, and clients: (1) the ownership of the practice and its relationship with the parent organization; (2) measures of performance used; and (3) the ways in which clients are defined.

Four classic models of faculty practice were identified in the early 1990s and can be seen in varying configurations today—the unification, collaborative, integrative, and entrepreneurial models.[1] Perhaps the earliest model, established in the 1970s, was the unification model in which the administration of the clinical agency and the school of nursing were unified such that faculty served as both clinicians and educators. In contrast to the unification model, the collaborative model used joint appointments to ascertain a faculty member's primary responsibilities within the school of nursing, but with an appointment within a specific clinical area. In this model, salary costs may be shared. A caveat for the NP considering this model is to negotiate specific responsibilities with each organization. Contracting for a.5FTE (half-time employment) appointment with a clinical agency in the face of teaching and research responsibilities can be daunting. The integrative model describes faculty and graduate students sharing patient care responsibilities. The most creative, yet potentially risky, model is the entrepreneurial model, in which faculty design their own practices, determining goals and objectives. Faculty provide care as part of their faculty responsibilities.

Exemplars

The entrepreneurial model is reflected in the West Virginia Rural Health Education Partnership Program (WVRHEP). This program evolved from the partnership between the State of West Virginia, the W. K. Kellogg Foundation, and the West Virginia School of Nursing to address the problem of critically limited primary health care in rural and medically underserved areas in the state. An academic practice was developed by an advanced practice nurse to provide prenatal and postpartum care at one of the WVRHEP health centers.[9] Several goals were realized keeping in mind the tripartite academic mission, for example, provide needed service to women in an underserved community, integrating students into practice, and using the practice to explore interventions to meet patient needs. Persily recognized the support of an infrastructure that encouraged retention of rural providers through interdisciplinary education.

A practice portfolio approach for faculty practice is currently used by several schools of nursing. Vanderbilt University School of Nursing (VUSN) has used this approach for over a decade, operating nurse-managed clinics at several sites in metropolitan Nashville and surrounding areas.[10] In this portfolio model, there are multiple practices with differing ownership, differing performance measures, and differing clientele. A comprehensive midwifery practice delivers at the Vanderbilt University Hospital. Each practice is clearly classified as equity, contract, and/or grant. Funding sources are most often combined with revenue largely dependent on the local reimbursement market for advanced practice nurses and patient volume. Credentialing and billing infrastructures are in place jointly through the school of nursing and the medical center. School health clinics are examples of grant-funded projects. Although these venues pose no financial risk, sustainability has been difficult. Contract practices include those with outside agencies and community physician practices in which faculty practice time is bought out, for example, the salary and benefits. Revenue generated by the nurse faculty member is kept by the agency or clinic that contracts with the school of nursing. Nurse practitioners maintain faculty rank with teaching, and scholarship activities are adjusted to reflect the practice appointment.

In 1994, the University of Pennsylvania School of Nursing established the Penn Nursing Network (PNN) as part of its strategic plan in an effort to integrate research, education, and clinical services to several client populations across the lifespan.[11] Practices were diverse, for example, the Collaborative Assessment and Rehabilitation for Elders (CARE) Program, Continence Program, Community and Neighborhood Midwifery Services, and the Health Corner in West Philadelphia. The infrastructure to support these enterprises included numerous functions supported by the school of nursing and university: administrative support, business planning (consultation, practice diversification), credentialing, finance (accounting analysis and projections, billing, regulations), grants management, human resources, information systems, legal and risk management, and marketing. Schools of nursing contemplating practice initiatives would be wise to consult with faculty experts from PNN. As noted by Swan and Evans,[11] "The clinical practice arm of a school of nursing's mission is actually a business with its own unique and specialized infrastructure needs (p 71)."

Facilitators and Barriers

In addition to the characteristics supporting successful practices described previously, Evans and Lang[4] identify readiness factors related to the development or expansion of academic nursing practice, which have been implied in the previous discussions. Readiness factors include mission and resources (people, educational, research, and organizational). Questions for the NP/school of nursing to ask are Is the practice compatible with the university's mission? Is there a critical mass of doctorally prepared faculty and staff to include advanced practice nurses (APNs)? Does a strong APN educational program exist? Is there continuous research funding? Are there resources for financial capital, administrative support? Are volunteer board members readily accessible?

The primary mission of academia has been education and the generation of new knowledge. Can there be a balance between the expectations in the face of scholarly endeavors? The history, mission and values, and resources of the respective school and parent university (to include geographic location) shape academic nursing practice. Questions posed by Evans and Lang[4] include the value the university places on the integration of missions and how the practice is measured and rewarded. Where does practice fit in the mission and vision of the school? Is it mentioned? What about the strategic plan, financial and operational plans?

The NP would be well served to explore these questions when contemplating practice opportunities within a school of nursing as well as networking with practice-active faculty within the parent organization and through professional organizations, for example, NONPF, AANP.

ACADEMIC NURSING CENTERS

As noted previously, faculty practice has been facilitated through academic nursing centers. The American Nurses' Association's (ANA) Nursing Center Task Force in 1987 offered the first comprehensive definition of nursing centers focusing on the control of practice by the nurse.

Nursing centers—sometimes referred to as community nursing organizations, nurse-managed centers, nursing clinics, and community nursing centers—are organizations that give the client direct access to professional nursing services. Using nursing models of health, professional nurses in these centers diagnose and treat human responses to actual and potential health problems, and promote health and optimal functioning among target populations and communities. The services provided in these centers are holistic and client-centered. And are reimbursed at a reasonable fee level. Accountability and responsibility for client care and professional practice remain with the professional nurse. Overall accountability and responsibility remain with the nurse executive.

Nursing centers are not limited to any particular organizational configuration. Nursing centers may be free-standing businesses or may be affiliated with universities or other service institutions such as home health agencies and hospitals. The primary characteristic of the organization is responsiveness to the health needs of the population.[12, p.1]

In her classic work, Barger[13] analyzed definitions used to describe nursing centers, also called *nurse-anchored, nurse-conducted,* and *nurse-managed centers.* Academic nursing centers are a subset of nursing centers with the purpose of providing educational experiences for students, a practice site for faculty, nursing services to the community, and a setting for faculty and students to conduct nursing research. The stated purpose of academic nursing centers has remained consistent over the past several decades; however, the emphasis on each of the purposes has varied.[14]

History of Academic Nursing Centers

The development of academic-based nursing centers (ANCs) began in the 1970s. In 1978, O. Marie Henry, D.N.Sc., R.N., in her address to the American Public Health Association, advocated for nursing centers in a variety of settings, for example, institutional, primary care, or community, to provide direct access to nursing care, to educate students, and to conduct research to improve both education and practice; nursing should be the primary focus.[12] Her ideas provided leadership at the federal level to support demonstration projects in schools of nursing, the popularity of these increasing throughout the subsequent decade. Funding for these centers was provided in part by federal government initiatives and private foundations (e.g., Robert Wood Johnson, W.K. Kellogg Foundation). The first federal award (from the United States Public Health Services [USPHS]), Division of Nursing Advanced Training Grant, was awarded to Arizona State University School of Nursing in 1977. The clinic is one of the few that continues today offering affordable health care for an underserved population, as well as serving as a clinical site for advanced practice nursing students and faculty and for research.[13]

Barger[14] explored the development of ANCs over the past three decades within the environment of evolving health policy and changing priorities and resources within nursing education. Certainly, academic nursing centers were well positioned in the early 1990s in the wake of health care reform, recognized as cost-effective and as integral to academia, providing educational experiences for students, practice sites for faculty, nursing services to the community, and settings for nursing research. Barger defines the current era of health policy as the "age of uncertainty and opportunity." As such, academic nursing centers must focus on quality issues as they continue to maintain a precarious balance between meeting the service needs of their clients and the needs of their academic base.[14]

The Institute of Medicine (IOM) 2001 Report, *Crossing the Quality Chasm: a New Health System for the 21st Century,* identified five core competencies across clinical disciplines that clearly impact academic nursing centers: (1) provide patient-centered care; (2) work in interdisciplinary teams; (3) employ evidence-based practice; (4) apply quality improvement; and (5) utilize informatics.[14]

Addressing the quality issue within the context of their experiences at the University of Texas Services ANC, Mackey and McNiel[15] defined measures for maintaining overall quality of a primary care ANC. These include a quality assurance program, financial stability, educational opportunities for students, research efforts, patient care processes, billing and insurance systems, administration and governance, marketing efforts, clinical records and information systems, credentialing and continuing education efforts for faculty and staff, facilities and environment, health education and wellness services, patient/corporate satisfaction feedback, and faculty and staff issues. The value added by ANCs over that of other primary care centers is the education afforded students and other faculty in the parent school of nursing.

Exemplars

Arizona State University College of Nursing (http://nursing.asu.edu/anc/index.htm) manages three nonprofit nursing centers with varied funding sources. The three centers include Community Health Services Clinic, noted previously as the first federally funded nurse-managed primary care center in the country; Breaking the Cycle Community HealthCare, which provides free or low-cost family planning services for uninsured adolescents and adults, and Escalante Community Center, serving low-income children, their families, and elderly adults. Each year, faculty mentor more than 200 undergraduate and graduate students in these centers. Services are provided to over 1000 people each month, bringing health care to clients in the neighborhoods in which they live, for example, a church, community center, and a retail strip mall.

The Michigan Academic Consortium, funded by the W.K. Kellogg Foundation, comprises four Michigan universities, their Schools of Nursing, and their eight ANCs. NP student feedback was analyzed over a 3-year period. Students reported value in being mentored by an NP and the ability to apply an understanding of their patients' economic, social, and cultural situations to treatment decisions.[16]

The Center for Integrated Health Care (IHC) represents a partnership between a free-standing community-based psychiatric rehabilitation center and the University of Illinois at Chicago College of Nursing.[17] People with severe and persistent mental illnesses (SPMI) receive care targeted for this vulnerable population by integrating primary and mental health care. Resources are shared between the partners, with the College of Nursing providing the business and quality assurance infrastructure. The major challenge for the IHC is financial sustainability. Currently the center is funded by a Division of Nursing grant and direct fee-for-service reimbursement, primarily from Medicaid.

A nontraditional ANC is one in the shape of a wellmobile. In 1994, the University of Maryland School of Nursing developed a full-service health clinic on wheels to meet the needs for community-based health care and educational experiences for NP students and faculty. This effort was established through a public-private partnership. With support from the Governor, an advisory board was developed and funds were raised to purchase the mobile unit; the purpose was to improve the health status of families and children in underserved communities. Funding was obtained through the Division of Nursing and private and public sources for the purchase of additional units. The value of strategic partnerships was identified especially in view of the financial viability of the program.[18]

At the forefront of the academic community nursing centers (CNCs) for over two decades, the University of Wisconsin-Milwaukee School of Nursing operates four centers in community-based organizations, for example, a homeless shelter, a low-income community. The identified client problems are complex. Partnerships were created with the neighborhoods in which the neighborhood center provided space, security, and transportation. Retrospective data over an 11-year period were analyzed, assessing the usefulness of the Lundeen CNC model to structure health care management of a population.[19] The type and volume of CNC services was influenced by shifts in CNC funding sources, staffing, neighborhood center programming, and socioeconomic changes in the community. Findings suggested that a computerized clinical documentation system that specifically tracks nursing practice is vital if nurses are to identify and be reimbursed for client care specific to nursing practice.

Facilitators and Barriers

As noted previously, the trajectory of ANCs follows that of federal funding, which is inconsistent at best. A distinguishing characteristic of academic nursing centers is that they serve as safety nets for vulnerable populations, often in high-risk communities. Hence sustainability becomes a primary goal and challenge. ANC program planning must include strategic, financial, marketing, organizational development and operations, and information management.[20]

CONCLUSION

Academic nursing practice, to include academic nursing center sites, must be viewed within the context of nursing education, health policy, and economic resources. The definition of academic nursing practice varies across settings reflecting the mission and values of the school and parent university. The challenge before the NP is that of integrating teaching, practice, and research while providing quality patient-centered care to diverse populations.

REFERENCES

1. National Organization of Nurse Practitioner Faculties (NONPF): *Faculty Practice Resource Center: Definitions & Models,* 2005 (website): http://www.nonpf.com/NONPF2005/FacultyPracticeResourceCenter/FPDef&Models.Htm. Accessed December 12, 2005.

2. Saxe JM, Burgel BJ, Stringari-Murray S, Collins-McBride GM, Dennehy P, Janson S, Humphreys J, Martinc H, Roberts B: What is faculty practice? *Nur Outlook* 52(4) 166-173, 2004.
3. Lang NM, Evans LE, Swan A: Penn Macy initiative to advance academic nursing practice, *J Prof Nurs* 18(2):63-69, 2002.
4. Evans LK, Lang NM, editors: *Academic nursing practice: helping to shape the future of healthcare,* New York, 2004, Springer.
5. Blair K, Dennehy P, White P: *Nurse Practitioner Faculty Practice: An Expectation of Professionalism,* NONPF (2005). Faculty practice resource center: Faculty practice statements (website): http://www.nonpf.com/NONPF2005/FacultyPracticeResourceCenter/FPStatements. Accessed December 11, 2005.
6. Lynaugh JE: Academic nursing practice: looking back. In Evans LK, Lang NE: *Academic nursing practice: helping to shape the future of healthcare,* New York, 2004, Springer, pp 20-37.
7. Evans LK, Swan BA, Lang NE: Evaluation of the Penn-Macy initiative to advance academic nursing practice, *J Prof Nurs* 19(l):8-16, 2003.
8. Sebastian JG, Stanhope M, Williams CA: Academic nursing practice models and related strategic issues. In Evans LK, Lang NE: *Academic nursing practice: helping to shape the future of healthcare,* New York, 2004, Springer, pp 38-65.
9. Persily CA: Academic nursing practice in rural West Virginia, *J Nurs Educ* 43(2):75-77, 2004.
10. Pilon B: Exemplar A: using a practice portfolio approach for faculty practice at Vanderbilt University School of Nursing. In Evans LK, Lang NE: *Academic nursing practice: helping to shape the future of healthcare,* New York, 2004, Springer, pp 58-59.
11. Swan BA, Evans LK: Infrastructure to support academic nursing practice, *Nurs Economics* 19(2):68-71, 2001.
12. American Nurses' Association: *The nursing center: concept and design,* Kansas City, 1987, American Nurses' Association.
13. Barger S E: Establishing a nursing center: learning from the literature and experiences of others, *J Prof Nurs* 11(4):203-212, 1995.
14. Barger SE: Academic nursing centers: the road from the past, the bridge to the future, *J Nurs Educ* 43(2):60-65, 2004.
15. Mackie T, McNiel NO: Quality indicators for academic nursing primary care centers, *Nurs Econ* 20(2):62-65, 73, 2002.
16. Tanner CL, Pohl J, Ward S, Dontje K: Education of nurse practitioner in academic nurse-managed centers: student perspectives, *J Prof Nurs* 19(6):354-363, 2003.
17. Marion LN, Braun S, Anderson D, McDevitt J, Noyes M, Snyder M: Center for integrated health care: primary and mental health care for people with severe and persistent mental illnesses, *J Nurs Educ* 43(2), 71-74, 2004.
18. Heller BR, Goldwater MR: The governor's wellmobile: Maryland's mobile primary care clinic, *J Nurs Educ* 43(2):92-94, 2004.
19. Hildebrandt E, Baisch MJ, Lundeen SP, Bell-Calvin J, Kelber S: Eleven years of primary health care delivery in an academic nursing center, *J Prof Nurs* 19(5):279-288, 2003
20. Esperat MC, Green A, Acton C: One vision of academic nursing centers, *Nurs Econ* 22(6): 307-312, 319, 2004.

THE ACADEMIC NURSING CENTER

A History of Federal Support

DAVID W. KELLY

*he federal government provided the first comprehensive federal authority to fund nursing education through the Nurse Training Act of 1964[1] by adding Title VIII to the Public Health Service Act. This Act provided the most significant nursing legislation in American history to date. A new era for nursing was dawning in which preparation of nurses was deemed important to the nation's welfare. The Nurse Training Act received widespread support from the nursing community and the public at large.

A NEW DAWNING

The Nurse Training Act was comprised of five different elements to be administered over a 5-year period. Each element provided an initiative to improve health care through the nursing education programs. The first program consisted of nursing school construction grants. The second component aimed to improve and expand educational programs in nursing schools through project grants for curriculum revision, faculty development, and experimentation with new and more effective instructional methods and teaching aids and audiovisual equipment.

A third element, available only to diploma schools of nursing, was designed to reimburse them for a portion of the costs of educating students whose enrollment could be attributed to the provisions of the Nurse Training Act. The fourth initiative of the Nurse Training Act provided for continuation of the Professional Nurse Traineeship Program. In the fifth element, provisions were made for a generous, long-term, low interest student loan program to enable more students to afford nursing school. The legislation also directed that a National Advisory

Council on Nurse Training be created to advise the Surgeon General on the Administration of the Nurse Training Act. A nationwide study of nursing and nursing education was mandated. Although over the years various sections were added, providing separate authorities for additional educational resources to support nurses, nurse midwives, nurse anesthetists, clinical nurse specialists, nurse practitioners, public health nurses, and nursing faculty; many of these original elements continue in practice today to support and guide nursing education and practice.

Over the first 5-year period, a total of $238 million dollars was allocated. The Federal Division of Nursing (Division of Nursing) provided consultation by staff to schools of nursing interested in applying for Nurse Training Act funds. Many institutions were hampered by obsolete or inadequate facilities. Schools that applied for construction grants also were encouraged to apply for funds to develop new educational methods. Examples of funded projects included development of a teacher evaluation instrument, a statewide continuing education program, and methods for using new instructional technologies such as closed-circuit television.

Passage of the Nurse Training Act sent a profound message to the nursing profession. Not only were nurses deemed critical to the heath of the nation but also their education was determined to be a worthwhile investment. This legislation would have a myriad of effects on nursing and nurses by directly increasing the numbers of nurses, making it easier for them to attend colleges and universities, and markedly improving the educational facilities and teaching methods.

By the late 1960s, new measures extended or modified the 1964 Nurse Training Act. Associate degree programs were growing at a rapid rate, and they could now qualify for federal support through accreditation by regional bodies. The Division of Nursing had funds officially earmarked to support its long-standing interest in reaching out to disadvantaged young people. Programs designed to facilitate minority access into nursing were rapidly initiated and funded to enhance the profession's diversity.

Legislation enacted in 1968[2] expanded the scope of project grants, the component of the Nurse Training Act that funded creative nursing ventures. Project grants allowed the Division of Nursing to fund innovative experiments to improve nursing education and patient care delivery. One such project allowed for planning and implementation of a new program for educating nurses for practice in expanded roles such as primary care.

EMERGING POSSIBILITIES AND CHALLENGES

The Nurse Training Act of 1971[3] broadened Title VIII authorities and presented the greatest investment yet in nursing education. This legislation included all of the conditions of the earlier enactment with important modifications. The mission of special project grants broadened, and funds were then specifically earmarked to encourage advanced nursing roles and to increase resources for underserved areas. Schools of nursing welcomed the new capitation grants authorized in the 1971 Act. Capitation allowed schools to accommodate larger enrollments, improved student-to-faculty ratios, and helped the financial stability of many schools. A new category of the Division of Nursing funding helped prevent many financially distressed nursing schools from closing. Programs and contracts to increase the number of nurses and to facilitate student diversity were supported. Special projects were funded to prepare former military corpsmen and medics as well as retiring policemen and firemen for a second career.

The focus on advanced practice nurses intensified in the 1970s. New graduate programs prepared clinical nurse specialists to meet the nursing needs of specialty populations such as burn victims. Graduate curricula were designed for nurse practitioners who could meet the primary care requirements of the disadvantaged in inner cities and other underserved areas. Early in the decade, the Division of Nursing began to fund certificate and master's degree nurse practitioner programs.

The first longitudinal study of nurse practitioners was commissioned by the Division of Nursing to estimate the need for future federal support by gathering data on the functions and utilization of nurse practitioners. This study also quantified the variability in and appropriateness of nurse practitioner preparation. A national perspective on their contributions to primary health care, particularly in medically underserved areas, was established as a result. The study demonstrated that nurse practitioners were a highly beneficial societal resource. Its results became the basis for funding for many years and facilitated the role's acceptance. It shaped the division's support for the role in the form of project grants, contracts, and consultation.

Rapidly changing treatment modalities, new roles for nurses, and shifting health care delivery patterns heightened the need for nurses to meet and plan the profession's response. During the 1970s the Division of Nursing supported many conferences on a wide variety of nursing topics. Nurses met in 1972 to discuss accountability for patient care in a changing health care environment. "The 'Decanal' Role in Baccalaureate and Higher Degree Colleges of Nursing" brought together nursing school deans to discuss the role of future nursing educational leaders.[4] Plus at other meetings, nursing research methodologies were critiqued, and participants evaluated team versus primary nursing on a variety of outcome measures. These conferences brought nurse leaders together and provided them with support to maintain momentum in the profession's ongoing development.

THE MALDISTRIBUTION OF PROVIDERS

By 1975, health care costs consumed almost 10% of the Gross National Product. Congressional attention had shifted from health care personnel shortages to the maldistribution of existing providers. This change in philosophy occurred in spite of data that suggested both shortages and maldistribution existed in the nursing arena. Congress recognized that not enough nurses practiced in rural and inner city areas. Shortages also existed in leadership, teaching, and advanced clinical practice.[5]

A crisis in elderly care began to evoke societal concern. Nursing homes had too few registered nurses; their personnel were under-trained and overworked. A series of governmental and privately commissioned reports analyzing nursing home failures and abuses were published in the middle and late 1970s.

The 1975 Nurse Training Act continued the provisions contained in Title VIII of the Public Health Service Act[6] and provided separate authorities for advanced nurse education. Armed with a new mandate, the Division of Nursing set to work implementing the 1975 legislation. The Act included specific authorities supporting the preparation of nurses with graduate preparation. Authority to meet the costs of planning, developing, and operating these programs was enacted. Special emphasis was placed on preparing gerontology nurses. Other legislation mandated reports to the Congress on the supply, distribution, and educational requirements for nurses. Included in subsequent reports were statistics regarding employment, compensation, specialty preparation, and foreign nurse graduates.

NURSE EDUCATION AND FACULTY PRACTICE

Faculty practice emerged as a major issue for nursing education in the late 1970s and early 1980s, and the nursing centers provided a venue to integrate service delivery with nursing education. Only after much debate, did the academic nursing centers and faculty-developed clinical sites become a viable alternative for facilitating faculty practice. These practice settings offered students a window into prevention and early intervention services, targeting individuals, families, and communities. Advance practice nurses, nurse practitioners, public health nurses, and mental health specialists were able to work with collaborating physicians to provide comprehensive primary care to vulnerable populations. The use of these nursing centers began as a part-time operation with little continuity of service or coordination of care.

This became reality only after nursing schools began placing an emphasis on faculty practice. The philosophy of the University of Rochester's Unification Model, for example, was that faculty clinical practice strengthened all components of the educational programs. One division-supported program, combining nursing education and health care delivery for the elderly, was established at the University of Lowell in Massachusetts. This gerontologic nurse practitioner program was designed to provide comprehensive care to the elderly and serve as a practice site for nurse practitioner students. Gerontologic nurse practitioner faculty was responsible for the project's direction and for providing services to clients as part of a joint practice arrangement with physicians. Students provided primary care to clients under faculty supervision. In a program evaluation, clinic attendees had a high degree of patient compliance with prescribed regimens and positive health care outcomes. Most nurse practitioner programs prepared clinicians who were readily accepted by the public and well prepared to meet their clients' health care needs; however, the Division of Nursing strove to further improve nurse practitioners' education.

The origins of federal funding for nurse practice arrangements can be traced back to a speech given by O. Marie Henry, U.S. Public Health Service, at an annual meeting of the American Public Health Association. In 1978, O. Marie Henry[7] spoke about the need to support settings in which the education of nursing students, the practice of patient care, and the research to improve both the education and practice would be planned and conducted by nurses. Henry said:

> "Nursing would be the primary focus of the centers—nurses would have the responsibility for the administration of the setting and its funds, and for coordinating all care provided to patients including that provided by other health disciplines."

With Henry's leadership, federal funding for demonstration centers in schools of nursing became available. The popularity of nursing centers in academic settings grew during the 1970s and 1980s, as nurse educators attempted to bridge the gap between service and education by providing clinical learning experiences for students in sites that faculty controlled.[8] Both the U.S. Public Health Service and private foundations launched a series of initiatives that made it financially feasible for schools of nursing to open these centers.

NURSE PRACTITIONERS AND PRIMARY CARE

Nurse practitioner programs contributed significantly to preparing nurses capable of providing primary care to the disadvantaged and geographically isolated. Between 1977 and 1979, the Division of Nursing funded nursing clinics in psychiatric day care centers, head start programs, prisons, and residential complexes for the elderly.[9] Services offered included physical examinations, treatment of minor illnesses, counseling, and primary prevention.

It was not only the disadvantaged who benefited from nurse practitioners. The first occupational health nurse practitioner programs brought health promotion and illness prevention into the workplace. Nurse practitioners, particularly those specializing in pediatrics and nurse-midwifery, were growing popular with the middle and upper classes.

Nurse-managed centers grew in visibility as one way to implement faculty practice, while simultaneously increasing opportunities for community-based experiences for students. With the increased federal emphasis on primary care, the U.S. Public Health Service, Division of Nursing, continued to offer special project grants to schools wanting to establish academic nursing centers and nursing practice arrangements. However, there was an emphasis on the provision of primary care services and an expectation that services would be available on a regular basis, with back-up services after hours.

The Division of Nursing also forged ahead in its support of doctoral preparation in nursing. Several conferences on doctoral education were supported in the late 1970s. Most of the nurse leaders attending were beneficiaries of nurse-scientist awards. Participants studied manpower requirements for doctoral-prepared nurses and debated the roles for which nurses needed doctoral degrees. Strategies to gain university support for doctoral programs were presented by the Division of Nursing. This national planning was deemed by many to be critical to the later expansion of doctoral programs in nursing.

Although the number of nurses with advanced degrees was growing, documents submitted to Congress by the Division of Nursing in 1977 showed that only 3.4% of registered nurses had graduate preparation.[10] As required by legislation, the reports summarized nursing manpower data. Highlighted in these communications was a call for more nurses with graduate-level preparation.

NURSE-MANAGED CENTERS

Academic nursing centers, nurse practice arrangements, and nurse-managed centers (nursing managed centers), whatever their name, have provided essential primary care services to the disadvantaged and geographically isolated through-out the United States in a cost-effective and professional manner. The concept of nurse-managed centers is often traced back to Lillian Wald and Margaret Sanger who led the way for nurses to provide health care to the community in the community. The nursing profession has evolved since then and today sets specific standards of practice for the profession. These include standards for advanced practice nursing, which allow for more independent practice. In federally funded nurse-managed centers, professional nurses are charged with the responsibility of managing the clinical and management functions of these settings. The scope of advanced practice has expanded to include both nursing and medical assessment, nursing and medical diagnoses, and disease management. In the health care arena, primary care encompasses primary prevention and patient education, which traditionally have been associated with nursing practice. Although economic principles require that health care be provided in a cost-effective manner, the financing of health care over the years has taken a larger percentage of both personal and governmental budgets. The confluence of these events provides strong rationale for the support of nurse-managed centers.

Evolution of Nurse-Managed Centers

The era from 1983 to 1992 was one of tremendous evolution for nurse-managed centers, as they responded to changes in federal health policy and transitioned from fledging, part-time operations to regular providers of primary care.[8] Nurse-managed centers that did not respond to these changes simply faded away. Others were able to capitalize on a health care environment focused on quality, access, and cost, and a few even developed multiple practice arrangements within the nursing school.

Many of the changes that influenced the operations of the nurse-managed centers were supported as amendments to the Public Health Service Act as modifications to the Title VIII legislation, Basic Nurse Education section. These legislative changes supported improvements in health care given by nurses, increasing educational opportunities for nurses, increasing access to primary care providers, increasing the diversity of the nursing workforce, addressing the population needs in health professional shortage areas and medically underserved communities, and by increasing nursing practice opportunities in communities.[11]

The Nurse Education Amendments of 1985 amended and extended Title VIII of the Public Health Service Act through fiscal year 1988. Section 3 of the Public Health Service Act reauthorized the Nursing Special Projects program to provide grants and contracts ... "demonstrate methods to improve access to nursing services in non-institutional settings through support of nursing arrangements in communities....."[11] In 1986 grant funds were awarded to support two unique nursing practice arrangements. They were located in two very different settings and focused on two very different populations. One was a correctional service center for male and female adolescents and the other was a clinic for the homeless. In both instances, primary health care services were planned and implemented by nurses.

By 1987, nine nurse-managed centers were funded through Nursing Special Projects demonstration grants. Sites included primary care nurse-managed centers, community-based centers, and nurse-managed centers for the homeless. All were located in urban areas and served racial and ethnically diverse medically underserved populations across the lifespan.

In 1988, the Nursing Special Projects program supported 13 nursing practice arrangements. These projects demonstrated and tested innovative methods to provide and improve access to nursing services for populations who historically lacked access to health care services (e.g., the homeless; inner-city and rural poor; public housing residents; and the elderly).

Programs and projects that improved minority representation in nursing and care to minority or vulnerable populations continued to receive the highest priority in legislative action. Funding was established through the Division of Nursing to encourage nurse-managed practices to improve access to primary health care in medically underserved communities. In 1990, the Division supported eight new and seven continuing nurse-managed center grants. These projects provided primary care services to an increasing number of special populations: non–English-speaking, noninstitutionalized mentally and physically disabled, immigrants, and persons with human immunodeficiency virus (HIV)/acquired immune deficiency syndrome (AIDS). The projects also reflected increasing emphasis on interdisciplinary education and practice, faculty practice plans, development of computer-based information systems, inclusion of nursing students as participants in clinic activities, and reimbursement strategies to ensure self-sufficiency. By the end of 1992, Nursing Special Projects supported 17 nurse-managed centers.

In its first report to the secretary of Health and Human Services and Congress, the National Advisory Council on Nurse Education and Practice called nursing,

"... a strategic asset for the health of the Nation."[12] For a number of reasons, nurse-managed centers have a strategic and growing role to play as cost-effective, community-based access points to quality health services. The philosophy of nurse-managed centers incorporates the education of patients, as well as health care professionals, in an environment that supports quality health care service delivery. Clinical practice sites in hospitals no longer provide adequate experiences to familiarize students with the changing health care delivery paradigm of community-based health services. Nurse-managed centers provide the opportunity for involvement of both undergraduate and graduate nursing students and provide sites for advanced practice faculty. Working within the community, nurse-managed centers become part of the community. Community health and advanced practice faculty are mentors and role models as they continually challenge themselves to provide newly identified services to clients and learning experiences for students.

FEDERAL FUNDING

Federal funding for nursing education, through authorities that responded to the changing needs of the health care delivery system, has supported programs for the education of both graduate and undergraduate nursing students. The Nurse Education Amendments of 1985 authorized the Nursing Special Projects Program to provide for grants and contracts to "... demonstrate methods to improve access to primary health care in medically underserved communities" and specified schools of nursing as the eligible grantees that would staff the project with faculty and students.[11] Amendments to the Public Health Service Act in both 1998[13] and 2004[14] continued to identify nurse-managed centers as an important priority, although with less specificity regarding administration and student involvement.

Nurse-managed centers provide ambulatory care alternatives to institutions. They allow creativity to provide models of practice that vary but usually include health maintenance and promotion services to a variety of populations. Since 1986, 121 nurse-managed center grants have been federally funded, with oversight by the Health Resources and Services Administration's (HRSA) Bureau of Health Professions, Division of Nursing. In fiscal year 2002, 18 nurse-managed center grants were funded, which provided 36 access points to care for underserved populations. Through this program, it has been estimated that nurse-managed centers provide 100,000 to 130,000 primary care encounters per year to high-risk and vulnerable clients. In addition, more than 2000 graduate and undergraduate nursing students participate in these clinical training sites each year. During a 5-year period, federally funded nurse-managed centers will provide more than 500,000 client encounters and educational experiences with underserved populations for thousands of students.

Currently, funded centers are located in both urban and rural areas. Service delivery occurs in school-based health centers, homeless shelters, correctional settings, residential domestic violence shelters, public housing for older adults and individuals with disabilities, and mobile health units, as well as more traditional primary care centers. Nurse midwifery, mental health, and primary care services are provided. The effect of disease management related to obesity, hypertension, diabetes mellitus, and asthma, as well as the effect of case management and health education, are monitored to determine outcomes related to therapeutic interventions. Accountability is a hallmark of nurse-managed centers.

Nurse-managed centers are currently funded for 5-year periods to provide support while other sources of funding are developed and third-party reimbursement mechanisms and contracts are established. It is in the best interest of the future of nurse-managed centers, the communities they serve, and the nursing profession to provide continuous services and demonstrate long-term outcomes. Since fiscal year 2000, a business plan has been included in the guidance for grant applicants, which emphasizes the importance of viewing nurse-managed centers as businesses and encouraging financial planning for sustainability.

Since the 1990s, the Division of Nursing has supported nurse-managed centers for a total of $66,693,864.[15] The federal contribution to the academic nursing center and nurse practice arrangement movement in the United States continues to be significant, and many of the nurse-managed centers currently in existence have benefited from HRSA funding. As of fiscal year 2004, there are 18 nurse-managed centers receiving continuation funding.[16] To help with plans for sustainability, the HRSA Center for Health Services Financing and Managed Care has established a technical assistance program for HRSA grantees in each State, regarding strategies to obtain third-party reimbursement. The fundamentals of coding, billing, and collections to improve revenues from third-party sources, such as Medicaid, State Children's Health Insurance Plans, Medicare, and private insurers are included. Increasing third-party revenues can help ensure the future viability of nurse-managed centers and possibly allow expansion of services.[17] Maximizing cost capture, when possible, will ensure grant funds go farther in increasing access to care for the most vulnerable populations.

Along with a strategy for third-party reimbursement and payer mix, development of a marketing plan including community links and advertising is encouraged. The need for a well thought out faculty practice plan, which is so important to faculty promotion, faculty income, and maintenance of clinical skills, must be well thought out and described. A key to success is the implementation of a well-planned management information system for patient data collection, billing, and outcome measurement. Consortia of nurse-managed centers are growing throughout the United States and are strategically planning for the viability of nurse-managed centers. Ultimately, collective data regarding patient outcomes and satisfaction will tell the story of the significant benefit of nurse-managed centers.

Today, the two major pieces of legislation that continue to influence nursing in the 21st century is the Health Professions Education Partnerships Act of 1998 (Subtitle B—Nursing Workforce Development), Public Law 105-392, and the Nurse Reinvestment Act of 2004, Public Law 107-205, which amended Title VIII of the Public Health Service Act. In 2004 the Public Health Service Act, Title VIII,

Section 831 was amended to address issues related to strengthening practice and retention and promote career advancement for nursing personnel in a variety of ladder programs. One such effort is to enhance patient care delivery systems through improving the retention of nurses and enhancing patient care that is directly related to nursing activities by enhancing collaboration and communication among nurses and other health care professionals, and by promoting nurse involvement in the organizational and clinical decision making processes of a health care facility.

The continued evaluation of nurse-managed centers and the demonstration of their benefits in the health care delivery system will be necessary to sustain their viability.

CONCLUSION

THE CHALLENGES AND OPPORTUNITIES FOR NURSE-MANAGED CENTERS ARE ENORMOUS IN TERMS OF SUSTAINABILITY AND ACCEPTANCE IN THE HEALTH CARE DELIVERY SYSTEM. AS DEMONSTRATED FOR THE PAST 30 YEARS, THE PUBLIC HEALTH SERVICE THROUGH THE DIVISION OF NURSING HAS PROVIDED SEED MONEY TO LAUNCH AND ENCOURAGE THE OPERATION OF THESE PRACTICE SETTINGS. PATIENTS KNOW AND TRUST NURSE PROVIDERS BECAUSE THEY LISTEN AND RESPOND TO THEIR NEEDS. COMMUNITIES SUPPORT NURSE-MANAGED CENTERS BECAUSE THEY FILL A GAP IN HEALTH CARE SERVICE DELIVERY. THERE IS A LONG HISTORY OF SUCCESS FOR THE POPULATIONS SERVED AND THE STUDENTS EDUCATED. IN CONCLUSION, IT IS IMPERATIVE THAT SUPPORT CONTINUES AT ALL LEVELS (E.G., CLIENT, STUDENT, FACULTY, COMMUNITY, STATE, AND FEDERAL), TO ASSIST THIS MODEL OF HEALTH CARE SERVICE DELIVERY TO GROW AND PROSPER.

REFERENCES

1. Public Health Service Act, Nurse Training Act of 1964, P.L. 88-581, 78 Stat 908, USC Congressional and Administrative News.
2. Public Health Service Act, Nurse Training Act of 1968, P.L. 90-490, 82 Stat 773, USC Congressional and Administrative News.
3. Public Health Service Act, Nurse Training Act of 1971. P.L, 92-158, 85 Stat 465, USC Congressional and Administrative News.
4. Salmon M: Division of Nursing, U.S. Public Health Service—50 years, *Image: J Nurs Scholarship* 29(4):302-303, 1980.
5. Health Resources and Services Administration, Public Health Service: *First Report to Congress, February 1, 1977*, Nurse Training Act of 1975, DHEW publication No. HRA 78-38, 1977, USDHEW (Available through National Technical Information Service [NTIS], Access Number HRP-0900501.).
6. Public Health Service Act, Nurse Training Act of 1975, P.L. 94-63, 89 Stat 354, USC Congressional and Administrative News.
7. Henry, OM: *Demonstration centers for nursing practice, education, and research.* Paper presented at the 1978 APHA annual meeting of the Association of Graduate Faculty of Public Health and Community Health Nursing, Los Angeles, Calif.
8. Barger S: Academic nursing centers: the road from the past, the bridge to the future, *J Nurs Educ* 43(2):60-65, 2004.

9. Kalisch P, Kalisch B: *Nurturer of nurses: a history of the Division of Nursing of the U.S. Public Health Service and its antecedents, 1798-1977*, unpublished manuscript, Washington, DC, 1977.

10. Roth A, Graham D, Schmittling G: *1977 National sample survey of registered nurses and factors affecting their supply*, Kansas City, MO, 1978, American Nurses' Association. (Available through NTIS, Access Number HRP-0900603.)

11. Public Health Service Act, Nurse Education Amendment of 1985, P.L. 99-92, 99 Stat 393, USC Congressional and Administrative News.

12. National Advisory Council on Nurse Education and Practice: *Nursing: a strategic asset for the health of the nation: First Report to the Secretary of Health and Human Services and the Congress*, Washington, DC, 2001, U.S. Printing Office. (Available through NTIS, Access Number BHP00191).

13. Public Health Service Act, Health Professions Education Partnerships Act of 1998 (Subtitle B—Nursing Workforce Development), P.L. 105-392, 112 Stat 3524, USC Congressional and Administrative News.

14. Public Health Service Act, Nurse Reinvestment Act of 2004, P.L. 107-205, 116 Stat 811, USC Congressional and Administrative News.

15. Bureau of Health Professions: *History of federally funded nursing practice arrangements 1985-2002*, unpublished report, 2004.

16. Clear J, Starbecker M, Kelly D: Nursing centers and health promotion: a federal vantage point, *Fam Comm Health* 21(4):1-14, 1999.

17. Hansen-Turton T, Kinsey K: The quest for self-sustainability: nurse-managed health centers meeting the policy challenge, *Policy Politics Nurs Pract* 2(4):304-309, 2001.

CHAPTER 16

FACULTY PRACTICE

JULIE C. NOVAK

❧

*F*or over 30 years, school of nursing faculty practice models or plans have been described.[1-4] Most early models were grant supported and often did not survive beyond the 5 years of foundation, state, or federal grant support. Over the past one to two decades, some faculty practice models have not only survived but developed integrated models of learning, service/practice, and discovery. They evolved from single source support to a mosaic of support, acquiring and generating multiple sources of revenue.

Faculty practice models developed by schools of nursing vary by definition, mission, philosophy, values, and region of the country. For the purpose of this chapter, faculty practice elements will include direct practice, indirect practice, and consultation. These models provide opportunities for integration of teaching/learning, research/discovery, and practice/community engagement while providing a potential revenue stream to the school with which they are affiliated.

Potash and Taylor[5] described three major categories of faculty practice plans (FPP) including the unification model, the collaborative model, and the entrepreneurial model. In this chapter exemplars are provided that incorporate elements of each of these models as featured in the faculty practice plans of three well established FPPs including Purdue University, the University of Texas–Houston, and the University of Wisconsin Milwaukee. At least a dozen other schools of nursing have had well established faculty practice plans for nearly two decades, for example, the University of California San Francisco, Michigan State University, the University of Michigan, the University of New Mexico, the University of Pennsylvania, the University of Rochester, the University of South Carolina, Vanderbilt University, and Yale University. Due to space constraints for this chapter, please refer to each of their websites for further information.

Furthermore, with the development of the Doctor of Nursing Practice (DNP), faculty practice plans/models will become more prevalent and more sophisticated. Thus the evolution of the DNP in nursing education and its effect on faculty practice also will be addressed.

DIRECT PRACTICE

Direct practice may include provision of care to individuals and families across a variety of settings. Direct practice models may be fee for service or capitated. Models may include nurse-managed clinics supported by federal, state, and foundation grants, patient revenues, Medicaid, Medicare, private insurers, and/or private donors. Faculty full-time equivalent (FTE) also may be purchased by private or community clinics, health maintenance organizations, hospitals, or industry. Advanced practice nurses including nurse practitioners, clinical nurse specialists, nurse anesthetists, and nurse midwives often find this integrated model of teaching and practice most satisfactory because clinical expertise is maintained while accruing hours for recertification. If well designed, this can be beneficial to the school of nursing because education and practice have the potential to be more relevant and more evidence-based. Faculty practice also can increase the financial viability of the school through revenue production while creating additional preceptorship sites for graduate students and capstone placements for baccalaureate students. These sites provide horizontal and vertical integration models of education. Horizontal integration includes the opportunity for a variety of faculty to serve as role models in a single site. This allows students to compare and contrast practice styles and to be mentored by a variety of faculty who possess different expertise and areas of specialization. Vertical integration is created through settings that may include a range of novice students to graduate students with varying levels of expertise.

Exemplar 1—Purdue University School of Nursing

The Nursing Center for Family Health, located on the lower level of the School of Nursing and in existence since 1980, is partially funded through the new Health Improvement Plan of the university. Health risk appraisals (HRAs) are completed by an outside vendor. This information is provided to the nursing clinic faculty and staff electronically with the client's permission and within HIPAA policy. Health screenings and telephonic, e-mail, or face to face follow-up counseling are provided through the faculty practice plan, the senior public health nursing course, and the adult nurse practitioner (ANP), pediatric nurse practitioner (PNP), and DNP graduate nursing student preceptorships/residencies. The program is funded by the university with the goals of primary, secondary, and tertiary prevention, improved employee quality of life and productivity, and ultimately reduced health care costs. The School of Nursing component of the 18,000 faculty, staff, retirees, and spouses is 5000 clients annually. The School is reimbursed $40 per client for the health screening. Telephonic counseling and costs of the program, for example, laptop computers and programs for interface with the outside vendor, are charged in addition to the $40 base. Third-party billing for additional programs related to health promotion, sports, school and camp physicals, women's health, lifestyle behavior change, and chronic disease management also supports the discovery, learning, and community engagement mission of the Nursing Center for Family Health.

Exemplar 2—Purdue School of Nursing Clinics and Contracts

Established in 1995, the Family Health Clinic of Carroll County (FHCCC) is supported by a mosaic of support from Purdue University, the state of Indiana Tobacco Control Trust Fund/Indiana State Department of Health (40%), patient revenues (26%), foundations (12%), private donors/gifts (11%), and Medicaid and Medicare billing (11%). As with many clinics and business in general, it took the first 5 years to consistently reach revenue neutral status. For the past 5 years, the clinic has been revenue positive (in the black).

The FHCCC incorporates both vertical and horizontal learning integration models. The FHCCC, located in rural Delphi, Indiana, 18 miles north of the Purdue main campus, provides appropriate, affordable, and accessible primary health care to individuals and families. The focus of the services is directed to uninsured or underinsured families living primarily in rural Carroll County, White County, and 10 other surrounding counties. Staffing includes one full-time staff nurse practitioner, three part-time faculty nurse practitioners (participating in the faculty practice plan), an RN, a clinic secretary, an office manager, and an interpreter. Senior nursing students have public health and capstone experiences in the FHCCC, and graduate students have preceptorships, cognate residencies, and clinical research projects in the FHCCC.

The clinic has grown and expanded its services over the past 10 years; client visits have grown 300%. The FHCCC maintains an open door policy; no one is denied services because of inability to pay. Objectives include meeting the health care needs of individuals, families, and communities across the lifespan. The clinic focuses on health promotion, health maintenance, and management of acute and stable chronic health problems with specific state funding sources for chronic disease management of diabetes, asthma, cardiovascular disease, and cancer. This value added service is reducing health care costs in the participating counties.

Child and adolescent health services include immunizations, health promotion, assessment, and supervision, developmental assessment and anticipatory guidance, diagnosis and treatment of acute illness, management of stable chronic conditions, and basic diagnostic laboratory testing. Women's health services include health promotion, annual pap and pelvic exams, breast health, mammogram referral, birth control, pregnancy testing, and pregnancy care, whereas men's health services include general health promotion, prostate and testicular cancer screening, and education. Counseling/coaching related to nutrition/exercise, obesity prevention/intervention, stress management, tobacco use prevention/cessation, STD prevention and treatment, and screening and diagnostic laboratory testing are also key components of the FHCCC. The clinic meets the needs of the growing Hispanic population, currently 27% of the patient population. Staff members each have some degree of Spanish fluency ranging from high school to Spanish for Healthcare Professionals (an elective in the School of Nursing) to full fluency. The clinic RN and nurse practitioners also provide case management and serve as a health information resource for the community.

Limited space had been a barrier to expansion of the FHCCC programs, with the number of annual client visits held at 3,200. With private foundation support, a new building is planned in 2007, incorporating other community services, for example, women, infant, children (WIC), senior public health nursing students, and a community room as a base for home health/public health nursing student visits and community education programs. This integration of public health nursing students and their professors will further strengthen the FHCCC community outreach, in-home care management, and continuity. The community room also will accommodate Community Advisory Governing Board meetings (an important component of faculty practice design, implementation, and evaluation) and staff meetings.

Faculty nurse practitioners who provide care at the FHCCC consistently report that the opportunity to teach and practice in an integrated model while maintaining their clinical expertise and certification is the reason that they maintain their faculty role. The added incentive of full-time or part-time summer employment, additional merit salary supplements, and travel support increases their satisfaction. In an era of lucrative opportunities in private practice, the healthcare system, and industry, maintaining faculty satisfaction, growth, and development is critical.

Exemplar 3: Trinity Nursing Center for Infant Health(TNCIH)—Purdue School of Nursing and Community Partners

To address access issues, area nursing faculty, a consortium of the three local nursing schools, created Nursing Schools United (NSU) in collaboration with a local church, foundation, and community agencies. The mission is to prevent families, newborns, and infants from falling through the cracks of the health care system. TNCIH is based at Trinity United Methodist Church in the lowest income neighborhood in Tippecanoe County. The need was based on the lack of space on local providers' Medicaid panels, the use of local ERs for primary health care, the fourth highest rates of child abuse and neglect in the state, and a waiting list of more than 300 clients and families at the local Head Start. Health and developmental assessment, immunizations, management of minor acute illness, and educational programs based on a needs assessment are the focus areas. Nursing students (AD, Diploma, BSN, MS, PNP, and DNP) and their respective faculty from the three programs developed an integrated service learning laboratory that focuses on community engagement and care that is evidence-based.

Evaluation of the model and parent/patient satisfaction will be measured quarterly in this new clinic. Foundation, university, private donors, and patient revenues based on a sliding scale provide a mosaic of support. Medicaid billing has been initiated and a collaborative federal grant will be submitted in 2007.

Exemplar 4: Indirect Care Contracts—Purdue School of Nursing

Indirect care is exemplified through population based models. For example, public health and community health faculty provide expertise to departments of health in areas such as county and statewide immunization programs, natural disaster preparedness, chronic disease management models, and/or homeland security assessment through gap analysis of all 92 counties in the state. In this model, a portion of the faculty member's contract is purchased for community assessment and planning, program design, implementation, evaluation and/or health policy development. Contracts range from 10% to 40% of the faculty member's salary.

Exemplar 5: Consultation

Consultation models overlap with indirect practice models. Consultation may include the provision of faculty experts for hospitals in the areas of better patient flow/scheduling models, operating room or critical care unit design, patient safety, cost containment, or organizational design. Because hospitals are challenged by the increasingly competitive health care market and realize they must improve their processes, share best practices, and improve efficiencies, a health care technical assistance program (HC TAP) was created by Purdue University. Through the Faculty Practice Plan, three nursing faculty members were subcontracted for 40% of their time during the academic year and full-time during the summer and fall to develop and co-lead 35 seed projects with individual hospitals and communities focusing on productivity, quality, safety, design, and cost. Patient safety, supply management, pharmacy processes, data management, organization of equipment for repetitive tasks in admissions, nursing stations, maintenance, patient rooms, and medical procedure rooms have been addressed. These seed projects are evolving into longer term projects involving four additional nursing faculty practice contracts. These contracts will purchase from 10% to 50% of faculty time. In many of these settings, graduate nursing students will take part in the projects.

Payment Models

In addition to direct purchase of faculty time based on the faculty member's base salary, time may be purchased at a higher rate based on hospital or agency salaries. If X is the faculty member's base salary and Y reflects grants and contracts that the faculty member brings to the school, then Z can be shared with the faculty in a salary bonus or placed in an account accessed by the faculty member for approved university purchases, for example, travel, supplies and equipment, a research assistant, and/or a teaching assistant.

For faculty practice to realize optimal financial benefit, advanced practice nurses must be named to provider panels. Being on a provider panel increases the billing opportunities to private insurers as well as federally funded programs. This will allow not only increased access and freedom of choice for patients but also add revenue options that lead to additional incentive payments to faculty.

Exemplar 6: The University of Texas–Houston (UT Houston)

One of the most sophisticated school of nursing faculty practice models was developed and implemented at the University of Texas–Houston. The faculty practice program links The University of Texas–Houston School of Nursing with community agencies to provide clinical and/or research services on a fee-for-service or contractual basis. UT Houston is a national leader and trendsetter in this concept of joining consultation with health care agencies.

Examples of these linked services include nurse practitioner prenatal clinics, cardiovascular rehabilitation services, group therapy for bipolar disorders, and emergency nurse practitioners for triage and urgent care. Benefits include the provision of a nursing expert in the clinical site without the cost of a full-time salary and benefits. Thus the faculty member contributes to the growth and development of the agency. The program offers not only a selected faculty member but also other RNs enrolled at the School of Nursing who are seeking professional learning experiences through various clinical projects. The program enhances capabilities to document clinical, cost, and quality outcomes and affords the opportunity to recruit the students after graduation.

An agency expresses a need for a certain service or set of services and determines how much time it will require. The School of Nursing matches the need with faculty expertise and arranges for the two parties to meet to discuss mutual interest. When an agreement has been reached, fees are calculated, the agreement contract is signed, and the services are initiated. Faculty members interview with the agency before final selection. A match between philosophies and working styles is very important to a successful outcome.[6]

Program Costs

Fees are calculated based on the level of expertise, taking into account the degree held and advance practice certification. Faculty are ranked as Consultants I, II, or III. Because the School of Nursing is a not-for-profit state agency, fees are used to cover only expenses, keeping costs for the agencies at a reasonable level and far below other means of obtaining these services. The contract is for a 12-month period and is renewable by mutual consent. Every agreement has an escape clause where either party, at any time, may give a 60-day notice of intent to cancel the contract. In case of emergencies, shorter notices are negotiated on an individual basis.

Revenues are dispersed according to a formula; 50% toward the Teaching Support Fund/replacement cost, 20% to the participating faculty member, 20% to the department or center, and 10% to the Dean's office.[6]

Exemplar 7: The University of Wisconsin–Madison (UWM) College of Nursing

The University of Wisconsin–Madison (UWM) College of Nursing has a variety of professional nursing activities that support its mission. Activities include the provision of direct health care, education, and/or consultation services to persons, families, agencies, and communities that support the faculty member's teaching and/or research responsibilities. The faculty practice program links the faculty with community agencies and/or institutions such as hospitals to provide clinical, educational, and/or research consultation services on a contractual basis. Some examples of services include development of community health education programs, health care research facilitation and/or consultation, provision of health care by nurse practitioners or clinical nurse specialists, community health assessments, strategic planning and program evaluation, and continuous quality management.

Benefits of the Faculty Practice Program include fostering collaborative relationships between UWM's College of Nursing faculty and community agencies/health care systems. Innovative, high-quality nursing services are provided to urban populations in outpatient and inpatient settings, contributing to the growth and development of the sponsoring agency/institution through the use of renowned nursing experts.[7]

Student Learning Opportunities

The UWM Academic Community Nursing Centers serve as innovative community-based clinical laboratories for undergraduate and graduate nursing students. The UWM philosophy contends that if communities are to improve their health status in the coming decades, it is imperative that the health care providers of the 21st century be educated about the special needs of urban communities. Furthermore, they must learn how to work with community residents and other community-based providers as partners.

UWM Academic Community Nursing Centers offer students a unique opportunity to increase cultural awareness, acquire cultural knowledge, and become culturally competent in providing health care to diverse populations. Undergraduate and graduate nursing students, under faculty supervision, participate in clinical learning experiences ranging from community screening activities to health program development and implementation. Thus students are prepared to help reduce health disparities in at-risk urban populations. Typical learning experiences include screening for cholesterol and hypertension, providing cancer prevention education and health promoting behaviors, home visits to provide case management and promote healthy lifestyles, primary care services such as employment physicals in a clinic setting, and school-based health services such as immunization clinics.[7]

Practice-Based Research Initiatives

The Institute for Urban Health Partnerships (IUHP) at UMW conducts ongoing research projects that explore innovative models of health care delivery and their effectiveness in reducing health disparities by improving health outcomes of at-risk populations. Sources of funding include the Health Resources and Services Administration (HRSA), Agency for Health Care Research and Quality (AHRQ), and a variety of foundations such as the Robert Wood Johnson Foundation, the American Cancer Society, and the Susan Komen Foundation. Recent research initiatives include The Midwest Nursing Center Consortium Research Network (MNCCRN). The MNCCRN is funded by the Agency for Health Care Research and Quality (AHRQ) as a Practice-Based Research Network (PBRN). The PBRN is a regional research network of academic nursing centers that includes 17 nursing centers in 8 academic institutions. Programs include Give it Up to Live it Up, a community-based exercise and nutrition project for populations at risk for diabetes and cardiovascular disease; Wellness for a Lifetime, a community-based exercise and nutrition project studying provider behaviors in supporting healthy lifestyles in eight participating MNCCRN nursing centers; Adolescent Pregnancy and Pregnancy Prevention Services, a longitudinal study that uses a life options model for adolescent pregnancy prevention and tests community-based case management strategies for parents; Automated Community Health Information System, development and testing of a system that helps assess a community's health that is used in collaboration with local health departments; and Outcomes of Advanced Practice Nurse Interventions in African-Americans with Type 2 Diabetes, identifying nursing interventions that help reduce complications from type 2 diabetes using the Omaha Classification System, and Anxiety, Depression, and Positive Functioning in Women with Heart Failure: Can Social Role Experiences Make a Difference? Other ongoing quality assurance/program management studies include analysis of cost effectiveness of case management as a primary care initiative, and analysis of client outcomes associated with nursing interventions as outlined in the Omaha Classification System.[7]

CHALLENGES TO FACULTY PRACTICE

In addition to funding constraints, the challenge of time constraints, lack of administrative support (particularly business expertise), and the lack of clarity regarding academic rewards (promotion and tenure) are the most significant barriers to faculty practice.[8] These issues must be addressed and a shared commitment to faculty practice must be realized in order to mitigate these challenges. If practice models are integrated and unified, if business expertise is provided, or nursing master's and doctoral programs provide a sub-specialization in business practices, and if practice/service/community engagement is clarified and valued in the promotion and tenure process, then these challenges are not insurmountable.

DNP DEVELOPMENT: IMPLICATIONS FOR FACULTY PRACTICE

The development of the Doctor of Nursing Practice (DNP) will enhance faculty practice program development. Twenty DNP programs have been established across the United States and 195 more are in various stages of development.[9]

The DNP program at Purdue University School of Nursing is the first in the Big 10/CIC and the first in Indiana. It is unique in that it delivers a curriculum from post-baccalaureate to the practice doctorate degree, with an emphasis on care of rural, underserved populations and the care of the rapidly growing Hispanic population in Indiana. The Nursing Center for Family Health (established in 1981), the Family Health Clinic of Carroll County (established in 1996), the new Nursing Schools United (NSU) Family Assessment Center and the federally funded Monon Nursing Health Center provides learning laboratories and the opportunity for integration. DNP students and their faculty create innovative program design for health care delivery, systems analysis, evidence-based practice, informatics, and health policy development.

The practice doctorate prepares individuals at the highest level of practice and is the terminal practice degree. The DNP program is designed to fill the growing need for expert clinicians who can strengthen health care delivery systems. Direct faculty practice in nurse-managed settings, indirect practice with populations of patients, and consultation with a variety of health care agencies, will serve as a model for DNP students in their cognate residencies and for graduates who will be prepared to change the face of health care. Graduates of the DNP program will ultimately affect the entire health care delivery system because of the unique focus on health care systems, leadership, and evidence-based practice. The degree represents the highest level of practice in nursing and incorporates the most independent and advanced nursing skills. The program is structured to prepare the students for cutting-edge roles in a changing health care system, knowing that the system will demand ever-higher levels of clinical skills and knowledge. Graduates will be experts in designing, implementing, managing, and evaluating health care delivery systems. At the same time, they will be prepared to provide leadership in maintaining the complex balance between quality of care, access, and fiscal responsibilities.[10]

Advanced practice nursing faculty who are master's prepared will have the option to complete the DNP program and its cognate residencies in nurse-managed clinics and other faculty practice sites. Transforming health care delivery recognizes the need for clinicians to design, evaluate, and continuously improve the context within which care is delivered. Removing barriers to advanced nursing practice is critical to finding solutions to the problems of a fragmented health care delivery system. Cost effective nurse-managed clinic delivery systems and sophisticated faculty practice initiatives provide excellent alternatives to a health care delivery system in the United States that is in turmoil and has been described as "broken." Nursing leaders at the highest levels have determined that a practice doctorate as the terminal degree is the best response to this crisis.[10]

Because of the information explosion and complexity of the health care delivery system, many master's programs in nursing are now exceeding 55 credits in order to prepare graduates for advanced practice roles. Within 15 years, it is projected that although bedside nurses still may come from a variety of educational programs leading to baccalaureate degrees and RN licensure, nurses in leadership positions and advanced practice roles must be prepared at the doctoral level. Nurses who currently hold master's degrees will have the option of obtaining a practice doctorate or they may choose to remain in their current clinical positions. These practice doctorates must have a skill and knowledge set that provides clear value added; faculty must be engaged in integrated models of practice, research, and education for these graduates to reach their full potential.

Nursing has many of the answers to the predominant health care dilemmas of the future, including (1) problems associated with normal human development, particularly aging; (2) chronic illness management across the lifespan; (3) health disparities associated with socioeconomic dislocations such as global migration, classism and sexism; and (4) the need for health promotion and disease prevention.[11]

Over the past several years, an upswing of interest in developing a viable alternative to the research-focused degrees—Doctor of Philosophy (PhD) and Doctor of Nursing Science (DNS, DNSc, DSN)—has occurred. In 2002, the American Association of Colleges of Nursing (AACN) charged a task force to examine the current status of clinical or practice doctoral development. It recommended that the practice-focused doctoral program be a distinct model of doctoral education that provides an additional option for attaining a terminal degree in nursing.

Informational shifts, demographic changes, growing disparities in health care delivery and access, and stakeholder expectations are all creating new demands on the nursing profession. The practice doctorate, with a focus on direct practice, health care leadership, and delivery systems offers nursing an exciting opportunity to meet these demands.[10] The DNP presents a clinical practice-oriented leadership development opportunity that allows the nurse to focus on evidence-based practice, defined as "the conscientious use of current best evidence in making decisions about patient care" and "a problem solving approach to clinical practice that integrates (1) a systematic search for and critical appraisal of the most relevant evidence to answer a clinical question; (2) one's own clinical expertise; and (3) patient preferences and values."[12] The nurse also focuses on research utilization and translation for the improvement of clinical care delivery, patient outcomes, and systems management. Such credibility is essential for getting funding from federal or private sources.

With growing emphasis on evidence-based practice (EBP), health care facilities are desperately looking for nurses with doctorates who can integrate systems approaches, provide leadership in interdisciplinary settings, bring "best practice" in patient care, ensure safe passage through the systems, and understand the importance of ongoing outcomes evaluation and efficacy of nursing practice. Nurse scientists need to be "linked" with nurses in practice settings to aid the translation of research into practice. Joint academic-clinical appointments are feasible and rewarding routes of faculty to connect research and practice through facilitation of EBP efforts. In fact facilitation is key to the success of translation efforts.[13] Integrated models of faculty practice provide settings for this translation to occur.

CONCLUSION

With the growth of Advanced Practice Nursing and the Doctor of Nursing Practice, the knowledge and information explosion, and the increasing complexity of health care, it is critical that faculty practice plans be created by schools of nursing. In order for practice and education to be evidenced-based and relevant, the discipline must encourage faculty practice and steer away from ivory tower models of the past. With the severe faculty shortage, professors who are encouraged to maintain their clinical expertise will experience greater role satisfaction. Finally, practice facilitates access to research populations, innovations, and policy makers. If nursing is to play a significant role in reengineering health care, then faculty members must be less insular and fully engaged in their discipline and their communities.

REFERENCES

1. Allison S: A framework for nursing action in a nurse-conducted diabetic management clinic, *J Nurs Adm* 3(4):53-60, 1973.
2. Grimes D, Stamps C: Meeting the health care needs of older adults through a community nursing center, *Nurs Adm Q* 4(3):31-40, 1980.
3. Lang N: Nurse-managed centers: will they thrive? *Am J Nurs* 83(9):1291-1293, 1983.
4. Ossler CC, Goodwin ME, Mariani M, Gilliss CL: Establishment of a nursing clinic for faculty and student clinical practice, *Nurs Outlook* 30(7):402-405, 1982.
5. Potash M, Taylor D: *Nursing faculty practice: models and methods*, Washington, DC, 1993, National Organization of Nurse Practitioner Faculties.
6. University of Texas- Houston School of Nursing (website): http://son.uth.tmc.edu/outreach/FacPractice.cfm
7. University of Wisconsin Milwaukee School of Nursing (website): http://cfprod.imt.uwm.edu/nursing/community/urban_health_education.cfm
8. Novak J: *Purdue University School of Nursing Faculty Survey*, West Lafayette, Purdue School of Nursing, 2005.
9. American Association of Colleges of Nursing. Doctor of Nursing Practice (DNP) Programs available online: http://www.aacn.nche.edu/DNP/DNPProgramList.htm. Accessed August 12, 2006.
10. Wall BM, Novak JC, Wilkerson SA: The doctor of nursing practice program development: reengineering health care, *J Nurs Educ* 44(9):396-403, 2005.
11. American Association of Colleges of Nursing (AACN): *White paper on the doctor of nursing practice*, 2004, AACN.
12. Sacket DL, Straus SE, Richardson WS, Glasziou P, Haynes RB: *Evidence-based medicine: how to practice and teach EBM*, ed 3, Edinburgh, 2005, Churchill-Livingstone.
13. Hopp L: Minding the gap: evidence-based practice brings the academy to clinical practice, Editorial, *Clin Nurse Spec* 19(4):190-192, 2005.

CHAPTER 17

RURAL HEALTH CENTERS

ALISON HUGHES

❧

*R*ural health centers provide primary care and preventive health services in rural and remote areas of the country. Rural residents make up about 20% of the total population of the United States, or 61 million people. Rural health centers are thus a critical part of the nation's health care safety net that serves rural and low-income Americans. Community health centers, federally qualified health centers, federally qualified health center "look-alikes," migrant health centers, rural health clinics, and free clinics all fall under the rubric, "rural health center."

The most important thing to understand about rural health centers is that their differences are tied to federal reimbursement systems and grant programs that govern the types of services offered. Except for the free clinics, which by virtue of their nature, do not bill for services, the clinics discussed herein are supplied with different billing numbers by the Centers for Medicare and Medicaid Services (CMS). The billing numbers determine the amount of reimbursement to be issued for a billable service. All billings are directed to a fiscal intermediary (FI) that is responsible for approving the billings and processing them to CMS. CMS publishes claims processing manuals that provide detailed directions on what services are billable, including patient encounters, payment calculation methods, payment determinations, and the like. Sections 329, 330, 340, and 340A of the Public Health Services Act (PHSA) make funds available only to community health centers, federally qualified health centers, and migrant health centers. Although not eligible for the PHSA grants, rural health clinics benefit from the enhanced reimbursement system through CMS and are eligible to apply for other federal funding.

Rural health clinics, community health centers, and free clinics are organized nationally through trade associations that actively advocate in Congress on issues pertaining to their interests. There is a useful link available through the Bureau of Primary Health Care that provides information on all clinics, except rural health clinics, and free clinics (http://ask.hrsa.gov/pc/).

COMMUNITY HEALTH CENTERS, FEDERALLY QUALIFIED HEALTH CENTERS, MIGRANT HEALTH CENTERS

These clinics are discussed together because they are governed by the same federal rules and regulations required by the Public Health Services Act grants mentioned earlier. Federally Qualified Health Center is a designation given to community health centers that receive Section 330 funding. Some community health centers are also migrant health centers because they serve the migrant population.

Community Health Centers

The first community health centers were established as part of President Lyndon Johnson's "War on Poverty" 40 years ago. The Economic Opportunity Act of 1964 established the Community Action Program that provided the first grant awards to the community health centers. By 1965 the first two grants were awarded to develop community health centers. At that time the health centers were referred to as "neighborhood health centers." The goal of the program was to provide quality health care to low-income individuals who lived in medically underserved areas of the United States. By 1966, six more neighborhood health centers were given grant awards, and by 1975, neighborhood health centers had evolved into community health centers as a result of Congress' community health center program. The 1980s saw the creation of Federally Qualified Health Centers to provide cost reimbursement to community health centers serving Medicare and Medicaid recipients.

The Health Centers Consolidation Act, passed by Congress in 1996, consolidated authority for community health centers, migrant health centers, health care for the homeless, and the public housing primary care program under Section 330 of the Public health Service Act. Today there are over 1000 community health centers located in 3600 rural and urban underserved areas.

The National Association of Community Health Centers is the national trade association that represents community health centers and migrant and homeless health centers. The Association's mission is to promote the provision of high quality, comprehensive health care that is accessible, coordinated, culturally and linguistically competent and community directed for all underserved populations. It represents its members' interests in Congress and with federal agencies.

One of the unique features of this group of health centers is their governance. The Section 330 grant program requires the centers to be governed by a community board comprised of a patient majority. In addition, community health centers must (a) be located in a federally designated medically underserved area (urban or rural); (b) have nonprofit, public, or tax exempt status; provide comprehensive primary health care services, referrals, and others services needed to facilitate access to care, such as case management, translation, and transportation; and finally, provide services to all in their service area, regardless of ability to pay; and (c) offer a sliding fee schedule that adjusts charges for care according to family income.

Another benefit to community health centers is the provision of medical malpractice insurance coverage under Federal Tort Claims Act. This means the Department of Health and Human Services will deem the clinicians to be federal employees for coverage for medical malpractice claims if credentialing and privileging requirements are met. Other benefits available to community health centers include access to the personnel resources of the National Health Service Corps, the J-1 Visa Waiver Program, access to reduced cost prescription and nonprescription medications through the 340B Drug Pricing Program, and to the Vaccines for Children Program.

The George W. Bush administration favors expanding services provided by community health centers. In 2002 the administration launched a 5-year initiative to expand health center capacity to 6.1 million patients. By 2005 this initiative was expanded further by providing an additional $63 million to help 105 targeted communities to extend health care services to low-income uninsured Americans.

Federally Qualified Health Centers

Federally qualified health centers are community health centers that receive federal grants through Sections 329, 330, 340 or 340A of the Public Health Services Act. Or they may be functioning as outpatient health programs or facilities operated by a tribe or tribal organization under the Indian Self-Determination Act (Public Law 93-638). As was mentioned earlier, FQHC status allows for cost reimbursement for services provided to Medicare and Medicaid beneficiaries.

Migrant Health Centers

The Migrant Health Act was enacted in September 1962 by Public Law 87-692, which added Section 310 to the Public Health Service Act. The Health Resources and Services Administration (HRSA) provides grants to community nonprofit organizations for a broad array of culturally and linguistically competent medical and support services to migrant and seasonal farm workers (MSFW) and their families. Migrant health centers are currently authorized under the Health Centers Consolidated Care Act of 1996, Section 330(g) of the Public Health Service Act. Like FQHCs, they are eligible to receive Section 330 funds and must meet the same requirements. However, they do not have to be located in a designated medically underserved area (MUA) or a medically underserved population (MUP) area.

The Community Health Center and Migrant Health Center (C/MHC) programs are designed to promote the development and operation of community-based primary health care service systems in medically underserved areas for medically underserved populations. They provide comprehensive primary health care services for migrant and seasonal farm workers and their dependents. The President's health care expansion initiative included migrant health centers in addition to the federally qualified health centers. In addition to their strong representation in Washington by the National Association of Community Health Centers (discussed previously), migrant health centers are also served through two other national entities, the National Center for Farmworker Health, and the National Advisory Council on Migrant Health.

The National Center for Farmworker Health in Buda, Texas, was established in 1974 for the purpose of enhancing the capacity of migrant health centers to provide access to care and eliminate health disparities between farm workers and the general population in the United States. The National Advisory Council on Migrant Health was formed in 1972 under the Federal Advisory Committee Act. It is composed of 15 members who make recommendations to the Secretary of Health and Human Services regarding the health and health care needs of migrant and seasonal farm workers in the Unites States.

Federally Qualified Health Center Look-Alikes

Federally Qualified Health Center (FQHC) Look-Alikes must meet the requirements of the Section 330 grant program, but do not receive the grants. They are, however, eligible for cost-based reimbursement under Medicaid and Medicare and may participate in the 340(b) Federal Drug Pricing program. These clinics must be fully operational at the time they apply for FQHC status and have Medicare and Medicaid billing numbers at the time of application. The look-alike designation is granted through the Department of Health and Human Services. Clinics applying for this designation may be public or private nonprofit entities. They must serve in whole, or in part, a designated Medically Underserved Area (MUA) or a Medically Underserved Population (MUP). They may not be owned, controlled, or operated by another entity.

RURAL HEALTH CLINICS

The clinics discussed previously serve both urban and rural populations, but rural health clinics are designated solely to serve rural populations.

The Rural Health Clinic Program was created in 1977 by Public Law 95-210 for the purpose of increasing access to health care in the nation's rural medically underserved areas and expand the use of midlevel practitioners (nurse practitioners, physician assistants, and certified nurse midwives) in rural communities. Although rural health clinics are not eligible to receive Section 330 grant funding like the community health centers, they do receive enhanced reimbursement from Medicare and Medicaid. The Health Care Financing Administration (HCFA) oversees the rural health clinic program. In 2004 there were over 3000 federally certified rural health clinics providing primary care services to over seven million people in 47 states, according to the National Association of Rural Health Clinics

Rural health clinics (RHCs) must be located in areas that are both rural and underserved. The areas must have current shortage area designations. Underserved is interpreted as a federally designated Health Professional Shortage Area (HPSA), a federally designated medically underserved area, or an area designated by the state's governor as underserved. In December 2003, CMS issued a new rule that requires that all rural health clinics must be located in "currently designated" shortage areas. The following URL leads to the federally designated HPSAs: http://bhpr.hrsa.gov/shortage/

RHCs are required to provide outpatient primary medical care services; employ at least one midlevel practitioner (a nurse practitioner or a physician assistant) for at least 50% of the time the clinic is open, meet health and safety requirements improved by Medicare and Medicaid, and must have a physician present on-site at least every 2 weeks and available by telecommunication for assistance at all times. Unlike community health centers, RHCs are not required to have a board of directors that represents the community served.

Hospitals located in rural areas may seek RHC designation for their clinics. Once the designation is approved, the hospitals are allowed to simultaneously share personnel between the RHC and the rural hospital without violating the co-mingling requirements. On the other hand, facilities may not be simultaneously operated as an RHC and a traditional fee-for-service Medicare practice. RHC practitioners who are "on the RHC clock" cannot bill Medicare Part B for covered services that would have otherwise been covered as RHC services. The key word here is "simultaneous."

Rural health clinics and community health centers are eligible to apply for federal funding through the Office of Rural Health Policy's Outreach and Network grant programs. The Office of Rural Health Policy Outreach Grant Program (http://ruralhealth.hrsa.gov/funding/outreach.htm) focuses on service delivery through creative strategies requiring the grantee to form a network with at least two additional partners. The Network Development Grant Program (http://ruralhealth.hrsa.gov/funding/network.htm) focuses on furthering ongoing collaborative relationships among health care organizations by funding rural health networks that focus on integrating clinical, information, administrative, and financial systems across members.

The purpose of the National Association of Rural Health Clinics (NARHC) is to improve the delivery of quality, cost-effective health care in rural underserved areas through the Rural Health Clinics Program (RHC Program). NARHC works with Congress, federal agencies, and rural health allies to promote, expand, and protect the interests of clinics in the RHC Program. Through the association, NARHC members become actively engaged in the legislative and regulatory process.

FREE CLINICS

Free clinics are private, nonprofit community based organizations that provide medical, dental, pharmaceutical, and/or mental health services at little or no cost to low-income, uninsured, and underinsured people. They are staffed by volunteer health professionals and community volunteers in partnership with other health providers. They are located in urban and rural areas of the country. Care is made possible through the donation of goods and services. Funding is generated at the local level. Free clinics are not eligible to receive Section 330 funds, but in March 2005, the Federal Tort Claims Act was extended to cover volunteer health care professionals working in free clinics. According to the National Association of Free Clinics, the country's free clinics serve over 3.5 million of the nation's uninsured and underinsured individuals. There are over 800 free clinics in 47 states.

The National Association of Free Clinics was formed in 2001 to support free clinics and the people they serve. The Association's goal is to unite these clinics into a "powerful voice for the uninsured" (NARHC website) through networking, monitoring, and providing input on national legislative and regulatory issues affecting free clinics, and providing education on the benefits free clinics bring to the health care system.

CONCLUSION

The sheer volume of activity underway by the many clinics described in this chapter would lead the reader to think that the health care needs of rural Americans are being adequately met. Not so. Rural health centers constantly face difficulties in recruiting health care providers to practice in rural and remote areas of the country. Recruiters face huge challenges in attracting the providers into rural communities, and the health workforce shortage promotes greater competition for providers.

The National Rural Health Association (NRHA) reported in a 2003 policy paper[1] that recruitment and retention of health care professionals is both challenging and expensive. The NRHA report focuses particularly on the shortage of physicians practicing in rural vs. urban areas. Further, in July 2001, the U.S. General Accounting Office reported on an emerging nurse shortage to the House Subcommittee on Health, Ways and Means.[2] This report points to a serious shortage of nurses that is expected as demographic pressures influence both demand and supply. The report notes that, "The future demand for nurses is expected to increase dramatically as the baby boomers reach their 60s, 70s, and beyond. The nurse workforce will continue to age, and by 2010, approximately 40% will likely be older than 50."

There are as yet many unresolved rural health issues and challenges. Existing federal efforts to support the provision of health care services through rural health center funding initiatives are commendable and far-reaching, but they are insufficient to fulfill the needs of a population that is living much longer than previous generations. The National Advisory Committee on Rural Health and Social Services[3] examines current rural health issues and makes recommendations to the Secretary of Health and Human Services. In its report entitled, "A Targeted Look at the Rural Safety Net," it points to the current vulnerability of the safety net of providers and recommends what it terms, "Mending the Net, Extending the Net." The report pieces together the interdependency of the safety net providers, and although it highlights access to hospital services, primary care, and workforce maintenance, it also points to critical ancillary issues that are important to the health care delivery system as a whole. Among the ancillary issues the report lists are (1) ensuring access to mental and oral health services; (2) improving and expanding the services of local public health departments; (3) recognizing and accounting for the uncompensated care provided by hospitals, free clinics, and physicians; (4) providing the capital necessary to build and maintain facilities; (5) extending care to isolated and underserved areas; (6) increasing health insurance coverage and providing affordable access to prescription drugs; (7) increasing access to transportation; and (8) improving reimbursement mechanisms to compensate for lifestyle and behavior change to improve health status. Rural health centers and their variants and the rural populations they serve could benefit tremendously through an injection of resources to help them strengthen all of these ancillary services.

REFERENCES

1. National Rural Health Association: *Healthcare Workforce Distribution and Shortage Issues in Rural America,* policy brief, March 2003 (website): http://www.nrharural.org/advocacy/sub/ policybriefs/WorkforceBrief.pdf. Accessed March 30, 2005.
2. United States General Accounting Office (GAO): Report to Chairman, Committee on Ways and Means, House of Representatives, Subcommittee on Health: *Nurse Shortage Due to Multiple Factors,* July 2001 (website): http://www.gao.gov/archive/2001/d01944.pdf. Accessed March 30, 2005.
3. National Advisory Committee on Health and Human Services: *A Targeted Look at The Rural Safety Net,* report to the Secretary of Health and Human Services, April, 2002 (website) http://ruralcommitteehrsa.gov/nacpubs.htm. Accessed March 30, 2005.

PART IV

SPECIAL CONSIDERATIONS

THE ELECTRONIC NURSE PRACTITIONER

Supporting Innovations in Care

SUSAN BRAGG LEIGHT

The whole of science is nothing more than a refinement of everyday thinking.

–Albert Einstein

*T*he utilization of information and communications technologies in health care since the 1950s has fundamentally changed the nature of clinical practice, record keeping, and overall health services management. Information technologies allow nurse practitioners to have a much better informed practice; they support the provision of real-time, patient-specific scientific information, and access to the best possible clinical evidence available delivered at the point of care.[1] Informational systems also allow for the appropriate accounting of fiscal and human resources expended in the treating of patients.[1]

Burgeoning telecommunications capabilities of the new millennium transform informational technologies that previously were computational and archival to ones that are now networked and global. Within the context of communications, connectedness, and our ease in accessing electronic resources, one might consider that "our world is now flat."[2]

TELEHEALTH INTERVENTIONS

The term *telehealth* is broadly defined as the integration of information and communications technologies to support the delivery of clinical services to patients, particularly in their place of residence or occupation. Telehealth has existed experimentally for more than 25 years; however, its use has been limited because before 2001, no third-party payer reimbursed for these services.[3] In 2001,

Medicare began to reimburse for telehealth office visits, consultations, and counseling at in-person rates, which has significantly boosted telehealth practice and development.[3]

Telehealth encompasses simple videoconferencing to very complex systems that include monitoring devices such as temperature, blood pressure, peak flow meters, and so on.[3] Some systems use videophones and ISDN lines (high-speed telephone networks) to allow patients and providers to interact in real-time across long distances while viewing images of each other.[1] Research studies on telehealth interventions have noted that it has distinct benefits: decreased cost; improved access; increased provider-patient communication, and improved compliance.[3] According to Dr. Schlachta-Fairchild, President and CEO of iTelethealth Inc., "Telehealth does not change the standards or scope of practice for health care professionals, merely the communications pathway by which the care occurs."[3]

Telehealth interventions have been shown to have positive patient outcomes. In a study of older at-risk home health patients, persons in the telehealth intervention (videophone-enhanced home health care) achieved improved functional status and enhanced activities of daily living as compared with those receiving usual care.[1] Those in the telehealth intervention were able to interact face-to-face with a clinician in a synchronous manner while viewing images of each other. Although the mechanism of effect was not explicated in the study; the author suggested that the visual cues that accompanied the auditory message allowed the clinicians to have enhanced supervision, emergency evaluation, and enriched interaction with clients.[1]

TELEHEALTH AND RURAL HEALTH CARE

Rural health providers face distinctive challenges in care delivery: relative isolation; limited communication with other health care providers; and lack of access to current health care information and continuing education opportunities.[4-6] Internet connectedness and videoconferencing capabilities are two strategies that can help providers in rural and underserved areas both improve their patient care and access state-of-the art health care information. The Missouri Telemedicine Network (MTN) established 21 videoconferencing sites in 16 Missouri counties along with the installation of a high-speed computer data infrastructure in outpatient practices within these counties.[5] Three of the counties were chosen as demonstration counties, and findings from the study yielded six themes related to care providers' receptivity to technologic change: turf; efficacy; practice context; apprehension; time to learn; and ownership.[5] These themes applied to the computer and videoconference aspects of telehealth and operated as perceived barriers or facilitators of change. "Turf" was a theme in the findings from those perceiving telehealth as a threat to livelihood or autonomy. Although some participants perceived the technology as a "good thing," others saw the connectedness to a big university as a threat to their sense of competency, autonomy, and livelihood.[5] "Efficacy" referred to whether the technology would fill a functional need in the practice, for example, in primary care "you basically know most of the stuff."[5] "Practice context" referred to the slower pace of rural areas to adopt technology in their clinical settings and "time to learn" speaks to the learning curve associated with the technology.[5] The theme "apprehension" referred to fear of the new technology and a generalized human aversion to change "Ownership" speaks to the professional and emotional investment in the technology; notably some administrators and stakeholders acknowledged the benefits of the technology and worked to adapt it to their needs and helping others "buy in" to the new technology.[5] Implications from this study noted that rural providers acceptance of telehealth is more likely to occur when there is organizational integration of the technology and a willingness to adapt to change, a perceived increased time efficiency, a sense of ownership of the technology, and the realization that change happens more slowly in rural communities.[5]

TELEHEALTH AND REMOTE DIAGNOSIS OF CERVICAL NEOPLASIA

Telecolposcopy and cervicography are two different diagnostic approaches that allow for the remote evaluation of women with possible cervical neoplasia. Telecolposcopy involves using real-time (video-like) digitized colposcopic images to examine the lower genital tract.[7,8] Local colposcopists use video-adapted colposcopes to capture and transmit these images via broadband cable or standard telephone lines. Computer and electronic supporting equipment is needed at both the transmitting and receiving end. Selected high speed systems will allow for synchronous (real-time) provider communication between an expert colposcopist and the local colposcopist.[7,8] Cervicography uses static, digitized colpophotographs that are taken with a 35-mm camera and developed at a central processing center. The final product resembles a magnified colposcopic photograph that is interpreted as negative, atypical, or positive. Cerviscopes (35-mm cameras) are used to acquire the cervigrams.[7,8]

In a study of 264 women comparing the accuracy of telecoposcopy and cervicography with on-site colposcopy in the remote evaluation of women with possible cervical neoplasia, it was demonstrated that telecolposcopy is at least as effective as cervicography in detecting cervical cancer precursors.[8] Although the differences were not statistically significant, computer-based telecolposcopy systems detected a higher percentage of women with CIN 2 or 3 (carcinoma in situ) than did cervicography. Additionally, telecoposcopy can provide immediate feedback to women whereas cervicography takes a minimum of several weeks to receive a report. However, on-site colposcopy had the greatest sensitivity for disease detection at either positive test threshold (CIN 1 and CIN 2).[8] Factors associated with this finding include the ability to manipulate the cervix, stereoscopic viewing, and longitudinal observation after acetic acid application.[8]

NURSE PRACTITIONER USE OF TELEHEALTH TECHNOLOGIES IN PRACTICE

Nurse practitioners and other advanced practice nurses have used telehealth technologies in a variety of ways during the past 10 years. Among the projects that have been implemented, Yancey et al.[9] described the use of computerized documentation of a rural intervention project for cancer care by nurse practitioners. Using a system based on the North American Nursing Diagnosis Association (NANDA) standards and modified with problems specific to patients with cancer, nurse practitioners tracked symptoms, complications, and the effectiveness of interventions.[9] Findings from the study noted efficient use of time for data input and retrieval, a standardized framework for nursing diagnosis, and uniformity of documentation between providers and locations.[9]

The Penn Nursing Network Information System Project, a clinical information system serving small nursing centers, was designed to allow researchers to pool small data sets useful for outcome evaluation or research. National protocols, such as those for asthma or hypertension, were incorporated into the system. The system used multiple classification choices and underwent continuous revision by clinicians to make it more useful to health care practitioners.[10]

A descriptive study to determine computer use by nurse practitioners in the San Francisco Bay Area found that for the 104 respondents, 83% used computers at work. "Obtaining client records from other agencies or departments" was rated the most useful computer application, followed by "internet searches" and "entering client record information."[11] Almost all nurse practitioners in HMOs (94%) accessed records from other agencies as compared with those in public clinics (57%) and private practices (25%). The authors concluded that nurse practitioners underused computer applications that had potential to improve client care in their practice.[11]

NURSE PRACTITIONERS, E-MAIL, AND PERSONAL DIGITAL ASSISTANTS

E-mail can be an important venue for nurse practitioners communicating with each other. E-mail discussion groups or mailing lists enable nurse practitioners to expand their communication to many participants and allow for discussions as diverse as forums for political action to clinical pearls.[3]

Personal digital assistants (PDAs) function as handheld computers, allowing the clinician to carry an up-to-date reference library in their pocket.[12] Examples of software programs available for PDAs include drug administration and dosage calculation programs; assessment and diagnostic tools such as STAT Cardiac Risk and the 5-Minute Clinical Consultant; and even global positioning software for rural-based or home–health APNs.[12] In addition, programs like "Patient Keeper" allow for documentation of patient outcomes, retrieval of lab results, and can be hot-synced to a desktop computer.[12]

INFORMATICS COMPETENCIES FOR NURSE PRACTITIONERS

Nursing informatics (NI) was defined in 1989 as a "combination of computer science, information science, and nursing science designed to assist in the management and processing of nursing data, information and knowledge to support the practice of nursing and the delivery of nursing care."[13] A key focus of nursing informatics is the development of solutions to represent, manage, and process health system information.[14]

As health care and nursing knowledge increase at a rapid rate, managing this information through the skilled use of technology becomes a basic core competency for practice. As such, nurse educators believe that informatics competencies need to be delineated for nurse practitioners and incorporated into both curricula and practice.[15] Common measures of performance for practitioners working in a managed care environment include such assessments as: benchmarking; patient outcomes research; best practice guidelines; and provider profiles/report cards.[15] Thus nurse practitioners need expertise in generating and managing both individual and aggregate level data, as well as technologic skill to administer an infrastructure that supports database management of population or large data sets.[15] In addition, the nurse practitioner with informatics competencies is able to support the retrieval and application of evidence from research protocols to clinical practice and to analyze the possibilities and limitations of systematically processed data, information, and knowledge.[15]

The informatics faculty at the Columbia University School of Nursing, together with the Nurse Practitioner program directors, developed a list of 32 informatics competencies needed for NP practice and education that encompassed three primary domains: computer skills; informatics knowledge, and informatics skills.[15] Examples of computer skill competencies included accesses shared data sets; extracts data from clinical data sets; and uses applications to aggregate and analyze data for forecasting.[15] Informatics knowledge competencies included supports efforts toward the development and use of structured languages; evaluates computer-assisted instruction (CAI) as a teaching tool; and is knowledgeable regarding optimal search strategies to locate clinically sound and useful studies from information sources.[15] Informatics skill competencies included converts information needs into answerable questions; uses data and statistical analyses to describe and evaluate practice; assists patients to use databases to make informed decisions; and designs and uses database reports.[15] Based on these informatics competencies, course assignments and content was developed to incorporate the needed knowledge and skills required. One-credit "intensives" were planned to concentrate on specific topics.[15] The author suggested that practicing NPs assess their level of proficiency for the proposed competencies and seek continuing education for those not mastered.[15]

RETHINKING TECHNOLOGY: INNOVATIONS IN ACCESS TO CARE

If you have not slept, or if you have slept, or if you have headache, or sciatica, or leprosy, or thunder-stroke, I beseech you, by all angels, to hold your peace, and not pollute the morning.

-Ralph Waldo Emerson

To access nonemergency health care, patients must gain access to a complex, ambulatory care system structured around a conventional "office appointment model".[16] This ineffective system does not accommodate the needs of diverse patients, which contributes to both the overuse and underuse of health care resources. Students in business school learn that consumers eventually get what they want (The Iron Law of Consumerism); who delivers the service and when they get it are the unknowns.[16]

The term *patient-centered access to care* refers to the ability to secure health care assistance as needed. The Institute of Medicine proposed six goals for improvements in the health care system in the 21st century: safety; effectiveness, patient-centeredness, timeliness, efficiency, and equitability.[17] The ability of a patient to secure the needed and desired health care services should enhance safety, effectiveness, and equity, which by necessity will require increased efficiency and will reflect enhanced patient-centeredness and timeliness.[16] Enhancing access requires systematic thinking and alignment of the goals of providers, patients, and payers.[16] In attempting to further develop these principles, the study authors[16] did a comprehensive literature review from 1985 using MEDLINE and Academic Health Reference Center databases. Findings from their search showed that implementing patient-centered access required embracing three principles, all of which have technologic implications: (1) work at the high end of expertise; (2) align care with need and preference; and (3) serve when service is needed.[16]

Work at the High End of Expertise

The labor-intensive nature of health care has led many to believe that making productivity gains is an impossible dream. Patient care access can be improved and costs can be decreased by rethinking who performs specific tasks; all members of the team, including the patient, need to work up to their level of training and expertise.[16] Health care professionals working below their level of expertise waste scarce resources, increase boredom and frustration, and impair access.[16]

Thus specialist physicians should do less of what generalist physicians can do; generalist physicians should do less of what nurse practitioners can do and nurse practitioners should do less of what nonclinical staff can do.[16]

Using information technology, a team approach to care and aligning skills with tasks illustrates this principle. Examples include electronic medical records, exam rooms with computer terminals, computerized decision support, e-mail patient communications to support nurse practitioners and nursing staff, and patients working at the highest possible level of expertise.[16]

Align Care with Need and Preference

The usual office visit does not take into account the diversity of patient needs. Although a conventional visit works best for those who need to be seen in person and whose problems can be addressed within the allotted scope of time, system overuse can occur when the appointment is used to ask several quickly answered questions or underused when a 20-minute appointment slot prevents the clinician from dealing with all the relevant issues.[16] Thus patient heterogeneity and preference dictate a more flexible service delivery model that offers alternative entry paths into the practice.

Examples of alternative access pathways include options such as group appointments with the care team, telephone appointments, and online communications. Group appointments are designed primarily as educational sessions but also allow for counseling, examination, referral, or prescriptions if needed. Group models for chronic disease management have documented improved health outcomes and satisfaction with these services.[18] In a study of 294 chronically ill older adults, comparing the effectiveness of a group outpatient model in a health maintenance organization with usual care, findings showed that the group model resulted in fewer hospitalizations and emergency room visits, increased patient satisfaction and self-efficacy, but had no effect on outpatient use or functional status.[18]

Telephone appointments have the potential to improve the quality of the clinician-patient encounter and the efficiency of the practice. Time would be reserved in the day for telephone consultations, and discussions would be less harried and more thorough.[16]

Currently, more patients are interested in e-mail communication with providers than vice-versa. Provider resistance to e-mail relates to preference for face-to-face communication, lack of reimbursement, confidentiality concerns, liability risks, fear of being overwhelmed by patient e-mails, and issues of out-of state licensure.[16] Some private health insurers are considering reimbursement for e-mail consultations, and the American College of Physicians has released a policy paper regarding reimbursement guidelines for e-mail consultations.[16]

Serve When Service is Needed

Enhancing patient access requires operational effectiveness, including determining optimum patient panel size, proper appointment length, and developing contingency plans for unanticipated demand.[16] Using a care team approach and nonvisit options such as telephone appointments and e-mail consultations also supports enhanced patient access.[16]

CONCLUSION

Information and communication technology is integral to contemporary health care. Nurse practitioners need to be vital forces in today's new technology-based delivery models and become tomorrow's informaticians. Will you be ready to meet the challenge?

REFERENCES

1. Brennan P F: Telehealth: bringing health care to the point of living, *Med Care* 37(2):115-116, 1999.
2. Walters D J: *Millennials: what to do?* Paper presented at the meeting of the Association of Deans and Directors of Nursing Education, Morgantown, WV, May 2005.
3. Segal-Isaacson AE: The electronic APN: new frontiers, *Nurse Pract* 27(Suppl 8-10):1214, 2002.
4. Buckwalter KC, Davis LL, Wakefield B J, Kienzle MG, Murray MA: Telehealth for elders and their caregivers in rural communities, *Fam Comm Health* 25(3):31-40, 2002.
5. Campbell JD, Harris KD, Hodge R: Introducing telemedicine technology to rural physicians and settings, *J FamPract* 50(5):419-424, 2001.
6. Leight SB: The application of a vulnerable populations conceptual model to rural health, *Public Health Nurs* 20(6):440-448, 2003.
7. Ferris DG, Litaker MS, Gilman PA, Leyva Lopez AG: Patient acceptance and the psychological effects of women experiencing telecolposcopy and colposcopy, *J Am Board Fam Pract* 16(5): 405-411, 2003.
8. Ferris DG, Litaker MS, Macfee MS, Miller JA: Remote Diagnosis of cervical neoplasia: 2 types of telecolposcopy compared with cervicography, *J Fam Pract* 52(4):298-304, 2003.
9. Yancey R, Given BA, White N, DeVoss D, Coyle B: Computerized documentation for a rural nursing intervention project, *Comput Nurs* 16(5):275-284, 1998.
10. Marek KD, Jenkins M, Westra BL, McGinley A: Implementation of a clinical information system in nurse-managed care, *Can J Nurs Res* 30(1):37-44, 1998.
11. Dumas JA, Dietz EO, Connolly PM: Nurse practitioner use of computer technologies in practice, *Comput Nurs* 19(1):34-40, 2001.
12. Enger JC: PDAs: a hands-down winner, *Nurse Pract* 27(Suppl 28):9, 2002.
13. Graves J, Corcoran S: The study of nursing informatics, *Image J Nurs Sch* 21(4):227-231, 1989.
14. Zytkowski ME: Nursing informatics: The key to unlocking contemporary nursing practice, *AACN Clin Issues Adv Pract Acute Crit Care* 14(3):271-281, 2003.
15. Curran CR: Informatics competencies for nurse practitioners, *AACN Clin Issues Adv Pract Acute Crit Care* 14(3):320-330, 2003.
16. Berry LL, Seiders K, Wilder SS: Innovations in access to care: a patient-centered approach, *Ann Intern Med* 139(7):568-574, 2003.
17. Institute of Medicine: *Crossing the quality chasm: a new health system for the 21ˢᵗ century*, Washington, DC, 2001, National Academy Press.
18. Scott JC, Conner DA, Venohr I, Gade G, McKenzie M, Kramer AM, Bryant L, Beck A: Effectiveness of a group outpatient visit model for chronically ill older health maintenance organization members: a 2-year randomized trail of the cooperative health care clinic, *J Am Geriatr Soc* 52(9):1463-1470, 2004.

Managing Quality of Care by Measuring Performance

IVO L. ABRAHAM • DEBORAH M. NADZAM • KAREN M. MACDONALD

Q uality management, the systematic effort to measure performance and take action to improve or maintain the quality of care, should be a core element of any clinical enterprise, from small solo practices to large health care systems. In this chapter, we introduce several concepts related to quality of care. We also describe a framework for performance measurement as a key tool to managing quality of care.

When talking about quality of care, one must adopt a broader perspective than just the actual delivery of care to patients and families. True, the actual care is at the core of quality management, however, a comprehensive program must also embrace the other factors that may have a direct or indirect impact: the context of care, from the organization of the practice setting to the community of which it is part; the use of clinical guidelines, protocols, and models of care; the regulatory and reimbursement environment; and the education and professional development, past and ongoing, of staff.

Is it possible to measure quality? Can we identify direct indicators of quality (as in: "this indicator shows we provide quality care"), or do we have to rely on indirect indicators (as in: "if indicator X drops, we can reasonably infer an improvement in the quality of care?")? What factors may influence our desired quality outcomes, whether these are unrelated factors (e.g., the pressure to see more patients in less time) or related factors (e.g., severity of illness)? How can we design evaluation programs that enable us to measure quality without adding significant burden and taking time away from direct patient care? How "scientific" should our quality monitoring be? Should it be as objective and rigorous as a research study? Is it necessary to go to the "extremes" of scientific rigor when the focus is on monitoring and changing quality of care in specific clinical settings? Should we benchmark the outcomes of our care to established guidelines or standards of care?

It would be ideal if this chapter could provide answers to all of these questions. However, it does not because currently there is no consensus on how to measure quality of care; there may never be. Furthermore, if the model of quality measurement were to exist, would it be relevant to all possible clinical sites; implementable without burdensome procedures and resource demands; and be sufficiently operational to enable quality improvement? Although it may not answer the question of how to measure quality of care, this chapter does provide guidance in the selection, development, and use of performance measures to monitor quality of care—as a springboard to quality improvement initiatives. After providing a definition of quality, we identify several challenges in the measurement of quality. We then introduce the concept of performance measures as the evaluation link between care delivery and quality management; and offer practical advice on how to measure performance. The chapter concludes with a review of common measurement problems.

MANAGING QUALITY OF CARE

Quality of Care: A Process, Not a State

The Institute of Medicine[1] (IOM) defines quality of care as "the degree to which health services for individuals and populations increase the likelihood of desired health outcomes and are consistent with current professional knowledge." Note that this definition does not tell us what quality is, but what quality should achieve. This definition does not say that quality exists if certain conditions are met (e.g., an increase in asthma-free days in adolescents with mild persistent asthma). Instead, it emphasizes that the likelihood of achieving desired levels of care is what matters. In other words, quality is not a matter of reaching something (as in: "we've got it!"), but rather the challenge, over and over, of improving the odds of reaching the desired level of outcomes (as in: "where are we and where do we go from here?"). Thus the definition implies the cyclical and longitudinal nature of quality: what we achieve today must guide us as to what to do tomorrow—better and better, over and over.

The IOM definition also stresses the framework within which to conceptualize quality: knowledge. The best knowledge to have is research evidence—preferably from randomized clinical trials (experimental studies), yet without ignoring the relevance of less rigorous studies (nonrandomized studies, epidemiologic investigations, descriptive studies, even case studies). Realistically, in nursing we have limited evidence to guide our care. Therefore, professional consensus among clinical and research experts is a critical factor in determining quality. Further, the knowledge element plays at three levels: to achieve quality, we need to know what to do (knowledge about best practice); we need to know how to do it (knowledge about behavioral skills), and we need to know what outcomes to achieve (knowledge about best outcomes).

The IOM quality of care definition contains several other important elements. "Health services" focuses the definition on care itself. Granted, quality of care is determined by such factors as knowledgeable professionals, good technology, and efficient organizations, yet these are not the focus of quality measurement. Rather, the definition implies a challenge to health care organizations small and large: organize yourself in such a way that knowledge-based care is provided and that its effects can be measured.

This brings us to the "outcomes" element of the definition. Quality is not an attribute (as in: "my hospital is in the top 100 hospitals in the USA as ranked by U.S. News & World Report") but an ability (as in: "only x% of my hypertensive patients have uncontrolled hypertension; however, when I switch them to another medication regimen, an additional y% will achieve hypertension control."). In the IOM definition, "degree" implies that quality occurs on a continuum from unacceptable to excellent. The clinical consequences are on a continuum as well. If our care is of unacceptable quality, the likelihood that we will achieve desired outcomes is nil. In fact, we probably will achieve outcomes that are the opposite of what is desired. As our care moves up the scale towards excellence, so will the odds that we will achieve (or, at least, get close to) the desired outcomes. Degree also implies quantification—trying to put a number to it. Though it helps to be able to talk to colleagues about, say, unacceptable, poor, average, good, or excellent care, these terms should be anchored by a measurement system.

A measurement system enables us to interpret what, for instance, poor care is by providing us with a range of numbers that correspond to "poor." In turn, these numbers provide us with a reference point for improving our care to the level of average: we measure our care again, look at whether the numbers have improved, and then check whether these numbers fall in the range of numbers defined as "average." Likewise, if we see a worsening of scores, we will be able to infer whether we have gone from, say, good to average.

Still dissecting the IOM definition, the reference to "individuals and populations" underscores that quality of care is reflected in the outcomes of one patient and in the outcomes of a set of patients. It focuses our attention on providing quality care to individuals while also aiming to raise the level of care provided to populations of patients.

In summary, the IOM definition of quality of care forces us to think about quality in relative and dynamic rather than in absolute and static terms. Quality of care is not a state of being, but a process of becoming. Quality is and should be measurable, and for this we need performance measures: quantitative tools that provide an indication of performance in relation to a specified process or outcome.

Quality of Care is in the Eye of the Beholder

If the IOM definition is indeed so helpful, why is there such divergence in operationalizing quality of care and designing quality management programs? For instance, clinicians wonder whether they, as individual practitioners, provide good care and how they can become better at what they do. They may also question whether they work for a good organization: one that consistently provides good care to all its patients, and challenges itself to find new and better ways of serving their patients. In contrast, health care organizations (from a solo practice to a large health system) worry about their relationship with their patients. Will they return? Will they refer family and friends? Managers worry about reimbursement, accreditation, and contracting—all of which are linked to the institutional level of quality of care. Purchasers and payers of health care try to find ways of balancing quality and cost. Providing the best possible care imaginable may be cost-prohibitive, yet too much cost management could have a negative impact on quality. Regulators and accreditors want assurances that safe care is being provided. For them, the issue is not one of top quality but rather of basic and necessary quality. Lastly, patients and consumers want assurances. They want the barriers to accessing care lowered. They expect their care to be safe. They hope that the care will make them better; or, at least, that suffering will be minimized.

Where do these divergent views on quality of care come from? It goes back to the process ("becoming") versus state ("being") issue. Quality improvement is a process of attaining ever better levels of care in parallel with advances in knowledge and technology. It strives towards increasing the likelihood that certain outcomes will be achieved. This "becoming" is the professional responsibility of those who provide care: clinicians, managers, and their organizations. In this respect, quality is what providers do. On the other hand, consumers of health care (patients, but also purchasers, payers, regulators, and accreditors) are much less concerned with the processes in place, but instead with the results of those processes: to them, quality is what consumers see and what they get.

Measuring Quality of Care

Challenges

Schyve and Nadzam[2] identify a number of challenges to measuring quality, several of which apply to care provided by nurse practitioners.

Stakeholders

The issue of quality of care being in the eye of the beholder points at the different interests of multiple users. Measurement and analysis methods must generate information about quality of care that meets the needs of different stakeholders. In addition, the results must be communicated in ways that are useful to each of the stakeholder groups.

Measurement Tools

We must have good and generally accepted tools for measuring quality. Notwithstanding their different needs, stakeholder groups must come together in their conceptualization of quality care so that relevant health care measures can be identified and standardized. A common language of measurement must be developed, grounded in a shared perspective on quality that is cohesive across yet also meets the divergent needs of various stakeholder groups.

Data Collection

Once the measurement systems are in place, data must be collected. This translates into resource demands and logistic issues as to who is to report, record, collect, and manage data.

Data Analysis

Data must be analyzed in statistically appropriate ways. This is not just a matter of using the right statistical methods. More importantly, user groups must agree on a framework for analyzing and interpreting quality of care data.

Addressing the Challenges

These challenges are not insurmountable. However, making a commitment to quality care entails a commitment to putting the processes and systems in place to measure quality through performance measures and to report quality of care results. In other words, once you decide to pursue excellence (i.e., quality), you must accept measurement and reporting—and overcome the various challenges. Let's examine how this could be done in your clinical setting as you try to improve the quality of care to patients. McGlynn and Asch[3] offer several strategies to address the various challenges in measuring quality of care.

Common Measurement Platform

The various user groups must balance competing perspectives. This is a process of giving and taking: proposing highly clinical measures to assist clinicians (e.g., asthma-free days), but also providing more general data for use by managers (e.g., use of inhaled corticosteroids versus leukotriene antagonists).

Accountability Framework

Committing to quality care implies that you assume several responsibilities and are willing to be held accountable for each of them: (a) providing the best possible care to older patients, (b) examining your own clinical knowledge and practice, (c) seeking ways to improve it, (d) agreeing to the evaluation of your practice, and (e) responding to needs for improvement.

Objectivity in the Evaluation of Quality

This requires adopting explicit criteria for judging performance—and building the evaluation process on these criteria. You, your colleagues, and your managers will need to reach consensus on how performance will be measured, and what will be considered excellent (and good, average, etc.) performance.

Routine Reporting
Once these indicators have been identified, you will need to select a subset of indicators for routine reporting. Select indicators that give a reliable snapshot of your and your team's care to patients.

Separate Quality and Finance
To avoid that (lack of) money drives (down) quality of care, it is critical to minimize the use of indicators for evaluating patients for financial or nonfinancial (risk management, accreditation…) purposes. Should you be cost-conscious? Yes, but cost should not influence your clinical judgment concerning what is best for your patients.

In summary, the success of a quality management program hinges on the decision as to what to measure. Good performance measures must be objective, data collection must be easy and minimally burdensome, statistical analysis must be girded by principles and placed within a framework, and communication of results must be targeted towards different user groups.

Conceivably, we could try to measure every possible aspect of our care—realistically, the planning for this will never reach the implementation stage. Instead, establish priorities by asking yourself: based on our clinical expertise, what is critical for us to know? What aspects of our care are high risk? What parts of our care are problem-prone; either because we have experienced difficulties in the past or we can anticipate problems as a result of lack of knowledge or resources? What (clinical) indicators would be of interest to other user groups: patients, the general public, management, payers, accreditors, and practitioners? Throughout this prioritization process, keep the bigger picture in mind: keep on asking yourself what questions you are trying to answer; and for whom?

MEASURING PERFORMANCE

Once you have decided what to measure, you must decide how to measure performance. There are two possibilities: either appropriate measures already exist, or you face the task of developing a new performance measure. Either way, there are a number of requirements of good performance measures that you will need to apply to the decision process.

What Are Good Performance Measures?

There are two ways to answer the question "is this a good measure"? First, you must decide the measure is of potential use to you and your organization. Once you've determined the usefulness of the measure, you should review its characteristics to determine whether it is a good performance measure in general (e.g., well defined, tested).

Usefulness

The process of selecting a performance measure begins with two sets of questions about its usefulness.

Usefulness of the Measure

What do I need to know? What is the measurement purpose of a given perform- ance measure? Do need and purpose match? If you cannot get to a "reasonable yes" on this first set of questions, the performance measure you are reviewing may not meet your objectives. By "reasonable yes" we mean that your assessment of the match between your need and the measurement purpose of the measure does not need to be 100%. Rather, in answering this question, you should evaluate to what extent the measure can be adapted to your needs, or to what extent you and your team can adapt to the measure.

Usefulness of the Measure's Output

How do I intend to use the performance measure? Can the measure be used this way? These questions about the usefulness of the output of the measure pertain to the relevance of the measure to your quality program. Does the measure give you performance results that you can apply to your efforts to improve care?

Characteristics of Good Performance Measures

Now that you have determined that a given measure will be of use to your organ- ization, you should evaluate key characteristics of the measure to ensure that it is adequately defined, tested, and operationalized.

Targets Improvement

The measure and its output must focus on improvement, not merely on the description of some aspect of care. It is not helpful to have a very accurate meas- ure that just tells you the status of a given aspect of care. Instead, the measure needs to inform you about current quality levels and relate them to previous and future quality levels. It needs to be able to compute improvements or declines in quality over time—so that you can plan for the future.

Precisely Defined and Specified

The measure needs to be clearly defined, including the terms used, the data elements collected, and the calculation steps to be made.

Validity

It is important that you obtain information about the validity of a measure. Validity refers to whether the measure "actually measures what it purports to measure"[4]

Sensitivity and Specificity

These concepts refer to the measure's ability to capture all true cases of the event being measured, and only true cases. You want to make sure that a performance measure identifies true cases as true and false cases as false; and does not identify a true case as false or a false case as true. Sensitivity of a performance measure is the likelihood of a positive test when a condition is present. Lack of sensitivity is expressed as "false positives": the indicator calculates a condition as present when in fact it is not. Specificity refers to the likelihood of a negative test when a condition is not present. "False negatives" reflect lack of specificity: the indicators calculate that a condition is not present when in fact it is.

Reliability
Reliability means that results are reproducible; the indicator measures the same attribute consistently across the same patients and across time. A measure is reliable if different people calculate the same rate for the same patient sample. The core issue of reliability is measurement error—the difference between the actual phenomenon and its measurement: the greater the difference, the less reliable the performance measure.

Interpretable
A performance measure must be interpretable; that is, convey a result that can be linked to the quality of clinical care. First, the quantitative output of a performance measure ("the number you get") must be scaled in such a way that users can interpret it. For instance, a scale that starts with 0 as the lowest possible level and ends with 100 is a lot easier to interpret than a scale than starts with 144 and has no upper boundary except infinity.

Risk-adjusted
Some patients are sicker than others are; some patients have more comorbidities; some patients are older and frailer… No doubt, you could come up with many more risk variables that influence how patients respond to nursing care. Good performance measures take this differential risk into consideration. They create a "level playing field" by adjusting quality indicators on the basis of the (risk for) severity of illness of your patients. Imagine that your patients are a lot sicker than those of another practice to which you are being compared. You and your team are at greater risk for having lower quality outcomes—not because you provide inferior care, but because your patients are a lot sicker to begin with and may not respond as well as less sick patients.

Easy to Collect
It might be helpful to use performance measures for which data are readily available, can be retrieved from existing sources, or can be collected with little burden. The goal is to gather good data quickly without running the risk of having "quick-and-dirty" data.

Within Your Control
Performance measures are indicators of quality. It is essential that these indicators reflect nursing practice and can be influenced by nursing care if you propose that they in fact do relate to nursing care. You cannot improve quality scores if the measures are based on variables outside your control.

Common Problems with Performance Measures

Just as much as you evaluate the strengths of a performance measure, you should review potential weaknesses.

Lack of focus: a measure that tries to measure too many things at the same time, or is too complicated to administer, interpret, or use.

Wrong type of measure: a measure that calculates indicators the wrong way; e.g., uses rates when ratios are more appropriate; uses a continuous scale when a discrete scale would be more informative (or vice versa); measures a process, when the outcome is measurable and of greater interest.

Unclear definitions: a measure that is too broad or too vague in its scope and definitions; for example, population is too heterogeneous, no risk-adjustment, unclear data elements, poorly defined values.

Too much work: a measure that requires too much clinician time to generate the data or too much manual chart abstraction.

Reinventing the wheel: It is okay to invent a better wheel by improving the materials, mechanics, and physics of the wheel. Likewise, it is okay to improve a performance measure; yet ask yourself, is this really an improvement or just a reinvention?

Measures events not within your control: You can only change what you do and what you can influence. Don't select a measure that focuses on a process or outcome that is out of your control to improve.

Trying to do research rather than quality management: Research entails data collection and analysis, but not all data collection and analysis is research— nor should it be. Stay focused! Don't try to change the world, which is what researchers (claim to) do. Instead, change your practice, your nursing care, and the health and well-being of your patients. You're more likely to succeed in improving the quality of care in your setting than researchers are likely to change the world.

Poor communication of results: Do you and your colleagues "get it" when you receive the quality of care results? If you don't, it may very well be that the way results are communicated is not effective.

Uninterpretable and underused: Uninterpretable results elicit responses of "what does this mean?" and "if I don't get it, what can I do with it?" These results will be of little relevance to your quality management program. Even worse is the "so what?" response: it means that you do not recognize the value of the measure to improving nursing care.

Using Existing Measures

Begin the process of deciding how to measure by reviewing existing measures. There is no need to reinvent the wheel—especially if good measures are out there. Review the literature, check with national organizations, and consult your colleagues. Yet, do not adopt existing measures blindly. Instead, subject them to a thorough review using the characteristics identified above. Also, contact health care organizations that have adopted these measures and review with them their experience.

Developing New Measures

It may be that, after an exhaustive search, you cannot find measures that meet the various requirements outlined above. You decide instead to develop your own in-house measure. Needless to say, the (daunting?) list of good and bad characteristics of performance measures should guide you and your team in your development efforts. Here are some important guidelines:

Zero In On The Population To Be Measured

If you are measuring an undesirable event, determine the group at risk for experiencing that event, and limit your denominator population to that group. If you are measuring a desirable event or process, identify the group that should experience the event or receive the process. Where do problems tend to occur? What variables of this problem are within my control? If some are not within my control, how can I zero in even more on my target population? In other words, exclude patients from the population when good reason exists to do so.

Define Your Terms

This is a painstaking but essential exercise. Try to be as precise as possible, even if it feels very "techy." It is better to measure 80% of an issue with 100% accuracy, than 100% of an issue with 80% accuracy.

Identify The Data Elements

Be clear about what you want to measure, how you will measure it, and how you will calculate the performance score. This is another painstaking but essential effort. The 80/100 rule applies here as well.

Test the Data Collection Process

Once you have a prototype of a measure ready, examine how easy or difficult it is to get all the required data.

CONCLUSION

There is no mystery to the process of performance measurement and quality management. However, it is hard work—from identifying what to measure, selecting the measures, collecting the data, analyzing and presenting results, and implementing change. To summarize, when finally determining the measures that are good for you and your organization, three things matter:

1. It works for your organization.

2. It is well defined, tested, and applied.

3. Quality improvement happens!

REFERENCES

1. Institute of Medicine, Kohn Lt, Corrigan LT, Corrigan JM, Donaldson MS, editors: *To err is human: building a safer health system,* Washington, DC, 2000, National Academy Press.
2. Schyve PM, Nadzam, DM: Performance measurement in healthcare, *J Strategic Performance Measurement* 2(4):34-42, 1998.
3. McGlynn EA, Asch SM: Developing a clinical performance measure, *Am J Prev Med* 14(3 suppl):14-21, 1998.
4. Wilson HS: *Research in nursing,* ed 2, Reading, MA, 1989, Addison-Wesley.

RISK MANAGEMENT

JANE M. DYER • MARIANN T. SHINOSKIE • DONNA BEHLER MCARTHUR

*A*pproximately 170,000 advanced practice nurses, referred to here as nurse practitioners (NPs), are represented in primary care, specialty practices, and acute care settings. NPs are licensed in 50 states plus the District of Columbia (DC) and may function independently in 27 states. NPs have some level of prescriptive writing authority in 50 states and the District of Columbia.[1]

Historically, NP education has not emphasized the business and legal aspects of practice; rather, students' clinical placements are targeted toward translating nursing theory into its practical application. Thus many new graduates who have met all the requirements for independent or collaborative clinical practices remain ill-prepared to anticipate potential pitfalls in contracting for employment in established health care settings and/or feel insecure in starting their own practices. The purpose of this chapter, therefore, is to identify those legal, business, and regulatory issues within the context of risk management. Simply stated, employment risk management is to job seeking what medical risk management is to patient safety.[2]

PRACTICE TYPES AND BENEFITS

NP practice includes three distinctive options: employment by a governmental agency, membership in a practice, and self-employment. Each carries with it both benefits and challenges; examination of scope of practice, schedule, salary, and benefits are all important considerations for deciding upon a position. Benefits can include, but are not limited to, health and dental insurance, other types of disability insurance, liability coverage (malpractice), and non-compete clauses.

EMPLOYMENT CONTRACTING

An employment contract is a document mutually important to NPs and their employers. The contract should clearly delineate the expectations and the responsibilities of each party. Negotiating a contract requires self-promotion by the NP and acceptance of the contract requires careful analysis of its terms. It is important to determine the value added, both in dollars and services, by incorporating an NP into an existing practice.

Benefits are often an area of negotiation. Organizations bound by limited salary structures may offer other incentives such as funding for educational meetings, professional licensing fees, and professional dues. An accepted part of employment negotiations is "If you do not ask for it, you will not get it." Practicing and refining negotiation skills with a colleague can be helpful and, depending on the flexibility of the terms, hiring an attorney to review the proposed contract may ultimately increase the value to the applicant.

Governmental agencies, such as local or state health departments and Veterans Administration Medical Centers, are known to be NP friendly. Such positions may offer opportunities to provide both direct patient care and administrative options. Government employment is virtually sure to include benefits such as salary, vacation, and health, disability, and liability insurance. State benefits may vary considerably based on location, responsibilities, and flexibility in negotiation. Applicants also will be served by understanding the actual job title: employees "at will" have different benefits and restrictions, for example, than do those employees hired by governmental or political groups.

Many of these concerns exist for employees or partners in a private group practice as well. An NP should review any employment package for an appropriate salary, benefits package, and language addressing either voluntary or forced termination. Of particular importance is awareness of any contract terms limiting the employees' right to continue to practice in the same local geographic area. Prospective employees should be alert to the potential consequences of a term commonly referred to as a *non-compete clause*. Although some jurisdictions have, through either judicial decision or by statute, limited the scope of allowable restrictions, the intent of the provision is to reduce NPs' professional options upon their departure from a practice. Contract language varies but may include terms precluding the practitioner from notifying current patients of a pending departure, recruitment of those patients into a new practice, and in the most extreme cases, establishment of *any* competing practice.

As noted, at the time of this writing, 27 states do not require physician involvement in NP practice; this flexibility provides NPs with exciting opportunities for entrepreneurship and a high level of independence. Of course, such NPs may be solely responsible for an understanding of, and compliance with, local, state, and federal regulations regarding practices.

Finding practice opportunities when relocating to a new community requires some ingenuity and networking. Suggestions include the following:

1. Talking with friends and colleagues who have contacts in the geographic or specialty area

2. Obtaining permission to use friends' and/or colleagues' names when talking with community residents knowledgeable about the practice

3. Consulting NP professional resources that include salary information

4. Exploring the Internet for information about the community, practice site and key names in the practice site.

LICENSING AND PRACTICE ISSUES

The practice of professions, including nursing, is regulated by each individual state. Although there is similarity among the states regarding the issues that are regulated, NPs should take individual responsibility for assuring compliance with the regulations in the states in which they practice. Commonly, state law (statutes) and professional/administrative rules (rules) address criteria for obtaining and maintaining licensure and the scope, limitations, and responsibilities attached to the licensure. Statutes are enacted by legislative bodies to establish the criteria for licensure and the scope of professional practice, and the rules generally expand the statutes, reflecting the collaboration between legislative bodies and representatives from the health care professions. The regulation of advanced nursing practice can most commonly be found in the state statutes/administrative codes under categories often referred to as either (or both) Professions and/or Health Care.

An exception to state control over areas of nursing practice is the delegation of professional responsibility to federal law. Generally, federal employees have reciprocal federal licensing in all states when working for the Federal Government. However, if they perform professional services outside of the scope of their federal employment, they are required to be licensed in the state in which the services are rendered.

NPs are required to have at least a general knowledge of the areas in which their practice is regulated and an appreciation of specific statutory prohibitions and/or requirements and the repercussions of failure to abide by them.

State Statutes Regulating Professions

Each state sets out criteria for professional licensure, including educational requirements, permissible scopes of practice, criminal background checks, prescriptive writing privileges, relationship to collaborating or referring practitioners, disciplinary processes, reciprocity of out-of-state licensure, and limitations, if any, on engaging in professional practice across state lines.

Typically, professional statutes have assumed that the practice will be limited to one state. However, changes in the provision of health care and the shortage of nursing professionals have required some degree of reassessment of that concept. The advancement of telehealth has given rise to requests that practitioners from one state be permitted to provide telemedical consultation for patients who, along with their referring providers, are physically located in a state in which the consulting physician is not licensed. Efforts are being made to enact legislation that would either remove the need for second licensure or ease the requirements for obtaining additional licensure.

Additionally, (resulting in part from the nursing shortage) many states (particularly those with large rural communities), have supported state legislation that provides reciprocity of nursing and NP licensure from state to state. This reciprocity is through collaboration with the RN/LPN and NP Compacts of member states. The NP applicant must satisfy each state's licensing and practice requirements.

LEGISLATIVE ASPECTS OF HEALTH CARE DELIVERY

A discussion of legislative issues impacting NP practice may seem overwhelming. Hopefully, this overview will offer the NP insight into basic concepts relevant to any practice setting. NPs are bound by federal and state statutes that expressly address health care–related issues. These laws establish specific requirements for, prohibitions against, or restrictions on the provision of certain health care practices, including dissemination of patient information. State laws also address mandatory reporting of certain aspects of health care that would otherwise be considered confidential.

Pertinent state laws may address such issues as authorization for decision making for medical/end of life decisions, informed consent, duties to report certain information to law enforcement agencies, criteria for mandating criminal background checks, treatment of minors, criteria for emancipated minors and permissible disclosure of health care information.

Some health care issues are addressed in both federal and state statutes. In those cases, the law that is most restrictive will apply. For example, if a state law protecting privacy of medical information is more restrictive than the Health Insurance Portability and Accountability Act (HIPAA), state law will be applied. Issues that are often addressed at both levels include privacy of patient information and medical records, treatment of special populations, such as the elderly or vulnerable neonates, and access to elective termination of pregnancy.

Specific Areas Governed by State Law

State law dictates certain parameters of clinical practice in addition to provisions addressing general oversight of health care professionals. Experience tells us that the majority of NPs learn to practice by adopting the culture in which they work. Thus they may or may not practice in a manner that is consistent with state law, either because their mentors are generally unaware of the statutory requirements or because they are not current with legislative changes. Additionally, NPs who relocate to another state, or who wish to practice in more than one state, must take into account the probability that the laws governing their practices will differ. The following examples serve as guidelines for potential state laws addressing issues about which NPs must be aware.

Scope of Practice and Prescription/Dispensing Authority

NPs must follow state law setting out the scope and limitations of their practices, including, if applicable, prescriptive writing privileges. Terms of such laws will address the degree to which NPs must have specific oral or written agreements with a collaborating physician and will articulate additional responsibilities for advanced practice to include prescribing and dispensing authority.

Statutory Authorization of Decision Making for Medical/End-of-Life Decisions

Living Wills

Living wills are enforceable documents (executed by individuals assumed to be legally competent at the time of the writing) setting out preferences for end-of- life decisions. Items addressed may include one or a combination of items, including, but not limited to no CPR, no artificial ventilation, cessation of current treatments such as medications, IVs and food/fluids. Copies of these documents should be kept by the authors' family members and care providers. In the event that families do not live in close proximity to the "patient," a copy should also be kept by a trusted local contact person who would be most likely to learn of any emergency situations that require immediate medical decisions.

Health Care Power of Attorney

The health care power of attorney creates the legal transfer of health-related decision making to a specifically designated person on behalf of persons who are either temporarily or permanently incompetent to do so. The health care power of attorney is designated by the potential patient and often lists a hierarchy of individuals rather than a single person so that if the primary representative is not available, the next in line will assume the responsibility. In the event of the "patient's" temporary incompetence, his return to competency restores the return of decision-making authority to him.

Legal Surrogacy

Surrogacy is a statutorily created hierarchy of health care decision makers in the absence of a competent patient, a legally binding health care power of attorney, and/or a living will. A common legal hierarchy is spouse (unless legally separated), adult child, or consent of majority of children, parent, domestic partner, adult sibling, close friend, or treating physician after consultation with an institutional Bioethics Committee, or concurrence by a second physician.

Informed Consent

The concept of informed consent, or consent for treatment, is a 20th century phenomenon spearheaded by violations of research ethics. Currently there are regulations governing informed consent requirements for human subjects.

The Patients Bill of Rights, approved by the American Medical Association in 1972, clearly articulates for both patients and providers the aspects of informed consent. Each state determines the scope of information required in consenting patients for routine and nonroutine health care. Specific requirements for valid informed consent in routine health care matters includes a clear, concise explanation, including the purpose of the treatment; potential risks and benefits and alternatives to treatment; a general consent for provision of all related health care, but not applicable to special procedures. Most nonroutine procedures (surgeries, invasive diagnostic tests) require written consent—signed by a competent adult patient or signed, for an incompetent patient, by a legally authorized representative or a statutory surrogate. The following are some additional aspects of informed consent:

- Minors typically may not consent for their own treatment unless:

    1. There is an emergency, which is generally defined as either an immediate need for care or a substantial risk to the life/health of the minor.

    2. The parent/guardian has not previously refused to consent for the same type of recommended care, and/or a delay in treatment would result in substantial risk to the minor's life/health.

    3. The minor is emancipated pursuant to statutory criteria which, in many states, requires a finding that the minor meets requirements such as complete financial independence and/or is living in a shelter.

    4. Pursuant to specific criteria set out by other state laws that may require treatment for sexually transmitted diseases or drug/alcohol abuse.

    5. In some states, even if they are not permitted to consent for their own care, statutes may permit minors to consent for the care of their child.

- Care for emergencies is implied, absent specific consent, if:

    1. There is an immediate need for the care.

    2. The patient has not previously refused recommended similar care.

    3. A delay in treatment would result in substantial risk to life/health.

- Refusals for treatment must be documented:

    1. By patient signature, or, if a patient is either unable or unwilling.

    2. Signed by a care provider with additional witness signature.

- Blood transfusion:

    1. Requires signature by the patient or an authorized legal representative.

    2. If a minor and parents refuse to consent, the law may require that the state office governing child protection be petitioned for a decision.

- Discharge against medical advice (AMA) requires signature of release form or signature by care provider and witness.

- Elective termination of pregnancy:

  1. State by state authorization; may limit access by age, term of pregnancy, source of funding.

  2. Minor provisions, which may affect not only abortion but also minor's access to pregnancy testing/care without parental consent (i.e., judicial bypass).

Legislative Review of Medical Administration

States reserve the right to delineate professional health care practice requirements, as well as the right to require statutory protections to health care institutions for limited functions. A typical statute addresses the review of certain medical practices. This review commonly requires that health care institutions create internal mechanisms, such as claims and litigation teams, quality assurance/sentinel event investigators, and professional practice committees whose responsibilities include the review of any suspicions or reports of questionable professional practices. To increase institutional compliance with these internal safety management processes, the statutes often include incentives to cooperate, such as providing legal protection against the release of patients'/NPs' identities and protection against the release of all communications surrounding those reviews. However, protection of the records is not absolute; legislatures may require that institutions report to the appropriate professional body any findings of professional misconduct that resulted in the practitioner's suspension of credentialing/privileging status. The additional level of protection granted in these circumstances is based on a legislative concern that if all records reflecting institutional review and discovery are to be available for use against the institution, there would be a disincentive to investigate and remediate those activities, which could result in increased risk to patients.

Items not statutorily protected from disclosure may include the dates of the occurrence at issue, the time and location of the proceedings and the fact that minutes of the proceedings were generated (but NOT the content). The extent to which the "effects" of the peer review/quality assurances processes are discoverable vary from jurisdiction to jurisdiction. Immunity may exist for some levels of participation, including members of the committee, administrators who assist in the peer review functions, and anyone who provides information for or testifies in the proceedings. Statutes may also protect the institution from subpoenaed testimony that is solely related to peer review processes and may protect hospitals from litigation brought by a practitioner because of the institution's post-review adverse actions against her/his privileges/credentialing.

Complaints to Professional Boards

Many states mandate reporting of health care practitioners who pose a threat to patients or institutions. In order to prevent a future conflict of interest, institutions should not provide legal or administrative support to the health care practitioner in question.

Confidential Medical Records

States generally legislate the protection of individual health care information from release to third parties. However, most states articulate circumstances under which medical information can be disclosed absent the authorization of the patient or his/her legal guardian. This includes release of information subject to mandatory reporting for public health and safety reasons, to report the suspicion of child abuse, or pursuant to a subpoena/court order. In medical malpractice cases, plaintiffs who file lawsuits alleging medical malpractice cannot protect themselves from the release of any medical records that reflect either the care that gave rise to the lawsuit or any care rendered either before or after the defendant's care necessitated by the incident at issue. Additionally, plaintiffs in "ordinary" negligence cases in which they claim injuries related to the incident (e.g., an automobile accident) cannot protect records that either showed prior treatment for the same complaints or care related to the physical sequelae they claim was caused by the incident. States may also disallow the unconsented release of medical records in furtherance of a public purpose, such as identifiable results of HIV testing or behavioral health records.

Criminal Background Checks

It is becoming more commonplace for states to require that several classes of workers, including health care providers, undergo prehiring criminal background checks. Even if the requirement does not cover all health care providers, such checks are almost uniformly required for practitioners who provide care to minors. Certain accrediting organizations, such as the Joint Commission on the Accreditation of Healthcare Organizations (JCAHO) have recently announced a new accreditation requirement mandating the performance of criminal background checks if the state statute requires such checks. The implementation of such guidelines may become problematic in training situations in which, for example, a student nurse from a program in a state that does not require background checks on all health care professionals desires to do a rotation in a facility located in a state that does have such requirements.

Medical Record Retention/Disclosure

States determine the requirements for retention of medical records, including electronic paper, audio, and/or video records and traditional paper records. As would be expected, because of the statute of limitations on filing lawsuits, the retention period for pediatric records is longer than that for adults.

Telemedicine

Because of shifting emphasis on methodologies by which health care is delivered, many states are now engaged, either through private enterprises or as a result of grant funding, in the provision of telemedical health care. One of the primary motivations for the advancement of telemedicine technology was the provision of specialized health care to rural areas and populations of restricted access patients, such as prisoners. Generally, telemedical care can be rendered for less overall cost and inconvenience than traditional care, which requires longer travel time and, for treatment of prisoners, entails safety risks and added costs. Because of the nature of rural communities, it may be that the nearest consultant, under whose care a patient might ultimately receive hospitalization and traditional care, would be an NP in another state. However, unless the state law in the patient's state provides for practice across state lines, such consultation would be unauthorized unless the consultant was licensed to practice in the state in which the patient was physically present. To that end, many states have contemplated, and some have enacted, statutes that provide for limited licensure at a reduced fee for out-of-state providers to serve as telemedicine consultants. Practicing outside such an arrangement could give rise to professional and legal problems no different than physically providing direct care in another state without being licensed in that state.

Statutory Duty to Report

For purposes of public health and safety, many states require access to and the use of patient information, without patient consent, in certain instances. Among those exceptions to required consent include mandatory reporting of certain sexually transmitted diseases, reporting of psychiatric patients who are deemed to be an immediate threat to a particular person, victims of either child or vulnerable adult abuse, and victims of sexual assaults.

Specific Issues Governed by Federal Law

Federal laws govern practices in all states, except that, if a corresponding state law is more restrictive than the federal law, the state law prevails. Not all state laws have federal counterparts. Examples of pertinent health care issues that are regulated by the federal government follow.

National Practitioner Data Bank

The National Practitioner Data Bank (APRNDB) was established to protect the public from unsafe health care practitioners by compilation and limited release of, as permitted, information regarding a health care provider's professional competency and conduct. Certain entities are required to report to the Bank any malpractice payments on behalf of any health care practitioner that were made in satisfaction of a medical malpractice claim. The required reporting includes any indemnity payment on behalf of a provider arising out of a settlement or a judgment of a malpractice claim, state licensing boards' disciplinary actions related to the professional conduct of a health care practitioner and any notice of any facility's disciplinary actions arising out of professional incompetence or misconduct that leads to either the restriction or surrender of the practitioner's credentialing, privileging, or licensure.

Access to specific Data Bank information is not available to the public; rather, it is information that can be accessed by health care institutions and state licensing boards for their evaluation of the appropriateness of professional licensing and institutional credentialing/privileging. However, the Data Bank does publish reports that are accessible to the public. The APRNDB 2003 report included data reflecting actions against medical doctors (MDs) and NPs (in this incidence referred to as APRN) through mandatory reporting of restrictions on, or loss of, professional licensure or institutional privileges/credentialing, adverse civil court judgements, and criminal convictions. Since the inception of APRNDB, nursing complaints constitute only 1.8% of **all** payments made and APRNs account for only 36.3% of the nursing claims. Among the APRN group, 20.9% of the nurse payments were on behalf of CRNAs (certified registered nurse anesthetists; nurse midwives were responsible for 6.7%;, nurse practitioners for 6.7% and advanced nurse practitioners 0.2% [3]

The APRNDB is currently reviewing indicators suggesting that, by removing the targeted individual identities and reporting in their place the corporate affiliation for/with whom they work, health care corporations are attempting to protect the practitioners. This results, to some extent, in sanitizing findings such that the very purpose of the Bank is weakened.

Emergency Medical Treatment and Labor Act

Commonly referred to as the "anti-dumping" statute, the Emergency Medical Treatment and Labor Act (EMTALA) requires that all hospitals with an emergency department and certain levels of urgent care centers that are Medicare participants provide medical screenings to determine the presence of an emergency. If an emergency is found, stabilization of the patient before discharge or transfer to another facility is required. There are severe sanctions, including monetary fines, for violations.

Limitations on Professional/Financial Arrangements

The federal government prohibits certain economic practices among health care consumers, providers, facilities, vendors, and payors through two specific federal statutes. These statutes increase the chances that clinical transfer/referral will be based on the best available practitioner rather than the self-interest of the referring practitioner.

Anti-Kickback Statute

42 U.S.C. 1320-a-7b(b), commonly referred to as the *anti-kickback statute*, prohibits practitioners, or their family members, from offering or accepting anything of value for the **purpose** of inducing a patient referral to a health care agency that receives Medicaid funding. Examples of exceptions to those restrictions include those to W-2 employees, purchasing agents, agencies known as "safe harbors" (which include hospitals or other receiving entities that replenish drugs/medical supplies used by first-responders during transport to facilities), payment pursuant to personal service and management contracts, managed health care plans that

offer increased coverage or reduced cost-sharing/premium amounts, investments in ambulatory surgical centers or multispecialty clinics and group practices and investments in underserved/rural areas. Penalties for violations include monetary fines, as much as 5 years of jail time and loss of Medicare/Medicaid provider status, state licensure, hospital privileges, and managed care contracts.

Stark (Self-Referral) Law 59 FR 65372

The Stark Law prohibits the referral of Medicare patients to any "Designated Health Services" if the referring party or his/her family member has any financial relationship with the second entity. The law disallows the referral of Medicare patients to any designated health services, as they are defined within the regulation, if the person/entity referring or any of his/her family members has a financial relationship with the designated health services such as compensation, ownership, or investment interests. An example of this would be if an NP practicing in a state referred all of her gynecologic patients requiring surgery to her husband's OB/GYN practice.

Health Insurance Portability and Accountability Act

As a result of the enormous publicity generated from the implementation of the most recently implemented patient privacy aspects of the Health Insurance Portability and Accountability Act (HIPAA), most NPs are more familiar with protecting the release of confidential patient information beyond the scope permitted in the law than they are with other federal/state statutes guiding their practices. Generally speaking, HIPAA applies to health care entities,(i.e., covered health care providers, health care clearinghouses, or health plans) that conduct certain health care transactions in electronic form.

The enactment of the HIPAA provisions covered three general standards: privacy, security, and transactions, each of which had required dates of implementation as well as definitions and guidance for implementation. In its most general interpretation, HIPAA requires the protection of personally identifiable health care information, patient notification of anticipated use of information unless specifically rejected by the patient, information about patients' ability to request a change of the medical record, the use of specific codes for billing in order to receive payment and security measures, through both technologic and procedural safeguards, to provide access only to those with a legitimate need to know.

Reports of noncompliance are accomplished by the filing of a complaint to the Department of Health and Human Services (DHHS). After review of the complaint, and upon request by, the institution must conduct an investigation and review within parameters set out by DHHS. The entity then must communicate its findings to DHHS and, if requested, make its institutional records available for review by DHHS.

The Office of Civil Rights (OCR) may charge $100/per violation, up to $25,000/year for multiple violations. One case arising out of one patient file may include several violations, each of which is assessed a separate amount. In addition to these monetary civil penalties, a finding of criminal offenses could result in incarceration for a maximum of 10 years and fines not to exceed $250,000.

Elder Abuse/Vulnerable Adult

The federal law mandates that each state provide programs to prevent abuse against adults who are deemed unable to advocate for themselves. The states are required to include services such as public education for the identification and prevention of abuse, neglect and physical/financial exploitation. Services contemplated under the act include provision and coordination of educational and outreach programs, development of reporting systems, collaboration of existing social service agencies, training for caregivers, both lay and professional, promotion of state legislation, and enactment of state mechanisms for gathering data on current status. Some associated duties required by the states include mandatory reporting by health care providers (including dentists and psychologists) or other classes of people (including police officers, social workers) of reasonably reliable information that a person responsible for the care of an incapacitated or vulnerable adult has caused harm to such adult. The reporting must be based on a reasonable belief that abuse or neglect of the adult or exploitation of his/her property has occurred or is likely to occur. In turn, the person's guardian or conservator must report such information, in person or by phone, within either 48 hours or, if involving a weekend or holiday, on the next working day. Mandatory reporting by an attorney or other legal guardian of unauthorized use or exploitation of an adult's property is required.

RISK MANAGEMENT

The United States may be seen as a litigious or blaming society where poor health outcomes are not readily accepted and health care providers are expected to be perfect. The number and type of lawsuits and the high monetary awards are often in the news. The availability of plaintiffs' attorneys and attitudes of potential jurors also may contribute to the current climate.[4] Malpractice is a concept that is especially difficult for NPs who pride themselves on "caring" for patients.

High-Risk Areas

Health care providers are very aware of the climate in which they practice. Although some may practice "defensive medicine", for example, ordering additional tests and procedures, others have found that the current climate has actually helped to improve provider-patient communication.[5] Managed care and decreasing reimbursements have placed more demands on health care providers, increasing the number of patients to be seen and decreasing the time spent with patients. NPs in a variety of specialties/practice settings are at increased risks for legal problems. For example, NPs employed in emergency rooms have transitional patient relationships; the potential for catastrophic outcomes if there

TABLE 20-1	

Behaviors to Help Prevent Legal Problems

Professional image	Sit when talking with patients and their families Respect confidences Listen carefully Involve patients in decision making Provide information clearly in understandable language Treatment Outcomes Risks and benefits
Good documentation	Document appropriately Write clearly and legibly, including NP's signature Fill in all blanks Document thought processes Use nonjudgmental terms Label a late entry as late Document all calls and consultations Explain any deviations from protocols
Do NOT	Alter, destroy, or lose a medical record Reference an incident report or other quality assurance activity in the medical record Vent emotions in the medical record

is a misdiagnosis or premature discharge, along with the high cost of previous malpractice suits involving emergency care. CRNAs and CNMs (certified nurse midwives), are also at high risk for malpractice suits again based on the potential for catastrophic outcomes. Approximately 400 NPs have had malpractice claims settled against them as reported in the National Practitioner Data Bank.[3] Suggestions to prevent legal problems are identified in Table 20-1.

In addition to the behaviors noted in Table 20-1, there are other activities in which NPs should participate to prevent liability. All organizations and group practices should have activities to address quality assurance, quality improvement, or risk management of health care provided. By participating in these activities, NPs will learn ways to decrease their liability and solve problems before they lead to malpractice suits. Local and national NP professional organizations offer a variety of other activities that can assist in reducing liability. Peer review activities may be available through these associations for NPs in solo practice. These organizations also offer educational sessions on updates of specialty topics and about reducing risk. NPs should attend these sessions and keep documentation of attendance. To reiterate, being knowledgeable of a state's statues governing NP practice and assuring that consulting physicians are also knowledgeable and participating in the legislative process are important NP responsibilities. Although many NPs may profess to be too busy to participate in these types of activities, they cannot afford not to participate.

Incident Reporting

Sometimes, in spite of everyone's best efforts, problems do occur. An NP's first efforts should be directed at immediately solving the problem. This demonstrates caring and does not demonstrate guilt. Assure that others providing care for the patient are aware of the problem and possible solutions. The NP should inform institutional administrators promptly. Everyone has a supervisor—even the NP in solo practice. An NP may have a supervising NP, office manager, medical director, or physician collaborator. Their organization may have a quality assurance or risk management group. NPs in solo practice carry malpractice insurance. Malpractice insurance carriers may need to be notified. An incident report should be completed. Never reference feelings of guilt, completion of proper reports, or notification of malpractice insurance carriers in the medical record.

Medical Malpractice

There are a variety of reasons for a medical malpractice lawsuit. Securing monetary compensation for someone who has experienced an adverse event is certainly one reason. There are noneconomic reasons as well. Perceived poor communication is often cited as another reason. Health care providers may be perceived as not listening, not answering questions, or not adequately explaining risks. Frustrated families may file a law suit in an effort to "find out what really happened." Providers may not recognize that patients and families have not understood information because of the terminology used or their emotional state. Patients and family may be dissatisfied or frustrated with what they perceive as poor care. Receiving a request for payment for that care may be a trigger for a lawsuit.

Being sued is one of the most stressful and negative events in an NP's professional career. Aspects of the actual case cannot be shared with colleagues, family, and friends, which contributes to feelings of isolation. However, it is important to inform family members of the existence of the case to allow them to be generally supportive. Discussions with insurers and lawyers, while confidential, are not always sources of support. An NP may choose to seek professional counseling during this period and should let their lawyers' know that they have done this. A third person should not be present during counseling, as this could result in loss of the privilege of confidentiality.

Litigation

As is evidenced on a daily basis, medical malpractice lawsuits create financial and psychologic costs to medical institutions and providers. Although this discussion is not intended to serve as a substitute for a thorough explanation of all the components of a lawsuit, and without even pretending to address the fallout of the psychologic costs to the professionals, a brief explanation of the process is warranted.

As set out earlier, each state defines certain parameters of medical malprac-tice lawsuits, including the statute of limitations (the time period within which a patient and/or the patient's family may file a lawsuit), what processes must be followed during the life of the lawsuit, and other pragmatic requirements. Often, the statute of limitations, which is a legislated cutoff for filing a lawsuit, starts to run at either the date the incident occurred or the date upon which the patient first could have known. An example of the difference is a surgery in which a renal artery was inadvertently cut and repaired during the surgery (which would start the limitation) versus the date upon which the discovery of a retained lap sponge in a postoperative abdomen (in which the date of the discovery, not the surgery, would toll the time period). Many states legislate shorter statutes of limitations for lawsuits against state agencies than those for private entities. Additionally, states commonly legislate a requirement for filing a legal notice of an intent to file no later than, for example, 180 days after the event occurred. Failure to comply with either the "Claims Statute" (intent to file) or the Statute of Limitations (cut-off for filing the lawsuit) can result in no remedy for the alleged malpractice. States also may enact laws that require, in medical malpractice cases, that any expert witness called by either side be experienced in the specific specialty at issue, or, for example, a law that prohib-its a lawyer filing the lawsuit from introducing into evidence that, subsequent to a bad outcome, the treating practitioners apologized to the patient for the unexpected result.

There are four required elements to professional negligence lawsuits, which include malpractice lawsuits. They are, with the most basic of explanations, duty, breach of standard of care, causation, and damages.

- *Duty:* sets out whether or not the practitioner being sued (the defendant) had a legally recognized duty to the patient. In its simplest form, this means that there is evidence that the practitioner saw the patient, provided some level of assessment and care, and created a records. States vary on whether a "curbside consult" gives rise to a "duty" between the original practitioner and a colleague who never saw the patient but provided an opinion "off the record" upon which the practitioner relied.

- *Breach of standard of care:* sets out, almost always by expert witness testimony, textbooks, and journal articles, a health care practitioner's failure to provide the professional standard for care. Although NPs are not charged with having the same standard as a consulting physician to whom they refer patients, they are charged with the standard of recognizing when care must be either shared or transferred.

- *Causation:* often described as "no harm, no foul" to indicate that even if one practices below the standard, if there is no definitive causal relationship between the breach of the standard of care and the harm incurred, the suit will be dismissed. This element also commonly requires an expert witness who, depending on the circumstances, may or may not be the same as the Standard of Care expert. For example, if a baby exhibits intermittent fetal heart rate decelerations that appear to resolve spontaneously, delivers vaginally, and at 2 years of age is diagnosed with cerebral palsy (CP), it is likely that the health care provider who managed the labor and delivered the baby would have one expert to testify that the intermittent decelerations were not an indication for an emergency delivery and, perhaps, a pediatric neurologist to argue against the decelerations being the cause of the CP. Technically, although it is legally possible to admit to the breach of the standard and be dismissed because no causal relationship was found, once a defendant health care provider admits to falling below the standard, the jurors may be unpersuaded that there was no relationship between the two.

- *Damages:* refers to the economic burden of having suffered the malpractice. In its most basic form, damages are calculated to compensate plaintiffs for the financial cost of the incident, including such items as medical bills, future medical care necessitated, loss of income (including the value of sick time/vacation time used), and long-term care. In most states, added to the plaintiff's recovery, in addition to the actual money damages, is "pain and suffering," for which a jury provides a sum that is meant to make the plaintiff/family whole for the overall adverse effects on their life that are not tied to a specific monetary amount. Tort reform, which has been adopted in many states in order to decrease what some say are exorbitant awards, are targeted primarily at capping the "pain and suffering" component. Typical caps range between $250,000 and $500,000.

CONCLUSION

Prevention is a concept familiar to NPs. Ultimately, no degree of information or safe practice will guarantee protection from malpractice claims against a health care provider; however, risk management will help the NP to avert clinical and/or business litigation. Succinctly put, know (or know where to access) the laws related to NP practice in your state(s), promote evidence-based practice, and be both physically and emotionally present when interacting with patients.

REFERENCES

1. Phillips SJ: A comprehensive look at the legislative issues affecting advanced practice nursing, 18th annual legislative update, *Nurse Pract* 31(1):6-8, 11-17, 21-28,2006.
2. Buppert C: *NP's business practice and legal guide,* ed 2, Boston, 2004, Jones & Bartlett.

3. National Practitioner Data Bank: *NPDB Summary Report*, 2005 (website): www.npdb-hipdb. com/pub/stats/2--3_NPDB_Annual_Report.pdf. Accessed March 5, 2005.
4. Laska L: Why Juries turn against doctors—some observations on big awards, *Med Liability Monitor* 20:4-6, 2004.
5. Symon A: Litigation and changes in professional behaviour: a quantitative appraisal, *Midwifery* 16(1):15-21, 2000.

APPENDICES

A. Contact Information for State Boards of Nursing and the District of Columbia, 265
   Compiled by Saowapa Dedkhard
B. Collaborative Agreements, 271
C. Sample Employment Contract, 285
D. Contract Negotiation for Nurse Practitioners, 291
E. Sample Advanced Practice Nurse Contract, 299
F. Sample Business Plan, 303
G. Glossary of Terms for Reimbursement, 311
   Gail P. Barker and Valerie S. Light
H. Practice Start-Up Timeline, 315
I. Resources for the Nurse Practitioner, 319
J. National Provider Identifier (NPI), 331
K. National Provider Identifier (NPI) Application/Update Form, 333

Contact Information for State Boards of Nursing and the District of Columbia

Compiled by

SAOWAPA DEDKHARD

%

Alabama Board of Nursing
770 Washington Ave., Suite 250
Montgomery, AL 36104
P.O. Box 303900
Montgomery, AL 36130-3900
Phone: (334) 242-4060
http://www.abn.state.al.us/

Alaska Board of Nursing
550 W. 7th Ave., Suite 1500
Anchorage, AK 99501
Phone: (907) 269-8161
http://www.dced.state.ak.us/occ/
pnur.htm

Arizona State Board of Nursing
4747 N. 7th St., Suite 200
Phoenix, AZ 85014
Phone: (602) 889-5150
http://www.azbn.gov/

Arkansas State Board of Nursing
University Tower Building
1123 S. University, Suite 800
Little Rock, AR 72204-1619
Phone: (501) 686-2700
http://www.arsbn.org/

California Board of Registered Nursing
1625 North Market Blvd., Suite N 217
Sacramento, CA 95834-1924
P.O. Box 944210
Sacramento, CA 94244-2100
Phone: (916) 322-3350
http://www.rn.ca.gov/

Colorado Board of Nursing
1560 Broadway, Suite 1350
Denver, Colorado 80202
Phone: (303) 894-2430
http://www.dora.state.co.us/Nursing/

Connecticut Board of Examiners for Nursing
Department of Public Health
410 Capitol Ave.
Hartford, CT 06134-0328
P.O. Box 340308
Hartford, CT 06134-0328
Phone: (860) 509-7624
http://www.dph.state.ct.us/

Delaware Board of Nursing
861 Silver Lake Blvd., Suite 203
Dover, DE 19904
Phone: (302) 744-4515; (302) 774-4516
http://dpr.delaware.gov/boards/nursing/index.shtml

District of Columbia Board of Nursing
Department of Health
Board of Nursing
717 14th Street, NW, Suite 600
Washington, DC 20005
Phone: (202) 724-4900, (877) 672-2174
http://hpla.doh.dc.gov/hpla/cwp/view,A,1195,Q,488526,hplaNav,
|30661|,.asp

Florida Board of Nursing
4052 Bald Cypress Way, BIN C02
Tallahassee, FL 32399
P.O. Box 6330
Tallahassee, FL 32314
Phone: (850) 245-4125
http://www.doh.state.fl.us/mqa/

Georgia Board of Nursing
237 Coliseum Drive
Macon, GA 31217-3858
P.O. Box 13446
Macon, GA 31208
Phone: (478) 207-2440
http://www.sos.state.ga.us/plb/rn/

Hawaii Board of Nursing
King Kalakaua Building
335 Merchant Street, Rm. 301
Honolulu, Hawaii 96813
P.O. Box 3469
Honolulu, HI 96801
Phone: (808) 586-3000
http://www.hawaii.gov/dcca/areas/pvl/boards/nursing/

Idaho Board of Nursing
280 N. 8th Street, Suite 210
P.O. Box 83720
Boise, ID 83720-0061
Phone: (208) 334-3110
http://www2.state.id.us/ibn/index.htm

Illinois Department of Professional Regulation
James R. Thompson Center
100 West Randolph, Suite 9-300
Chicago, IL 60601
Phone: (312) 814-2715
http://www.idfpr.com/

Indiana State Board of Nursing
Professional Licensing Agency
(Attn: Indiana State Board of Nursing)
402 W. Washington Street, Room W072
Indianapolis, IN 46204
Phone: (317) 234-2043
http://www.state.in.us/pla/bandc/isbn/

Iowa Board of Nursing
River Point Business Park
400 S.W. 8th Street, Suite B
Des Moines, IA 50309-4685
Phone: (515) 281-3255
http://www.state.ia.us/nursing/

Kansas State Board of Nursing
Landon State Office Bldg.
900 SW Jackson Street, Suite 1051
Topeka, KS 66612
Phone: (785) 296-4929
http://www.ksbn.org/

Kentucky Board of Nursing
312 Whittington Parkway, Suite 300
Louisville, KY 40222-5172
Phone: (502) 429-3300
http://kbn.ky.gov/

Louisiana State Board of Nursing
3510 N. Causeway Blvd., Suite 601
Metairie, LA 70002
Phone: (504) 838-5332

Temporary Address:
5207 Essen Lane, Suite 6
Baton Rouge, LA 70809
Phone: (225) 763-3570
http://www.lsbn.state.la.us/

Maine State Board of Nursing
161 Capitol Street, # 158 State
House Station
Augusta, ME 04333-0158
Phone: (207) 287-1133
http://www.state.me.us/boardofnursing/

Maryland Board of Nursing
4140 Patterson Ave.
Baltimore, MD 21215-2254
Phone: (410) 585-1900
http://www.mbon.org/main.php

Massachusetts Board of Registration in Nursing
239 Causeway Street
Boston, MA 02114
Phone: (617) 973-0800
http://www.mass.gov/dpl/boards/rn/

Michigan Board of Nursing
Michigan/DCH/Bureau of Health
Professions
Ottawa Towers North
611 W. Ottawa
Lansing, MI 48933
P.O. Box 30193
Lansing, MI 48909
Phone: (517) 335-0918
http://www.michigan.gov/mdch

Minnesota Board of Nursing
2829 University Avenue SE, Suite 200
Minneapolis, MN 55414-3253
Phone: (612) 617-2270
http://www.nursingboard.state.mn.us

Mississippi Board of Nursing
1935 Lakeland Drive, Suite B
Jackson, MS 39216
Phone: (601) 944-4826
http://www.msbn.state.ms.us/

Missouri State Board of Nursing
3605 Missouri Blvd.
Jefferson City, MO 65109
P.O. Box 656
Jefferson City, MO 65102
Phone: (573) 751-0681
http://www.pr.mo.gov/nursing.asp

Montana State Board of Nursing
301 South Park
P.O. Box 200513
Helena, MT 59620-0513
Phone: (406) 841-2340
http://www.discoveringmontana.com/
dli/bsd/license/bsd_boards/nur_board/
board_page.asp

Nebraska Board of Nursing
Dept. of Health and Human Services,
Nursing and Nursing Support
301 Centennial Mall South

Lincoln, NE 68509-4986
P.O. Box 94986
Lincoln, NE 68509-4986
Phone: (402) 471-4376
http://www.hhs.state.ne.us/crl/nursing/
nursingindex.htm

Nevada State Board of Nursing
5011 Meadowood Mall Way, Suite 201
Reno, NV 89502-6547
Phone: (775) 688-2620
http://www.nursingboard.state.nv.us/

New Hampshire Board of Nursing
21 South Fruit Street, Suite 16
Concord, NH 03301
Phone: (603) 271-2323
http://www.state.nh.us/nursing/

New Jersey Board of Nursing
124 Halsey Street
Newark, NJ 07102
P.O. Box 45010
Newark, NJ 07101
Phone: (973) 504-6430
http://www.nj.gov/lps/ca/medical/
nursing.htm

New Mexico Board of Nursing
6301 Indian School Road, NE, Suite 710
Albuquerque, NM 87110
Phone: (505) 841-8340
http://www.state.nm.us/nursing/

**New York State Department of
Education, Board of Nursing**
Education Bldg.
89 Washington Ave.
Albany, NY 12234-1000
Phone: (518) 474-3817
http://www.op.nysed.gov/nurse.htm

North Carolina Board of Nursing
3724 National Drive, Suite 201
Raleigh, NC 27612
P.O. Box 2129
Raleigh, NC 27602-2129
Phone: (919) 782-3211
http://www.ncbon.com/

North Dakota Board of Nursing
919 South 7th Street, Suite 504
Bismarck, ND 58504
Phone: (701) 328-9778
http://www.ndbon.org/

Ohio Board of Nursing
17 South High Street, Suite 400
Columbus, OH 43215-7410
Phone: (614) 466-3947
http://www.nursing.ohio.gov/

Oklahoma Board of Nursing
2915 N. Classen Boulevard, Suite 524
Oklahoma City, OK 73106
Phone: (405) 962-1800
http://www.ok.gov/nursing/

Oregon State Board of Nursing
800 Oregon Street N.E., Suite 465
Portland, OR 97232-2162
Phone: (971) 673-0685
http://www.oregon.gov/OSBN/

Pennsylvania State Board of Nursing
2601 N 3rd Street
Harrisburg, PA 17110-2004
P.O. Box 2649
Harrisburg, PA 17105-2649
Phone: (717) 783-7142
http://www.dos.state.pa.us/bpoa/
cwp/view.asp?a=1104&q=432883
&dsftns=30628

Rhode Island Board of Nurse Registration and Nursing Education
105 Cannon Building
Three Capitol Hill
Providence, RI 02908
Phone: (401) 222-5700
http://www.health.ri.gov/hsr/professions/nurses.php

South Carolina State Board of Nursing
110 Centerview Drive
King State Building, Suite 202
Columbia, SC 29210
P.O. Box 12367
Columbia, SC 29211-2367
Phone: (803) 896-4550
http://www.llr.state.sc.us/pol/nursing/

South Dakota Board of Nursing
4305 South Louise Ave., Suite 201
Sioux Falls, SD 57106-3115
Phone: (605) 362-2760
http://www.state.sd.us/doh/nursing/

Tennessee Board of Nursing
425 Fifth Avenue North
1st Floor—Cordell Hull Building
Nashville, TN 37247-1010
Phone: (615) 532-5166
http://www2.state.tn.us/health/Boards/Nursing/index.htm

Texas Board of Nurse Examiners
333 Guadalupe, Tower 3, Suite 460
Austin, TX 78701
Phone: (512) 305-7400
http://www.bne.state.tx.us/

Utah State Board of Nursing
Heber M. Wells Bldg., 4th Floor
160 East 300 South
Salt Lake City, UT 84111
Phone: (801) 530-6628
http://www.dopl.utah.gov/licensing/nurse.html

Vermont State Board of Nursing
81 River Street, Heritage Building
Montpelier, VT 05609-1712
Phone: (802) 828-2396
http://www.vtprofessionals.org/opr1/nurses/

Virginia Board of Nursing
6603 West Broad Street, 5th Floor
Richmond, VA 23230-1712
Phone: (804) 662-9909
http://www.dhp.virginia.gov/nursing

Washington State Nursing Care Quality Assurance Commission
Department of Health
HPQA Nursing Commission
310 Israel Road SE
Tumwater, WA 98501-7864
P.O. Box 1099
Tumwater, WA 98507-1099
Phone: (360) 236-4700
https://fortress.wa.gov/doh/hpga1/HPS3/Nursing_Home_Admin/default.htm

West Virginia Board of Examiners for Registered Professional Nurses
101 Dee Drive, Suite 102
Charleston, WV 25311-1620
Phone: (304) 558-3596
http://www.wvrnboard.com/

Wisconsin Department of Regulation and Licensing
Board of Nursing
1400 E. Washington Ave.
P.O. Box 8935
Madison, WI 53708
Phone: (608) 267-2112
http://drl.wi.gov/boards/nur/index.htm

Wyoming State Board of Nursing
1810 Pioneer Avenue
Cheyenne, WY 82002
Phone: (307) 777-7601
http://nursing.state.wy.us/

COLLABORATIVE AGREEMENTS

$\mathcal{E}$xamples of collaborative agreements or guidelines that must be addressed in collaborative agreements are usually found through state boards of nursing. Some state boards have specific forms that must be completed for the collaborative agreement. Others provide guidelines for what constitutes an agreement but are less clear about how the agreement should actually be constructed. It should be noted that each collaborative practice has unique characteristics and is governed by specific state laws. Nurse practitioners (NPs) should enter into an agreement consistent with the guidelines of the state where they intend to practice (see Appendix A for state board of nursing contact information). It is also advisable to consult an attorney familiar with collaborative agreements to assist in developing the agreement, particularly if the state does not provide specific forms to be completed. The following are a few starting places for information. The list is not inclusive of all states simply because states vary with respect to requirements for collaboration.

These contacts and examples are samples *only* and do not reflect legal recommendations because the editors of this text are not attorneys. The reader is advised to seek legal counsel when preparing a collaborative agreement to assure consistency with state nurse practice regulations.

 ALABAMA STATE BOARD OF NURSING

Application for Approval to Practice in Alabama as Certified Registered Nurse Practitioner (CRNP) or Certified Nurse Midwife (CNM)

http://www.abn.state.al.us/main/downloads/applications/AP%20APPS/CRNP-CNM-Application.doc

 MARYLAND BOARD OF NURSING

Nurse Practitioner Written Agreement

http://www.mbon.org/adv_prac/np_agreement.pdf

MICHIGAN NURSES ASSOCIATION

http://www.minurses.org/apn/NP%20Collaborative%20A.doc

NORTH CAROLINA BOARD OF NURSING

New Nurse Practitioner Rules and the Collaborative Practice Agreement: A Guide for Implementation

http://www.ncbon.com/NewNPRules.asp

PENNSYLVANIA BOARD OF NURSING

Application for Certified Registered Nurse Practitioner (CRNP) Prescriptive Authority (includes 2-page standardized form that is required for the application)

http://www.dos.state.pa.us/bpoa/lib/bpoa/20/nurs_board/crnp_application_
for_prescriptive_authority.pdf#search='pennsylvania%20board%20of%20nursing
%20collaborative%20agreement'

SOUTH DAKOTA BOARD OF NURSING

http://www.state.sd.us/doh/nursing/cnpagree.pdf#search='nurse%20practitioner
%20collaborative%20practice%20agreement'

Another document to consider reviewing was prepared by the Minnesota Medical Association: *Questions and Answers for Physicians Entering into Prescribing or Collaborative Agreements with Advanced Practice Registered Nurses,* which describes some questions physicians also may have about collaborating with NPs. Knowing physicians' questions or potential questions about collaboration is important from the perspectives of negotiating and establishing positive working relationships. This document is available online at http://www.mnmed.org/Protected/Questions&Answers.pdf#search='nurse%20practitioner%20collaborative%20agreements'

A sample collaborative agreement also may be found through professional organizations. One such example is through the National Organization of Nurse Practitioner Faculties (NONPF) at http://www.nonpf.com/fpcollabagreesample. htm. The sample agreement is as follows:

COLLABORATIVE PRACTICE AGREEMENT

It is the intent of this document to authorize the nurse practitioner(s) at the _____ clinic(s) to practice under these protocols without direct supervision, as specified in the Medical Practice Act, Texas Civil Statutes, Article 4495b, section 3.06(d)(5) and (6). This document sets forth guidelines for collaboration between the supervising physician(s) and the nurse practitioner(s).

Development, Revision, and Review

The protocols are developed collaboratively by the nurse practitioners, delegating medical director, and supervising physicians. These protocols will be reviewed annually and revised as necessary.

Approval

The protocols will be approved annually on the initial approval date by the nurse practitioners, medical director, and supervising physicians. The Statement of Approval will be signed by all of the above parties recognizing the collegial relationship between the parties and their intention to follow these protocols. Signature on the Statement of Approval implies approval of all the policies, protocols, and procedures in this document. Nurse practitioners and physicians who join the staff mid-year, or who cover the practice, also signify approval of the protocols. It is the task of the medical director to see that the written approval of all the above parties is obtained.

Setting

The nurse practitioners will operate under these protocols at the (Name of Institution) clinics listed below:

    Clinic 1: (name and address)
    Clinic 2: (name and address)

Supervision

The nurse practitioners are authorized to practice under the protocols established in this document without the direct (on-site) supervision or approval of the supervising physicians. Consultation with the supervising physicians, or their designated back-up, is available at all times, either on-site or by telephone when consultation is needed for any reason.

Consultation

The nurse practitioners are responsible for providing health services to clients of the (name of clinic or agency). The nurse practitioners will provide health promotion, screening, safety instructions, management of acute episodic illness and stable chronic diseases. Referrals will be made, as needed, to other health care providers.

Physician consultation will be sought for all of the following situations and any others deemed appropriate. Whenever a physician is consulted, a notation to that effect, including the physician's name, must be recorded in the patient's medical record.

Consultation will occur:

- Whenever situations arise that go beyond the intent of the protocols or the competence, scope of practice, or experience of the nurse practitioners.

- Whenever the patient's condition fails to respond to the management plan within an appropriate timeframe, based on the provider's clinical judgment.

- For any uncommon, unfamiliar, or unstable patient condition.

- For any patient condition that does not fit the commonly accepted diagnostic pattern for a disease/condition.

- For any unexplained physical examination or historical finding or abnormal diagnostic finding.

- Whenever a patient requests.

- For all emergency situations after initial stabilizing care has been initiated.

Medical Records

The nurse practitioners are responsible for the complete, **legible** documentation of all patient encounters using the SOAP format.

Education and Training

The nurse practitioner must possess a valid Texas license as a Registered Nurse and be recognized by the Texas Board of Nurse Examiners as a Nurse Practitioner.

Evaluation of Clinical Care

Evaluation of the nurse practitioners will be provided in the following ways:

- A minimum of a monthly review by the supervising physicians of a minimum of 10% of patient charts. A written record of the review is to be kept.

- Annual evaluation by the supervising physicians based on written criteria.

- Informal evaluation during consultations and case review.

- Periodic chart review as part of chart audits by the Quality Assurance Committee.

Practice Guidelines

The nurse practitioners are authorized to diagnose and treat common medical conditions under the following current guidelines (including, but not limited to):

Barker, LR, Burton, JR & Zieve, PD. (1999). *Principles of Ambulatory Medicine*, 5th ed., Williams & Wilkins or comparable current edition of medical references available on-site at the respective clinics

OR

Other published, accepted sources of medical information, as agreed upon by the collaborating parties and/or identified below:

OSHA guidelines
CDC guidelines for immunizations
Uphold, CR & Graham, MV (1998). *Clinical Guidelines in Family Practice*, 3rd ed. Gainesville, FL.: Barmarrae Books, Inc.

Drug Prescriptions

Nurse practitioners at this facility shall be authorized to prescribe dangerous drugs (excluding controlled substances) as authorized by the Texas Board of Nurse Examiners (BNE) under Rule 222, Advanced Practice Nurses Limited Prescriptive Authority and the Texas Board of Medical Examiners (BME) under Rules 193.2-193.4 and 193.8, Delegation of Prescriptive Authority. Authority shall be delegated by the Medical Director of the Methodist Health Care Ministries and supervision of prescribing activity shall be conducted by the Medical Director and supervising physicians as indicated in the Rules. It is the responsibility of the nurse practitioners to obtain prescription ID numbers from the appropriate Board. The Medical Director shall inform the BME, in writing, of his intent to delegate prescriptive authority as required in the Rules.

References for prescriptions will be the current *Physician's Desk Reference* and/or the *Nurse Practitioner/Physician Monthly* or *Quarterly Prescribing Guide.* Additionally, there may be limitations placed on prescriptions to an approved formulary for the MHCM.

Collaborating Parties: Statement of Approval

We, the undersigned, agree to the terms of this Collaborative Practice Agreement as set forth in this document.

_____ Medical Director
_____ Supervising Physician
_____ Supervising Physician
_____ Supervising Physician
_____ Nurse Practitioner
_____ Nurse Practitioner
_____ Nurse Practitioner

Approval Date _____
Renewal Date _____
Renewal Date _____

Another example of collaborative agreements may be found at the Michigan Nurses Association website. Scroll through the collaborative agreement section under frequently asked questions to find several examples of collaborative agreements: http://www.minurses.org/apn/apn-npfaq.shtml#collab.

The sample agreements found on the Michigan Nurses Association website are as follows:

COLLABORATIVE AGREEMENT SAMPLE A

1. The undersigned nurse practitioner and physician agree to the following collaborative practice agreement for provision of health care services to clients at (location, address)_____.

[1.A] 2. The health care services provided by the nurse practitioner will include health maintenance, management of acute episodic illness, and stable chronic illness.

[1.B] 3. (Doctor) and (nurse practitioner) agree that the latest edition of (resource) and others will be the reference texts to define referral and consultation criteria.

[3] 4. As collaborating physician, (doctor) agrees to:

  (a) Be available for record review and co-signature (when appropriate) on (scheduled time).
  (b) Be available for telephone consultation on a 24-hour basis.
  (c) Be on-site for consultation on (schedule time).
  (d) Delegate prescriptive privileges via mutually developed formulary.

[3] 5. As collaborating nurse practitioner, (nurse practitioner), agrees to:

  (a) Utilize mutually developed practice protocols.
  (b) Prescribe, as delegated, from the formulary, and consult, when needed, for those medications not approved in the formulary.
  (c) Maintain accurate records of all consultations.

[4] 6. (Doctor) and (nurse practitioner) agree to review all resource/referral guidelines, protocols and practice goals, and objectives.

[6] 7. (Doctor and Nurse practitioner), as parties to the collaborative agreement, are responsible and accountable for performing in accord with the collaborative practice agreement, and within their separate and distinct scope of practice as defined by the Michigan Public Health Code.

[2] 8. Agreed to by _____ (Doctor)
  _____ (Nurse practitioner)
  Approval date _____ Review date _____
  Review date _____

COLLABORATIVE AGREEMENT SAMPLE B

The undersigned nurse practitioner and physicians agree to the following collaborative practice agreement for provision of health care services at (location, address).

The health care services provided by the nurse practitioner will include the following: health maintenance, management of acute episodic illness, and stable chronic illness.

(Doctors) and (nurse practitioner) agree that the following reference texts will be used to define referral and consultation criteria: (resources listed) as well as others mutually determined.

(Doctors) and (nurse practitioner) agree to review these reference texts annually.

As collaborating physicians, (doctors) agree to be available for consultation as necessary. Documented evidence of consultation will include a progress note entry or referral letter.

Periodic oral reports reviewing the mutual goals of this collaborative practice will occur.

(Doctors) and (nurse practitioner) acknowledge that each professional has separate accountability for his/her own scope of practice.

Agreed to by:

(Doctor) _____ Date: _____

(Doctor) _____ Date: _____

(Nurse practitioner) _____ Date: _____

COLLABORATIVE AGREEMENT SAMPLE C

The undersigned nurse practitioner and physician agree to the following collaborative practice agreement for provision of obstetrical and gynecological services at (location, address).

The services to be provided independently by the nurse practitioner include:

Health maintenance
Low-risk obstetrical care
Well-woman gynecology
Management of acute obstetrical and gynecological illnesses
Management of stable, chronic gynecology illnesses

Services to be provided interdependently include:

High-risk obstetrical care
Gynecology surgical care

We agree to meet periodically (at least monthly) to review cases and discuss management plans. In addition, the following reference texts will be utilized to assist with consultation and/or referral criteria: (resources listed)

Documented evidence of consultation will occur in the following situations:

Non-stress tests
Abnormal lab values
Abnormal VSN results

And others as determined by the nurse practitioner. Consultation will be reflected in the progress notes. Counter signature of the note by the physician will occur when a prescription is written by the nurse practitioner.

We agree that an annual review of our mutual goals and objectives will occur.

We agree that each of us has separate accountability for our respective scope of practice.

(Nurse Practitioner) _____ Date: _____
(Physician) _____ Date: _____

COLLABORATIVE AGREEMENT SAMPLE D

The undersigned nurse practitioner and physician agree to the following collaborative practice agreement for the provision of health care services at (location, address).

The services to be provided by the nurse practitioner include:

Health maintenance of teens and adults
Management of acute and chronic illness

We agree to meet at least monthly to review cases and discuss management plans. In addition, the following reference texts will be utilized by the nurse practitioner to define consultation and/or referral criteria: (resources listed)

Documented evidence of consultation as needed will be reflected in:

Progress notes
Countersignature by the M.D. of progress notes when a prescription is written
   by the nurse practitioner

An annual evaluation of our mutual goals and objectives will occur.

We agree that each of us has separate accountability for our respective scope of practice.

(Nurse Practitioner) _____ Date: _____
(Physician) _____ Date: _____

COLLABORATIVE AGREEMENT SAMPLE E

The undersigned nurse practitioner and physician agree to the following collaborative practice agreement for provision of health care services to clients at (location, address).

Care services provided by the nurse practitioner will include health maintenance, management of acute/episodic illnesses, and management of stable chronic illnesses.

(Doctor) and (nurse practitioner) agree that the Protocols for Nursing Practice as mutually developed will be the guide to define advanced practice including consultation and referral criteria.

Both parties mutually developed and agree to this document per our signatures. As collaborating physician, _____ agrees to:

- Be available for record review when appropriate

- Be available for telephone consultation during clinic hours

- Review mutually developed practice protocols annually

- Delegate prescriptive privileges as outlined in the protocols

  As collaborating nurse practitioner, _____ agrees to:

- Follow mutually agreed upon protocols as described above

- Review mutually developed practice protocols annually

- Prescribe, as delegated, from the protocol, and consult when needed for those medications not approved in the protocol.

- Document consultation and referral with physician in progress notes.

  Both parties agree to ongoing development of this relationship and evaluation at regular intervals, both formally and informally.

  Both parties will mutually review the objectives of this relationship, discuss the protocols, and practice concerns every six months.

  Each party is responsible and accountable for performing to a full and appropriate extent his/her role and function in accord with the collaborative practice agreement, the individual's professional level of knowledge and expertise, legitimate legal practice regulations as defined by the Michigan Public Health Code, and policies of the agency.

Agreed on this day _____
(Nurse Practitioner) _____ (Physician) _____

MODEL FOR PRESCRIPTIVE AUTHORITY DELEGATION OF CONTROLLED SUBSTANCES

I, (Physician), delegate to (Nurse Practitioner) the authority to write prescriptions for Controlled Substances in Schedules (specify #) (be sure of requirements for 2, 4, and/or 5 as part of her/his practice at (address).

**NOTE: A separate document is needed at each practice site. ** Effective (Date).

(Exception and limitations)
or
(None)

If appropriate, indicate any drugs and their Schedule for which NP cannot write scripts, or any limitations. An example would be to exclude a class of drugs that the physician would not himself/herself prescribe.

This authorization agreement will be reviewed, and revised as needed, annually.

Agreed to by
(Physician) _____ (License #) _____ (Date) _____
(Nurse Practitioner) _____ (License #) _____ (Date) _____

Annual Review

(Comments, "No Changes," or indicate revisions) _____
_____

Agreed to by:

(Physician) _____ License #: _____ Date: _____
(Nurse Practitioner)_____ License #: _____ Date: _____

Annual Review

(Comments, "No Changes," or indicate revisions) _____
_____

Agreed to by:

(Physician) _____ License #: _____ Date: _____
(Nurse Practitioner) _____ License #: _____ Date: _____

This is a sample collaborative agreement to meet prescriptive authority regulations.

COLLABORATIVE AGREEMENT FOR ADVANCED NURSE PRACTITIONER

Prescriptive Authority

This collaborative agreement, dated _____, is made and entered into by and between [state name of the Nurse Practitioner], registered professional nurse in advanced practice, hereinafter referred to as [state name such as Ms. Nurse Practitioner], and _____, MD, a licensed [name of state where licensed] physician (license #_____), hereinafter referred to as [state name such as Dr. _____].

Whereas, Ms. Nurse Practitioner is recognized by the [insert name of the State Board of Nursing] as a nurse in advanced practice (license #_____), and;

Whereas, the [insert name of the State Board of Nursing] may authorize qualified nurses in advanced practice to prescribe prescription drugs in accordance with the provisions of [insert state code. An example is West Virginia Code §30-7-15a, 15b, 15c, and §30-15-1 through 7c], and;

Whereas, in order to qualify for prescriptive authority, an advanced nurse practitioner must enter into a written collaborative relationship with a licensed physician for prescriptive practice as required by [insert state code. An example is West Virginia Code §19-8-3 Application and Eligibility for Limited Prescriptive Authority of the West Virginia Code], and;

Whereas, Dr. _____ has agreed to serve and act as a collaborative physician pursuant to [insert state code. An example is West Virginia Code §19-8-3], which requires the following [example from West Virginia Code]:

Mutually agreed upon written guidelines or protocols for prescriptive authority as it applies to the advanced nurse practitioner's practice

3.1.2.2. Statements describing the individual and shared responsibilities of the advanced nurse practitioner and the physician pursuant to the collaborative agreement between them

3.1.2.3. Provision for the periodic and joint evaluation of the prescriptive practice

Provision for the periodic and joint review and updating of the written guidelines or protocols

Therefore, in consideration of the mutual covenants and agreements contained herein, the parties agree as follows:

Ms. Nurse Practitioner and Dr. _____ have reviewed and accepted the protocols outlined and published in the following references as clinical guidelines for advanced nurse practitioner practice for the diagnosis and prescription of therapeutic measures as they apply to advanced nurse practitioner practice under [Cite state code. An example is Title 19 "Legislative Rules," Section 8, "Limited Prescriptive Authority for Nurses in Advanced Practice," for the West Virginia Board of Examiners for Registered Professional Nurses].

Uphold, Constance & Graham, Mary B. (2004). *Clinical Guidelines in Family Practice*. 4th ed. Gainesville, FL: Barmarrae Books.

Burns, C., Brady, M., Blosser, C., Starr, N. & Dunn, A. (2004). *Pediatric Primary Care: A Handbook for Nurse Practitioners*. 3rd ed. St. Louis: Saunders.

Should one of the above published protocols recommend treatment with any drugs excluded from [Insert state code. An example is West Virginia Prescriptive Authority, the West Virginia Code §19-8-6 Drugs Excluded from Prescriptive Authority] then state code shall be followed and the advanced nurse practitioner shall not prescribe any drugs as excluded by the code.

Ms. Nurse Practitioner and Dr. _____ shall jointly review the above referenced protocols at least biannually and at any other time as mutually agreed upon for updating or any other necessary modifications.

Joint evaluation of advanced nurse practitioner practice shall be conducted at least every 6 months and as needed and mutually agreed upon by Ms. Nurse Practitioner and Dr. _____. At a minimum, this review shall involve a random review of client charts for which the advanced nurse practitioner has provided treatment that includes prescription drugs.

Although the collaborative physician, Dr. _____, or his sole designee, shall be available for phone consultation as needed, client care remains the responsibility of the advanced nurse practitioner, Ms. Nurse Practitioner, unless referred to the collaborative physician for care. Emergency situations that may arise during the advanced nurse practitioner's practice should be managed through the utilization of 911 and appropriate emergency support measures such as CPR, and referred to the appropriate tertiary setting of choice. Referrals for specialty evaluation are made on the basis of client needs, choice, and within guidelines of the client's health plan or third party payer.

This collaborative agreement will remain in accordance with the [Insert state code. An example is Title 19, Series 8, Legislative Rules, "Limited Prescriptive Authority for Nurses in Advanced Practice," for West Virginia Board of Examiners for Registered Professional Nurses]. Should Ms. Nurse Practitioner or Dr. _____ terminate this collaborative agreement, it shall be the responsibility of Ms. Nurse Practitioner, the advanced nurse practitioner, to immediately notify the [insert name of State Board of Nursing].

This collaborative agreement expires on _____

_____   _____

Signature (Nurse Practitioner)   Date

_____   _____

Signature (Collaborating Physician)   Date

SAMPLE EMPLOYMENT CONTRACT

*E*MPLOYMENT AGREEMENT (the "Agreement") made as of May 1, 2004, by and between EMPLOYER, INC., a Maine corporation with its principal place of business in Portland, Maine ("EMPLOYER") and EMPLOYEE, an individual resident of Portland, Maine (the "Employee").

PURPOSE AND EMPLOYMENT

The purpose of this Agreement is to define the relationship between EMPLOYER and Employee. EMPLOYER hereby employs Employee, and Employee hereby accepts employment by EMPLOYER, upon all of the terms and conditions of this Agreement.

DUTIES

Employee shall serve EMPLOYER by providing women's health services to EMPLOYER'S clients, and shall further perform such similar duties as may be assigned to Employee from time to time by EMPLOYER. EMPLOYER anticipates that it will schedule Employee to work approximately sixteen (16) hours per week, with additional hours added according to practice demands and both parties' mutual consent.

Employee shall (i) devote Employee's attention and best efforts to the duties hereunder, including the promotion of the success of the business of EMPLOYER; (ii) perform such duties in a reasonable, prompt, honest, and faithful manner (only by mutual consent will [1] Employee accept work as an NP for another entity and [2] EMPLOYER hire an additional NP); and (iii) not participate actively in any other business during the term of Employee's employment under this Agreement without EMPLOYER'S consent.

Employee acknowledges that Employee owes full loyalty to EMPLOYER, and shall not engage in any activity or enter into any transaction that would constitute a conflict of interest with the duties and loyalties owed to EMPLOYER.

EMPLOYER is employing Employee based on Employee's representations that she is a licensed and certified R.N., M.S. and F.N.P. Employee shall, upon EMPLOYER'S request, provide proof of such professional certifications. At Employee's sole expense, Employee shall also take any and all such steps (including, without limitation, timely acquisition of continuing education units) as are necessary to maintain said professional license throughout the term of this Agreement (and any extensions thereto).

CONTRACT AT WILL

The term of Employee's employment under this Agreement will commence on May 1, 2004 (the "Commencement Date"), and continue through April 30, 2005 (the "Initial Term"). Either party may terminate this contract by giving written notice of no less than sixty (60) days to the other of a desire to terminate. This agreement will automatically extend for twelve (12)-month periods commencing on the first anniversary of the Commencement Date and each subsequent anniversary thereof. Unless either party gives written notice to the other of a desire not to extend the term of this Agreement at least sixty (60) days before the end of the Initial Term or any extension, the Agreement will automatically be extended for successive additional twelve (12)-month periods commencing on the first anniversary of the Commencement Date and each subsequent anniversary thereof.

Employee's employment under this Agreement may be terminated prior to the end of the Initial Term or any extension thereof as provided below:

Upon the death of Employee, this Agreement will automatically terminate, and the only obligation EMPLOYER will have under this Agreement will be to pay Employee's personal representative, administrator, or executor Employee's unpaid salary base through the date of the Employee's death;

EMPLOYER may terminate Employee's employment hereunder at any time without notice for cause. Upon such termination for cause, the only obligation EMPLOYER will have under this Agreement will be to pay Employee's unpaid base salary through the date of termination. For purposes of this Agreement, "for cause" shall mean:

- Employee's disability
- Breach of conduct as defined in the employee policy manual
- Any other conduct by Employee generally recognized under applicable laws as cause for termination
- A sale of all or substantially all of the assets of Company
- A staff reduction or reorganization resulting in the elimination or substantial redefinition of Employee's position with EMPLOYER
- A termination or substantial curtailment of the business of EMPLOYER within the area or division in which Employee works

For purposes of this Agreement, "disability" shall mean any physical or mental condition which prevents Employee, after EMPLOYER has made such accommodations as may be required by law, from performing Employee's full duties to EMPLOYER for any cumulative period of three (3) months during any six (6)-month period.

Notwithstanding the above, before terminating the employment of Employee for any of causes (3.2.2.1) through (3.2.2.6) above, EMPLOYER shall give Employee ten (10) days' written notice and an opportunity to cure, except that if the nature of Employee's conduct is such that EMPLOYER may be materially harmed if it so postpones terminating Employee's employment, then EMPLOYER need not give Employee an opportunity to cure and may terminate Employee's employment immediately.

COMPENSATION

Employee shall be compensated at the rate of $35 per hour, payable weekly or in accordance with Company's payroll policies. EMPLOYER shall withhold state and federal taxes to the extent required by applicable law. Hourly compensation shall be subject to review at 6 months and then annually thereafter.

EMPLOYEE BENEFIT PLANS; FRINGE BENEFITS

Employee shall be entitled to benefits as per EMPLOYER stated policies that hold for any other EMPLOYER employee.

EXPENSES

If EMPLOYER requires Employee to incur any travel, entertainment, or similar expenditures for the benefit of the Practice during the term hereof, it will reimburse Employee for such expenditures on the basis of vouchers submitted by Employee which have been approved by Employee's supervisor. Employee is responsible for all expenses of her professional liability insurance. During the term of this Agreement (plus extensions thereto), Employee shall maintain professional liability insurance coverage and with coverage equal to or greater than that of the other Nurse Practitioner.

PROPERTY OF COMPANY

All records, files, client lists, or plans, developed or created by Employee during the term of this Agreement, individually or in conjunction with others, which may directly or indirectly relate to the practice of EMPLOYER or any of its affiliates shall be the property of EMPLOYER.

RESTRICTIVE COVENANTS

Nondisclosure. Employee acknowledges, covenants, and agrees that:

During employment by EMPLOYER under this Agreement, Employee has and will come to have knowledge and information with respect to confidential plans, projects, practice methods, operations, techniques, clients, client lists, employees, financial condition, policies, and accounts of EMPLOYER and its affiliates with respect to their practice ("Confidential Information"),

During the term of Employee's employment and for one (1) year, Employee will not divulge, furnish, or make accessible to anyone (other than in the regular course of Employee's performance of services for the benefit of EMPLOYER, its successors, assigns, and affiliates) any knowledge or information with respect to any Confidential Information, and

All organizational or administrative papers and records, including all memoranda, notes, plans, data, or other documents, and any and all copies thereof, whether made by Employee or not, reasonably related to EMPLOYER'S practices are the sole and exclusive property of EMPLOYER. Employee shall not remove from the Practice's premises any such written information concerning the Practice's business.

Solicitation. Employee agrees that at all times during the term of employment under this Agreement and for a period of twelve (12) months after the termination of employment with EMPLOYER under this Agreement or otherwise, Employee will not, directly or indirectly, for or on behalf of any other practice solicit, divert, take away, or accept the medical records of any of the clients of EMPLOYER that were served by EMPLOYER during the term of employment or any prospective clients of EMPLOYER that EMPLOYER actively served within one (1) year prior to the termination of this Agreement for the purpose of selling the services provided by EMPLOYER during the term hereof to any such client or prospective client. Employee further agrees that Employee will not, within the foregoing period of time, directly or indirectly, attempt or seek to cause any of the foregoing clients of EMPLOYER to refrain from seeking care from EMPLOYER.

Interference with Employees. Employee agrees that during employment under this Agreement and for a period of twelve (12) months after the termination of Employee's employment with EMPLOYER under this Agreement or otherwise, Employee will not, directly or indirectly, for or on behalf of any other practice request or induce any other employee of EMPLOYER or its affiliates to terminate employment of such persons with EMPLOYER or its affiliates.

Remedy for Breach. The parties recognize that the services to be rendered under this Agreement by Employee are special, unique, and of an extraordinary character, and that in the event of a breach of this Agreement by Employee or EMPLOYER, then either party shall be entitled to institute and prosecute proceedings in any court of competent jurisdiction, either in law or in equity, to obtain damages, or to enforce the specific performance of any terms, conditions, obligations, and requirements of this Agreement, or to enjoin the party who breached the Agreement from continuing those actions which cause a breach of this Agreement, or to take any or all of the foregoing actions. Nothing herein contained shall be construed to prevent the pursuit of any other remedy, judicial or otherwise, in case of any breach of this Agreement by either party.

Effect of Termination. Expiration of the term of Employee's employment under this Agreement or termination of Employee's employment either by EMPLOYER or Employee shall in no way limit or restrict Employee's obligations under this Section 8 which shall remain in full force and effect for the remaining periods set forth in such Section.

PARAGRAPH HEADINGS

Paragraph headings contained in this Agreement are for convenience only and shall in no manner be construed as a part of this Agreement.

AMENDMENT

This Agreement may be amended or modified only in writing signed by both parties.

COUNTERPARTS

This Agreement may be executed in two or more counterparts, each of which shall be deemed to be an original but all of which together shall constitute one and the same instrument.

WAIVER

The failure of either party hereto in any one or more incidences to insist upon the performance of any of the terms or conditions of this Agreement, or to exercise any rights or privileges conferred in this Agreement, or the waiver of any breach of any of the terms of this Agreement shall not be construed as waiving any such terms and the same shall continue to remain in full force and effect as if no such forbearance or waiver had occurred.

APPLICABLE LAW

This Agreement shall be construed according to the laws of the State of Maine.

SEVERABILITY

In the event any term of this Agreement shall be held invalid or unenforceable by any court of competent jurisdiction, such holding shall not invalidate or render unenforceable any other term contained in this Agreement.

ENTIRE AGREEMENT

This Agreement embodies the entire understanding of the parties with respect to Employee's employment with EMPLOYER and incorporates any previous agreement, written or oral, relating to such employment.

ASSIGNMENT AND SUCCESSORS

Employee's rights under this Agreement shall not be assignable by Employee.

This Agreement may be assigned by EMPLOYER and shall inure to the benefit of and be binding upon EMPLOYER, its successors and assigns.

MEDIATION

If a dispute arises under this Agreement which the parties are unable to resolve through direct negotiations, the parties agree to engage jointly the services of a professional mediator and to participate in good faith in such mediation. If the dispute is not resolved as a result of such mediation within thirty (30) days after such mediation is commenced or such longer period to which the parties may agree, each party shall be free to pursue any legal or equitable action as it considers appropriate. IN WITNESS WHEREOF, EMPLOYER has hereunto caused its corporate name to be signed and sealed, and Employee has hereunto set her hand, all being done in duplicate originals, with one original being delivered to each party as of the day and year first above written.

EMPLOYER, INC.

By:_____
EMPLOYER

_____
Employee

(From Hamric AB, Spross JA, Hanson CM: *Advanced practice nursing: an integrative approach,* ed 3, St. Louis, 2005, Saunders.)

CONTRACT NEGOTIATION FOR NURSE PRACTITIONERS

AUTHORED BY AMERICAN ACADEMY OF NURSE PRACTITIONERS

COMMITTEE ON PRACTICE: CHAIR, MARGARET FRIEL, STAFF LIAISON,

JAN TOWERS, LENORE RESICK, MARY JO GOOLSBY, EVELYN JACKSON,

NORANN PLANCHOCK, SUE TANNER, BARBARA WEIS

Preparation is very important to the nurse practitioner hoping to conduct a successful interview and negotiate an employment contract. When preparing for an interview, it is helpful to utilize one's personal, professional, and community network to gather information about health care practices in the area. It is important to be prepared to discuss the financial benefits a nurse practitioner can offer to the practice as well as improved quality of care, higher patient satisfaction and more flexibility for the physician. Spending a day observing a practice site can help you make decisions regarding your participation in that practice.

A professional resume should be prepared and submitted at the time of the interview. Written employment contracts are important, providing protection for both the nurse practitioner and the employer. Prior to signing a final agreement, the services of an attorney with experience writing medical or nurse practitioner contracts should be retained. In addition, the following factors should be considered.

1. **Nurse Practice Act**
   Do your homework first regarding the state practice act.
   a) Make sure you are familiar with the scope of practice in the state and the steps needed to be legally licensed and to renew your license.
   b) Be familiar with the regulations pertaining to nurse practitioner practice in your state where you will be practicing.
   c) Know the parameters of prescriptive authority in your state.
   d) Know the collaboration (if any) requirements with physicians.

2. **Practice Setting**
   Before scheduling an interview seek answers to the following questions:
   a) What type of practice is this? Family? Specialty? Rural health?
   b) Does this practice employ other nurse practitioners?
   c) Does the practice accept Medicaid patients, Medicare patients?
   d) Is this practice supportive of the role of the nurse practitioner?
   e) What is the reputation of the practice in the community?
   Questions to be considered during interviews or negotiations are:
   a) How much autonomy will you as a nurse practitioner have?
   b) Will the nurse practitioner be recognized as a primary care provider?
   c) Will you be able to practice at your full scope of practice?
   d) What is the practice mix? Physicians, other providers, support staff?
   e) What is the practice's philosophy of patient care? Does the practice support patient education, health promotion, and disease prevention? Does it participate in community outreach?
   f) Is the practice site supportive of clinical research? Precepting students? Participation in teaching or presenting papers or posters at conferences?
   g) Will there be opportunities for hospital admissions? What is the reputation of the hospital where you would be admitting patients?
   h) What percent of your time will be directed toward administrative duties and what will they entail?
   i) Are there organization policies in place such as grievance procedures?
   j) What are the expectations for taking call? Working evenings or weekends? Making hospital rounds?
   k) Are there any special skills or training required for this job? (e.g. suturing, ACLS)
   l) Is patient satisfaction evaluated?
   m) What method of performance evaluation is in place for the NP?
   n) What kind of support staff would be suitable for you?

Personal Inventory

The following is a comprehensive tool that may be used to evaluate your needs and desires in an employment or contractual arrangement.

PERSONAL EMPLOYMENT ASSESSMENT

1. I plan to join a _____ practice.
   (Type)
2. I prefer a payment plan of salary only _____, salary with productivity based pay _____, hourly contract _____.
3. I am willing to take call _____, willing to work evenings _____, willing to work week-ends _____, willing to make hospital rounds _____.
4. I am willing to travel _____ miles to my practice site.
5. Rate the following in order of importance from 1-9 with 1 being the most important and 9 being the least:
   - a. Autonomy of Practice _____
   - b. Ready access to physician _____
   - c. Ready access to laboratory _____
   - d. Rural Setting _____
   - e. Urban Setting _____
   - f. Working with other NPs _____
   - g. Working alone _____
   - h. Autonomy of Patient Scheduling _____
   - i. Compensation _____

6. Rate the following (1) must; (2) would like to have; (3) not necessary
   - a. Benefits _____
   - b. CEU Allotment _____
   - c. Paid time off for attending professional meetings _____
   - d. Malpractice Insurance _____
   - e. Retirement _____
   - f. Profit Sharing _____
   - g. Professional dues paid _____
   - h. Flexible scheduling _____
   - i. Disability insurance _____
   - j. Paid personal days _____
   - k. Paid sick days _____
   - l. Paid vacation   2 weeks _____ 3 weeks _____ 4 weeks _____
   - m. Paid health insurance   Personal _____ Family _____
7. I am most comfortable working with those who exhibit the following characteristics:
   _____
   _____
8. My greatest strength is _____
9. An area of weakness that I plan to change to a strength is _____
10. I plan to renegotiate my contract in _____

Modified with permission from Wilson, Shala, ANP-C, CS (2001) Personal Employment Plan

3. **Negotiation Tips**

Negotiation Strategies include the following:

    a. The goal to negotiation is to create a "win-win" situation. Each of you has something to offer: they a job, and you, your expertise. Look to see how you both can mutually benefit. That way each of you wins.

    b. If possible don't make the first offer; it is better to know what they're offering in order to present a counter offer.

    c. If the first offer seems generous and it is to your liking, take time to think it over.

    d. Know what will be the least you need in order to accept the job and what is considered your walk away point.

    e. Salary negotiations go hand in hand with your benefit package and hours of employment.

4.   Negotiating Compensation

    Determining Worth of Service: When negotiating contracts, it is important to determine both the amount of income that the nurse practitioner may bring into the practice and the associated cost to the practice. While there will be variability among practices due to the specialty, the location and the outstanding debts of the practice, the following guidelines will help you determine what compensation you might be able to contract.

    The federal government focuses on three elements when determining compensation for medical services provided: cost of service (the cost of compensating the clinician providing the service); the practice overhead (includes utilities, rent, supplies, payment to support staff, etc); malpractice insurance. While the formula used for Medicare reimbursement has been based on a percentage of 48% service, 48% overhead and 4% malpractice insurance, these percentages may vary from practice to practice. (See attached example from one primary care practice.)

    a. Ask for the percentage of practice income that goes for overhead expenses. Be sure to ask what the practice includes in the category of "overhead" expenses.

    b. Generally a private practice will wish to net some profit from your participation. A general figure is 15-20%. Determine if that is the case in the practice you are considering. Is this included in the overhead cost quoted to you?

    c. Determine if a percentage of your gross receipts are expected to be used for physician consultation. (Seasoned nurse practitioners may expect to pay 10-15% of their gross receipts for this service.) Is it included in the overhead cost quoted to you?

    d. It will be important to be able to access your productivity data within the practice.

Determine how this will be accomplished in the practice site you are considering.

DETERMINING ARNP WORTH OF SERVICE

The data in this example was provided by a nurse practitioner employed in an internal medicine practice in a small city in Kentucky. The income projected is based on the amount actually received by the practice for the nurse practitioner visits. Twenty five percent of the patients have Medicare; 65% have a HMO or PPO; and 10% have commercial insurance.

The nurse practitioner saw 18 patients per day. Two were new patients; sixteen were established patients. Of the established patients, two were Level 2 visits, seven were Level 3, three were Level 4, and four were annual physicals (Level 5). There were also charges for two EKGs and three microscopic urinalyses.

The nurse practitioner generated income of $1075 per day - $5375 per week – and $258,000 per year (assuming 48 weeks worked).

The following chart illustrates the costs incurred by the internal medicine practice to employ the ARNP. Overhead costs include additional supplies and equipment needed, plus two full-time employees at $10 per hour to support the nurse practitioner (a nursing assistant and clerical help).

COST TO PRACTICE TO EMPLOY ARNP

Salary	$80,000
FICA	6,120
Health Insurance	4,000
Malpractice Insurance	504
Continuing Education	2,000
401K	3,200
Professional org/license	150
	95,974
Overhead	54,446
Expense to Practice	150,420
Income Generated by ARNP	258,000
Profit to Practice	**$107,580**

Patient Care/Practice Expectations
  a. Determine the number of patients the nurse practitioner is expected to see, remembering that a new graduate will need more time in the first six months of practice. It will also help to find out what the most frequently billed CPT codes are for the practice and the amount received for those codes.
  b. If you are expected to take call or make hospital rounds, determine what percent of the other practice provider's salaries are attributed to this activity. You would expect to receive a like percentage if you take rotation with other providers.
  c. If you are to be salaried and your clinical and administrative schedule requires longer days or evening hours, you may wish to negotiate a half-day off/week to compensate for this time.

Bonus/Productivity Payment
  a. Negotiating a bonus payment system may be important, particularly as the nurse practitioner develops a large patient base. Bonus formulas can be based on productivity, quality, profit or patient satisfaction. If a patient satisfaction based formula is agreed upon, using a satisfaction tool is helpful in determining the bonus formula.
  b. A productivity-based bonus may be appropriate if the nurse practitioner is on at least a 50% fee-for-service system. Formulas are usually based on number of patient visits per year. Quality based bonus payments may be more practical under a capitated system where profit is measured by maintaining high quality care in as few visits as possible. In this case bonuses should be awarded for meeting or exceeding quality standards.

Profit Sharing
  When negotiating profit sharing, it is important that the language regarding the determination of the profit share is clear. It is important to negotiate the right to access the company audit and a method for handling disputes.

5. **Benefit Negotiations**
  The following benefits as a salaried employee should be included:

   a. Health Insurance. Health insurance is an ever-rising cost of business. If you need family coverage make sure that it is a part of your benefits, even if you would have to pay the additional costs. Some employers also have dental and eye coverage for their employees.

   b. Vacation. Vacation benefits should include at least three to four weeks a year.

   c. Sick Leave. Sick leave is generally two weeks or one day per month per year.

   d. Travel. Ask about travel allowance if house calls or travel to other clinics is expected.

   e. Continuing Education. Continuing education allowance and paid leave. One to two conferences per year is not inappropriate; be sure to include enough in allowances to allow for airfare, room and food for at least one national conference. (An allowance of $1500 to $2500 for this purpose is not unreasonable.)

   f. Malpractice Insurance. With malpractice insurance coverage, ask if it is an occurrence or claims made type of policy and ask the amount of coverage. Negotiate for a malpractice policy that is an occurrence policy for at least $1 million per claim and $3 million aggregate.

   g. Fees. Membership in professional organization; licensure, and DEA fees should be paid.

   h. Subscriptions. Office subscription to appropriate nurse practitioner journal.

   i. Retirement Plans. Retirement plans including employer's contribution and years when vested needs to be determined.

   j. Disability Insurance. Disability insurance is a benefit you may want to negotiate, especially if you are the major income producer in your family.

6. Contract Restrictions

   a. Some employment contracts include a clause regarding restrictions on competition. A restrictive covenant restricts an employee from setting up a practice within a specified geographic area for a specified number of years. After leaving the practice the concerns of losing business if an NP moves to another practice nearby has made this inclusion a greater demand.

      1.) Restrictive covenants are considered legal and can be enforced as long as they are reasonable. If this covenant is challenged in a court of law, the judge will determine the outcome. The judge will consider the needs of the public versus the harm to the employer.

      2.) The restrictive covenant may be a fact of life, so decide if this is an area that as a NP you may be willing to give up realizing that you may have to trade-off other practice opportunities in order to get a reasonable contract.

   b. A contract may include language regarding termination clauses. A contract may list specific reasons for termination with cause such as should the NP become disabled, lose their license, be convicted of a felony, etc. A termination without cause contract doesn't give the NP any job security and is not considered prudent for a NP.

   c. Avoid contracts that include clauses that give the employer or contractor the right to make modifications at their discretion without notice.

   d. Avoid contracts that do not have renewal clauses.

   e. A lawyer knowledgeable in contract law should be consulted.

References

1. American Academy of Nurse Practitioners.
   Web access http.//www.aanp.org/contracting.htm
2. American Nurses Association (2000), Negotiations 101, CE Workplace Advocacy Alternative Dispute Resolutions, An Overview.
   Washington, DC: American Nurses Association
3. Apcock, G (1995). Negotiating an employment contract. <u>Nurse Practitioner</u>, 20(6), 22-23.
4. Buppert, C. (1997). Employment agreements: cause that can change an NP's life. <u>The Nurse Practitioner</u> 22(8), 108-119.
5. Buppert, Carolyn. Nurse practitioner's business practice and legal guide Chapter 10 <u>The Employed Nurse Practitioner</u>, Chapter 10, 277-305.
6. Campbell, K. (1993). Evaluation a private practice for employment. <u>Journal of Pediatric Health Care</u>. September-October 240-241
7. Giovino, J. M. (1999). You can't always get what you want…but sometimes you can, <u>Family Practice Management</u> Dec. 1-5.
8. Henry, P. (1995). The nurse practitioner's guide to practice agreements. <u>Nurse Practitioner Forum</u> Vol 6, No. 1, 4-5
9. Herman, JA. Selph A, Knox M, Nussbaum, J, Franklin R. (1998).
   Negotiating for ACNPs: creating a powerful position. R. Kleinpell and M. Piano, eds. <u>Practice Issues for the Acute Care Nurse Practitioner.</u>
   New York: Springer
10. Mangan, D. (2001). Shape a contract you'll be glad you signed. <u>MedicalEconomics</u>. January 8, 79-84
11. Millers, S. (2000). Negotiating your salary. <u>Patient Care for Nurse Practitioners 72</u>.
12. Porter-O'Grady, T. (1996). Consider this ……The business of partnership.
    <u>Advanced Practice Nurse Quality</u>. Volume 2, 81-82
13. Wilson, S. (2001). Personal Employment Plan

SAMPLE ADVANCED PRACTICE NURSE CONTRACT

Employment Agreement Between Central City Health Systems and Carol Jean Cusack, Pediatric Nurse Practitioner

C arol Jean Cusack, hereinafter referred to as "PNP," agrees to employment and duties of pediatric nurse practitioner at Central City Health Systems, hereinafter referred to as "CCHS." The clinical practice of the named practitioner will be limited to the primary care of and minor urgent treatment of children patients of CCHS, seen within the context of the family care philosophy espoused by CCHS, in a collaborative relationship with W. Harvey Doe, MO, FAAP and Mary Beth Jones, MD.

Schedule: PNP accepts employment for 40 hours per week scheduled Monday through Friday 9:30 AM to 5 PM at the CCHS practice site. PNP will be expected to make AM hospital rounds In the newborn nursery at Central City Hospital, said rounds to include education of parent of newborns born in the last 24 hours to patients of the CCHS practice. This obligation at Central City Hospital will occur before the 9:30 AM hour. This schedule may be modified with mutual agreement by both parties. In situations where the final patient has not been seen by 5 PM on any given day, PNP may agree to stay overtime (not to exceed a total of 48 hours per week) for an additional payment of $35.00 per hour. There are no weekend work or call hours required during this contract period.

Salary: The base salary shall be $55,880.00 annually, payable in equal increments of $1/24$ on the first and third Thursdays of each month. Adjustments to this salary base will be made at the minimum of 5% annually, coinciding with the initial date of employment. CCHS will pay additional $5.00 per patient in excess of 5000 patients at the end of the calendar year, the payment being made as a bonus check on December 20. All other adjustments in salary, except as outlined above, will be negotiated at the end of the annual performance evaluation and will commence with the first pay check of the following month.

OTHER EMPLOYMENT BENEFITS

Health Insurance—PNP agrees to participate in the medical and dental options of Monmart Health Insurance Plan at the rate of $23.42 per pay period, to be matched equally by CCHS. Details of health insurance coverage will be described in a separate contract with Monmart Health Insurance Plan.

Retirement—CCHS agrees to contribute $150.00 per month toward PNP's retirement plan beginning after the first 90 days of employment by CCHS, so long as the retirement plan in effect conforms to the guidelines of the U.S. Internal Revenue Service.

Paid Leave—CCHS agrees to pay 8 days salary for leave due to illness and an additional 2 days salary for "unspecified" leave annually. If all 10 days are not used by December 31, CCHS agrees to compensate PNP in dollars or time off at the discretion of PNP. Any dollar amount will be paid in the first pay check of January.

Paid Holidays—CCHS agrees to pay for the following holidays when the practice is closed: January 1, Martin Luther King Day, July 4, Labor Day, Thanksgiving Day, the day after Thanksgiving, Christmas Eve, and Christmas Day. CCHS further agrees to pay for a holiday on PNP's birthday each year.

Vacation—CCHS agrees to paid time off for PNP for vacation 10 days annually (2 work weeks) after the first 6 months of employment. After 2 years, paid vacation will increase to 15 days and after 4 years, paid vacation will increase to 20 days per year. Paid vacation will not increase thereafter.

Continuing Education—CCHS agrees to 5 days paid time off for PNP's participation in continuing education courses and will pay a maximum of $1500.00 annually for tuition. Other expenses related to continuing education will be the obligation of PNP.

Malpractice Insurance—CCHS will pay for an occurrence-based insurance policy in the amount of $3 million per occurrence, $5 million total claims per year. Insurance carrier may be chosen by PNP. The total amount of said policy will be paid on the day this contract commences and annually thereafter for the duration of employment. It is the obligation of PNP to submit necessary documentation for said payment to office manager in advance of the due date each year.

Professional Licensure and Recertification—CCHS agrees to pay the fees associated with renewal of the RN license every 2 years in accordance with Board of Nursing policy and renewal of PNP certification as designated by the certifying organization, not to exceed a maximum of $350.00 in a 3-year period. PNP is obligated to provide documentation to enable such payments in advance of the due date.

Loan Repayment—In lieu of a first-year bonus, except as otherwise specified in this agreement, CCHS agrees to repay the educational loan of $2680.60 in

PNP's name at First National Bank. The full amount is due on the day after the 90-day probationary period for PNP ends.

CONTRACTUAL AGREEMENT

A probationary period shall extend from the day this agreement commences to 90 days thereafter, during which time either party may terminate this agreement with a 72-hour notice; thereafter, a 30-day written notice of such termination shall be required by either party. CCHS reserves the right to compensate PNP for 3 days' salary in lieu of 72-hour notice or with 1 month's salary in lieu of the 30-day written agreement.

PNP will receive a written performance evaluation from the collaborating physicians at the end of the probationary period, 6 months and annually or as otherwise requested by either party. PNP will receive a copy of the criteria for performance evaluation in advance of such evaluation.

This employment agreement renews itself automatically on a monthly basis until either party serves notice to terminate in accord with procedures designated in this agreement, or employment of PNP may be terminated with cause with a 24-hour notice in the event of conviction of a felony, loss of license to practice as an APN, or gross negligence that compromises the safety of CCHS patients or staff.

_____

Signature of PNP

_____

Date

_____

Signature of CEO of CCHS

_____

Date

(From Robinson D, Kish CP: *Core concepts in advance practice nursing,* St. Louis, 2001, Mosby.)

Sample Business Plan*

A Business Plan for a Not-For-Profit Venture Presented to the Central State Medical Center Foundation by Ann Logue, RNC, MSN, CNS, and Frances Holden, RN, MSN, CNS for Seed Funding for Central City Parent Support Group

EXECUTIVE SUMMARY

Last year in this city, 151 childbearing couples were discharged from a hospital without their baby because of a stillbirth, early pregnancy loss, or newborn death. These individuals went home to face one of the most devastating of personal tragedies without continuity of care from the health professional community. With a support group in place, this would not have been the case. Healthy grief resolution might have been facilitated and complicated grief quickly identified and referred for appropriate therapy. This plan is for a group that will belong to the community. It has no direct hospital affiliation but does enjoy the support of all three hospitals in the city.

The Central City Parent Support Group proposes to serve local couples and their peers in the counties contiguous to Montgomery by providing a professionally led, mutual self-help support group that meets monthly but allows ongoing access to the group network via telephone. The meeting place on the St. Mary's Medical Center campus has been donated. The APNs who will serve as co-leaders are volunteering their time and expertise, as are other members of the professional team. All team members have academic and experiential preparation appropriate to meet the mission of the proposed support group— to provide continuity of planned grief intervention for couples experiencing perinatal loss, with the ultimate goal of healthy grief resolution.

Financial assistance in the form of "seed money" is being requested from the Community Service Account of the Foundation of Central State Medical Center for a total 3-year amount of $2357.50, all of which will be devoted to either a lending library for group members or to marketing the enterprise. The first year's projected budget is $1857.50, which would have been an investment of $12.30 for each of the 151 couples who suffered perinatal losses in Montgomery last year.

The addition of this postvention (post-event intervention) service will add a primary prevention measure that has the potential to affect the mental health of hundreds of childbearing families annually and to make subsequent childbearing emotionally easier.

THE BUSINESS AND THE MARKET

The Central City Parent Support Group is a professionally led, voluntary, confidential, mutual self-help group without cost, composed of couples and their significant others who have experienced a perinatal loss. *Perinatal loss* refers to a loss associated with stillbirth, miscarriage, or other early pregnancy losses (e.g., ectopic pregnancy, elective medical termination), or newborn death. This is not a therapy group. Group members who need therapeutic intervention beyond the scope of the group's co-leaders will be referred to appropriate providers for such intervention.

There is no other support group of this type in the city of 619,000 or in its contiguous counties. One group in this city, Compassionate Friends, serves the needs of parents grieving the loss of a child of any age. However, perinatal loss has some unique components, and its grief-counseling model is different than those for other losses. The Central City Parent Support Group will meet the unique needs of a particular population not being addressed by the existing group.

National statistics on perinatal loss indicate that the stillbirth rate is 1.2%, early known pregnancy loss is 20% or greater, and the newborn death rate is 1.6%. See Table F-1 for a translation of those statistics in reference to Central City.

TABLE F-1			
Perinatal Loss Statistics for Central City: 1996-1998*			
TYPES OF LOSS	1996	1997	1998
Stillbirths	24	21	27
Early pregnancy loss at less than 20 weeks gestation	96	107	116
Newborn deaths	9	6	8

*Does not reflect losses in situations without hospital admission. Data provided by hospital liaison personnel.

This data represents 634 total losses; when both members of the childbearing couples are considered, this accounts for 1268 parents experiencing perinatal loss in the last 3 years. These data do not begin to reflect grandparents or others who might profit from grief support, nor do they represent losses that occur without a requisite hospital admission or those that occurred in contiguous counties within commuting distance of a support group. If, as empirical study suggests, 10% of affected individuals attend a support group, the numbers show the value of a perinatal grief group in the city.

As an open self-help group, couples can enter at any point in their grief experience and stay for as long as needed. Consequently, the group will continue to evolve over time. As they begin to heal, the couple in the group will serve as a self-help network to other couples and as panel members for training health care professionals and medical and nursing students to better understand perinatal loss and grief resolution.

OBJECTIVES

The purpose of the Central City Parent Support Group is to provide continuity of planned grief intervention for couples experiencing perinatal loss, with the ultimate goal of healthy grief resolution. To that end, the objectives are as follows:

- Provide emotional support while creating a context for learning about how to cope with the profound grief associated with perinatal loss.

- Enable individuals who have experienced perinatal loss to come together in a safe, nonjudgmental, and confidential forum for the purpose of sharing their mutual concerns.

- Provide an atmosphere where group members can develop sensitivity to the needs and feelings of others and come to recognize the universality of emotion, even as they are being supported in gaining insight into their own loss.

After the initial 6 months, the effectiveness of the group method as a post-vention strategy for grief resolution will be monitored by member survey. This data and the numbers of participants will be documented and shared with obstetrical services at the area hospitals. Data will be presented only in aggregate form to protect individual confidentiality of group members. Annual evaluation will commence on the 1-year anniversary date of the group's formation.

In the second year and thereafter, nursing and medical students will be allowed to observe the group with permission of the participants and a vow of confidentiality. No more than two students will be allowed to attend any session. Student requests for experience in the group will be managed by Ann Logue.

MANAGEMENT

Group Co-leaders

Ann Logue, RN, MSN, CNS: Holds a Master's degree in nursing with specialization in perinatal nursing and is nationally certified as a CNS and a perinatal grief counsellor and coordinator; has 14 years of clinical experience in hospital and community settings with obstetrical patients and families and currently works as a clinical specialist in the perinatal services division of Central State Medical Center; has served as a consultant on varied aspects of obstetrical care, authored two articles, presented at numerous professional conferences, and served as a clinical faculty member for both nursing and medical students; MSN thesis topic dealt with *The Lived Experience of Losing a First-Born Child*; has had graduate level coursework in group dynamics.

Frances Holden, RN, MSN, CNS: Holds a Master's degree in nursing with a specialization in mental health/psychiatric nursing and is nationally certified in that area of specialization; has 17 years of clinical experience with populations experiencing emotional crises and mental illness; currently employed as a certified CNS at Central State Medical Center where she is the mental health liaison nurse for the hospital; has served as a clinical faculty member for both medical and nursing students, authored several manuscripts related to emotional crisis and mental health, and served as consultant and presenter on related topics; has also taught courses in group dynamics and led support groups over her years of clinical practice; also brings personal perspective to her role as group leader, having experienced a perinatal loss herself.

Referral Team

In the event that group members need intervention beyond the scope of professional practice of the APN co-leaders of the support group, the following individuals have agreed to accept referrals. Compensation for services will be negotiated with individuals who need ongoing intervention with these health professionals, but a one-time referral visit will be granted at no cost. All have also agreed to serve as consultants to the group and to provide 30-minute didactic sessions on occasion to the group.

John Lacosse, MD: Psychiatrist with 31 years of clinical experience; currently serves as chief of Mental Health Services, Central State Medical Center

Susan Gill, MSW: Licensed social worker assigned to the Maternity Pavilion at St. Mary's Medical Center; has 6 years of clinical practice experience, with a focus on social work interventions for childbearing families.

Patty Micheli, MD, FACOG: Board-certified OB/GYN with 8 years of clinical practice; holds associate professor rank in the medical school at Central State University and has a private practice in the city with privileges at all hospitals serving obstetrical patients.

Other Personnel

John Paul Sorbin, CPA: Group volunteer; will provide annual review of financial records of the group.

Lydia Chastain, RNC, BSN, OB/GYN nurse manager, St. Mary's Medical Center: Group volunteer; will serve as hospital liaison with the support group

Betty Lou Jones, RN, OB/GYN nurse manager, Langley Community Hospital: Group volunteer; will serve as hospital liaison with the support group.

Geraldine Wentworth, RNC, MSN, patient care coordinator of Perinatal Services, Central State Medical Center: Group volunteer; will serve as hospital liaison with the support group.

SERVICE DESCRIPTION

When the mysteries of birth and death coincide in the case of perinatal loss, couples are forced to shift quickly from preparing for a normal, happy childbirth to dealing with the life-shattering loss of a baby. All three hospitals in the city—St. Mary's Medical Center, Langley Community Hospital, and Central State Medical Center—have effective inpatient grief support programs in place that are based on national standards of care. Even smaller hospitals in the contiguous counties have similar programs, thanks to the perinatal outreach efforts of Central State Medical Center. However, at present, there is no continuation of planned intervention for these couples—no planned follow-up with health care providers until the medical check-up after miscarriage or childbirth at an interval of 4 to 6 weeks. Sending grieving couples home after perinatal loss without postvention negates what we know empirically to be true: that their journey of grief is just beginning. Moreover, research indicates that for some this journey will last up to 24 months.

When a couple experiences such a loss, emotional healing comes not from forgetting, but from remembering. A grief support group will facilitate the kind of remembering that enables healing and serves as a measure of primary prevention of mental health problems. This co-led self-help group will provide a monthly forum for couples to connect with professionals capable of facilitating grief resolution and with others who share the singleness of perinatal grief. The leaders will bring a practical wisdom borne of advanced education and their collective clinical experience to promote healthy coping with loss.

The group leaders will use the caring model, which involves caring without obligating others to reciprocate; nurturing; and personally committing to be present in the group setting and at other times by telephone. They will assume responsibility for helping couples gain the usual benefits of a grief support group: (1) instillation of hope that they can heal; (2) recognition that certain emotions are universally experienced by grieving couples; (3) information about how to adjust to loss, cope with holidays and other events, help family members cope, and plan for another pregnancy; (4) problem-solving related to grief and loss; (5) cohesion associated with a newly evolving network of peers; (6) expression of emotions in a cathartic way; and (7) examination of existential questions about life and loss.

MARKET ANALYSIS

The market for the Central City Support Group is patients of childbearing age and their family members in a six-county area who have sustained a perinatal loss and seek the services of a self-help group as a way of resolving their grief. The one support group in this area, Compassionate Friends, has as its mission serving patients who have lost children of any age. It is not perceived to be a directly competitive service because it does not deal exclusively with the unique needs inherent in situations of perinatal loss.

MARKETING STRATEGY

The support group will meet monthly on the third Tuesday evening of the month, from 7:30 PM until 9:00 PM in the Women's Center reception room of Building C at St. Mary's Medical Center. This space, provided free of charge, is a comfortable, homelike reception area designed for women awaiting non–pregnancy-related diagnostic tests. It is not used in the evenings. The location is distant enough from the obstetrical service and Lamaze classrooms that patients will not encounter painful reminders while going to and from meetings. There is free adjacent parking in a well-lighted lot. Restrooms, public telephones, and snack machines are located nearby.

Prospective group members will learn about the group in the following ways:

- Printed notices will be provided in the packet of materials given to couples experiencing perinatal loss in all hospitals in the city and all those served by the perinatal outreach program of Central State Medical Center. Verbal referrals will be made by hospital staff members working with these couples.

- A reminder of the group meeting will be printed monthly in the Support Group section of the *Montgomery Telegraph and News*.

- Co-leaders will be interviewed about the group 2 weeks before the first meetings on the television programs "Mornings with Dell" on WGIX.

- Notices about the support group will be sent to all obstetricians in the city and five surrounding counties, along with a professional letter from the co-leaders asking for referrals.

- Notices about the support group will be sent to all mortuaries in the city and five surrounding counties, along with a professional letter asking that notices be provided to appropriate patients.

- Notices about the support group will be sent to all outpatient surgical centers in the area where patients experiencing early pregnancy loss might receive care.

- Co-leaders will provide 1-day sensitivity training sessions and participate in week-long training sessions annually for health professionals who care for this patient population. Written announcements about the group will be included in conference materials.

- The support group will be listed with the national RTS Bereavement Services office at LaCrosse Lutheran Hospital, Gundersen Clinic Ltd., LaCrosse, Wisconsin, as a potential referral site.

- The support group will be mentioned in all written public-service materials related to perinatal or obstetrical services at the city's three hospitals that provide such care.

FINANCIAL PROJECTIONS

There is no charge for participation in the support group; co-leaders are volunteering their time, as are other professionals. The meeting space is being provided without cost.

The financial needs for the first year reflect the purchase of books, pamphlets, and teaching materials for a lending library and storage for these library resources. Multiple copies of some of the items will be purchased. Other first-year needs include letterhead stationery and envelopes, note cards, and business cards. Financial needs during the second and third years will be upkeep of the lending library and replacement of the expendable supplies noted above ($250.00 per year). Funds are being requested in the following amounts from the Foundation of Central State Medical Center's Community Service Account. Funds will be maintained in the First National Bank of Montgomery.

TABLE F-2

Budget: Year One

ITEM	COST
Multiple copies of books and pamphlets for lending library	$1400.00
Lockable wooden bookcase for storage of lending library materials (to be housed in Women's Center reception area)	150.00
When a Baby Dies video	150.00
Stationery with letterhead (250 sheets)	32.50
Envelopes with logo (250)	44.00
Business cards (100)	18.50
Teaching kits on facilitating healing	62.50
TOTAL	$1857.50

SUMMARY

The Central City Parent Support Group is a voluntary, self-help group led by APNs with specialization in caring for this patient population. This is a group that belongs to the community; it does not have a hospital affiliation as such, but it does enjoy support from all hospitals in the city. The group will meet on a monthly basis in a donated space conducive to the group's purpose; group membership will be free. The primary mission of the group is helping couples experiencing the life-shattering experience of perinatal loss to resolve their grief in healthy ways. A secondary mission is to provide expertise and a forum for teaching prospective health care professionals about the unique dimensions of this kind of loss and how to intervene to facilitate healthy grief resolution. The requested funds are being devoted to marketing the group and providing a lending library for members on topics related to perinatal grief and coping.

---

*NOTE: Not included in this business plan are the Appendices for the CVs of the principals involved, details of the budget, and a copy of the letters and announcements in the marketing section.
From Robinson D, Kish CP: *Core concepts in advance practice nursing*, St. Louis, 2001, Mosby.

GLOSSARY OF TERMS FOR REIMBURSEMENT

GAIL P. BARKER • VALERIE LIGHT

Bundled services:

Clinical services are bundled together and billed at one price to a third party. An example of this might be a transplant. A package price is negotiated with a third party payer and only one claim is sent for all clinical services involved in the transplant. Payment for bundled services is distributed to the various clinical departments based on a prorated formula.

HCPCS*:

Healthcare Common Procedural Coding System. This is a unique 5-digit numeric or alpha-numeric code that describes a clinical service performed. There are three levels of HCPCS codes:

Level I—Current Procedural Terminology (CPT). A CPT is a unique five-digit code that describes the clinical service performed. A CPT describes "what" took place. Today most payers use the universal CPT codes developed by the American Medical Association.

Level II—National Codes. Alpha-numeric national codes are used primarily to report most medical services and supplies. Level II also includes modifiers. A modifier is a two-digit code added at the end of a procedure code (CPT) that can either affect payment or provide information only. More than one modifier can be appended to a CPT on a claim form. Modifiers are used to further describe services rendered. Two common modifiers are:

26—professional [interpretive] service

TC—technical or facility service

Level III—Local Codes. Alpha-numeric codes that are maintained by individual state Medicare carriers. Level III codes were scheduled to be eliminated as part of the implementation of HIPAA, which requires a standardization of procedure codes. However, the elimination has not yet been implemented (as of August 2006).

ICD-9-CM:

International Classification of Disease, 9th Revision, Clinical Manual. This is a three- to five-digit system that is used to code morbidity data for disease classification. If the CPT code describes "what" service took place, the ICD-9 code describes "why" the service took place. Today most payers in the United States use the universal ICD-9 codes to justify why a service (CPT) took place. ICD-10 is scheduled to be introduced in the next few years.

RBRVS:

Resource-Based Relative Value System. This is the basis for the physician Medicare fee schedule. It is made up of three parts: (a) work relative value, (b) practice expense relative value, (c) malpractice relative value unit. Each of these values are multiplied by the respective geographic adjustment factor and then added together to equal the aggregate relative value unit (RVU) for a specific area [(WRV × GAF) + (PERV × GAF) + (MRV × GAF)]. Each RVU is then multiplied by the national conversion factor. This calculation represents the reimbursement amount for each service (CPT) performed. Every CPT is assigned a different value resulting in a distinct reimbursement for each service.

Managed Care:

Managed care is the management of health care through quality and cost.* There are several types of managed care, and today managed care represents the most common health care payment method in most regions of the United States. The most popular managed care plans are listed below. In almost all cases managed care services are provided by practitioners enrolled in networks, and when patients stay within network, after co-insurance and deductible amounts (if applicable) are met, they are not billed for the balance of charges.

- **FFS (discounted fee for service):** reimbursement is derived from an agreed upon fee schedule (frequently established based on RBRVS). A practitioner or provider group agrees to accept the fee schedule for each clinical service performed. Service plans and preferred provider organizations (PPOs) generally operate under a fee-for-service structure.

- **HMO (health maintenance organization):** second most popular managed care option; based on a mutually agreed upon "capitated" monthly fee. This is generally a per-member–per-month (PMPM) amount that is paid to the provider regardless of the services performed. The PMPM is calculated based on demographic information such as gender and age. The concept is the practitioner and insurance company benefit if fewer health care services are provided; the patient benefits when premiums do not increase. HMOs can have open or closed panels. Open panels allow private practitioners to "join" the network and to see patients in their offices. Closed panels restrict services to only those providers who exclusively practice in the HMO. There are two basic types of HMO plans, traditional HMOs and open access HMOs. Traditional HMOs restrict service delivery (with some exceptions) to those providers who are part of the network. Primary care providers (PCPs) generally direct the care of the patient and authorize services to other [network] providers. With the exception of an emergency, if a patient self-refers or sees a provider outside of the network, he or she is responsible for the cost. In the open access model, members may access any network provider without an authorization from the PCP. What differentiates an open access HMO from a PPO is that providers share the cost risk in an open access HMO.

- **POS (point of service):** third most popular method; combines plans and allows members to choose which plan they will use at the time of service. A patient can self-refer and go "outside" of the managed care network for a higher out-of-pocket cost or stay within the network for a lower cost.

Third-Party Payer:

An organization that pays a patient's medical claims on their behalf. Two examples are insurance companies and correctional institutions. The patient generally pays a monthly premium for this coverage when it is an insurance company.

* Bench S, Magnani R, Parkinson J, editors: *2006 Professional: HCPCS, Level II,* Salt Lake City, 2005, Ingenix.

Practice Start-Up Timeline

❧

NINE MONTHS BEFORE PRACTICE START-UP

- Select a geographic location.
- Obtain contracts from third-party payers and hospitals you wish to join.
- Determine start-up costs of a practice and your net worth.
- Develop a business plan.
- Investigate sources of capital investment in your practice.
- Obtain loan applications, speak to various loan officers and submit applications.
- Determine when telephone books are printed and submit listing information for your practice.
- Open a business checking account.
- Obtain state nursing license, advanced practice license, and federal DEA number.
- Investigate potential physician collaborators if needed in your state.

SIX MONTHS BEFORE PRACTICE START-UP

- Investigate practice locations for rent or purchase.
- Inquire about zoning laws and signage requirements regarding your type of practice.
- Determine utility requirements for your practice and the sources and cost.
- Determine office layout, design, and necessary structural improvements.
- Determine needed office and medical equipment and determine cost of leasing versus buying.

- Explore and select business consultants, specifically a lawyer, accountant, banker, insurance broker, and medical biller.

- Determine form of the practice, such as solo practice, partnership, or corporation, and have your attorney draw up all legal documents for your signature.

- Evaluate all contracts *with your attorney* before signing.

- Investigate medical practice systems that include scheduling, billing, and records keeping.

- Apply for federal Medicare and Medicaid provider numbers and obtain fee schedules.

- Obtain CPT book and ICD-9-CM and the HCFA 1500 insurance claim forms.

- Formalize a collaborative agreement with an area physician if required by law.

- Apply for an office laboratory license or a CLIA waiver.

- Apply to managed-care provider panels for provider status.

- Apply to local health-care institutions for hospital privileges.

THREE MONTHS BEFORE PRACTICE START-UP

- Arrange for professional malpractice insurance for providers and liability insurance for the practice and equipment.

- Arrange for health and disability insurance for yourself and employees.

- Arrange for telephone service installation and an answering service for the practice, beeper service, and call-forwarding service.

- Order signage for the practice.

- Investigate and arrange for the acceptance of credit cards as a payment option.

- Design and order announcements for the opening of your practice.

- Apply for your federal and state EIN through your local IRS office and state labor department.

- Review federal and state tax requirements with your accountant and obtain booklets describing federal, state, and city tax withholding requirements.

- Develop a policy and procedure manual for the practice.

- Develop job descriptions for all employees.

- Begin advertising and interviewing for office personnel.

- Arrange for needed services such as biomedical waste management, specimen pick-up, janitorial services, laundry services, and ground maintenance and snow removal.
- Order clinical supplies and set up an inventory control system.
- Order business supplies such as state prescription pads (if mandated), appointment cards, business cards, letterhead stationary and envelops, stationery supplies, deposit stamp for checks, petty cash vouchers, purchase order forms, telephone message pads, and patient referral forms and disposition forms.
- Order office equipment and arrange for delivery.
- Determine office hours.
- Determine fee schedule.
- Develop advertising information such as a booklet of services for patients, press release announcing opening of practice, and introduction letters to local health care providers, pharmacy and medical equipment suppliers, and pharmaceutical representatives in your area.

ONE MONTH BEFORE PRACTICE START-UP

- Set up your office.
- Arrange for utility start-up including telephone, gas, electric, and water.
- Hire a medical biller and obtain your Medicare, Medicaid, and MCO provider numbers.
- Hire office personnel and train them with respect to office policies, telephone procedures, appointment scheduling and collection of fees, and use of the medical office system.
- Establish the office cash-flow procedures and a petty cash fund.
- Install your office sign.
- Accept patient appointments.
- Place announcements, advertisements, and press releases in local newspapers and distribute to local community groups and area professionals.

OPENING DAY

Congratulations, you have started an independent APN practice!

From Joel LA: *Advanced Practice Nursing: Essentials for Role Development,* Philadelphia, 2004, FA Davis. *CLIA,* Clinical Laboratory Improvement Amendments; *CPT,* current procedure terminology; *DEA,* Drug Enforcement Agency; *EIN,* employee identification number; *ICD-9-CM,* International Classification of Diseases, Ninth Revision, Clinical Manual; *IRS,* Internal Revenue Service; *MCO,* managed care organization.

RESOURCES FOR THE NURSE PRACTITIONER

CARDIOVASCULAR

- American College of Cardiology: *http://www.acc.org/*
- Society of Interventional Radiology: *www.sirweb.org*
- National Heart, Lung, and Blood Institute: *www.nhlbi.nih.gov/*

CASE STUDIES

- Association of Cancer Online Resources: *www.acor.org*
- Case Study RX: *https://eval.medinfo.ufl.edu/cgi-bin/eval.cgi?dr=casestudyrx*
- Johns Hopkins Medicine—Allergy &Clinical Immunology: *www.hopkinsmedicine.org/allergy/*
- Karolinska Institutet: Clinical Case Studies, Grand Rounds: *www.mic.ki.se/Medcases.html*
- Medical Simulations, Online Interactive Continuing Education Case Studies: *www.medicalsimulations.com/*
- University of Pittsburgh School of Medicine, Center for Continuing Education in the Health Sciences and the Department of Pathology: *https://secure.opi.upmc.edu/pathcme/index.cfm*
- University of Virginia Health System: *www.healthsystem.virginia.edu/internet/pediatrics (search words: case studies)*

CLINICAL RESOURCES

- Agency for Healthcare Research and Quality: *www.ahcpr.gov*
- Doctor's Guide: *www.docguide.com*
- eMedicine from WebMD: *www.emedicine.com*
- FDA Health Professional Site, online reporting of health issues: *http://www.fda.gov/ oc/oha/default.htm*
- HealthWeb: *http://healthweb.org/*
- Mayo Clinic: *www.mayoclinic.org*
- MedlinePlus: *www.nlm.nih.gov/medlineplus*
- National Heart, Lung, and Blood Institute—Clinical Practice Guidelines: *www. nhlbi.nih.gov/guidelines*

DERMATOLOGY

- American Academy of Dermatology: *www.aad.org*
- Electronic Textbook of Dermatology: *www.telemedicine.org/stamford.htm*
- Dermatology Image Atlas, Johns Hopkins University: *www.dermatlas.com/derm/*
- National Psoriasis Foundation: *www.psoriasis.org/*
- University of Iowa, Department of Dermatology: *http://tray.dermatology.uiowa. edu:80/Home.html*

DRUG INFORMATION AND THERAPIES

- The Stanford Health Library: *http://healthlibrary.stanford.edu/*
- Medscape Today: *www.medscape.com*
- U.S. Food and Drug Administration: *www.fda.gov/default.htm*

E-JOURNALS AND CONTINUING EDUCATION

- American Academy of Nurse Practitioners/AANP SmartBrief: *www.aanp.org*
- Advance for Nurse Practitioners: *http://nurse-practitioners.advanceweb.com/main.aspx*

- EMedicine (from WebMD): *www.emedicine.com*
- Family Practice News: *www.efamilypracticenews.com*
- Hardin MD, The University of Iowa: *www.lib.uiowa.edu/hardin/md*
- Medscape Med Students: *www.medscape.com/medstudents*

ELDERLY

- National Institute on Aging, Alzheimer's Disease Education & Referral Center: *www.nia.nih.gov/alzheimers*
- The American Geriatrics Society: *www.americangeriatrics.org/*
- National Conference of Gerontological Nurse Practitioners: *www.ncgnp.org/*
- National Institute on Aging: *www.nih.gov/nia*
- The Stanford Health Library/Senior Health: *http://healthlibrary.stanford.edu/resources/internet/bodysystems/seniors_intro.html*

EMERGENCY/ EMERGENCY PREPAREDNESS

- American Red Cross, Disaster Services: *www.redcross.org*
- American College of Emergency Physicians: *www.acep.org/webportal*
- CDC/Bioterrorism/Emergency Preparedness & Response: *www.bt.cdc.gov/bioterrorism*
- Department of Health & Human Services (DHHS)/Agency for Toxic Substances & Disease Registry: *www.atsdr.cdc.gov*
- US Department of Homeland Security/National Disaster Medical System: *http://www.oep-ndms.dhhs.gov/*
- US Environmental Protection Agency (EPA)/Office of Emergency Management/Chemical Emergency Preparedness & Prevention Office: *www.epa.gov/ceppo/*
- Federal Emergency Management Agency (FEMA)/Plan Ahead/Protect Your Family and Property: *www.fema.gov/plan/prepare/index.shtm*
- National Institutes of Health (NIH): *www.nih.gov/*
- U.S. Department of Labor/Occupational Safety & Health Administration (OSHA): *www.osha.gov/*

ENDOCRINOLOGY

- American Association of Clinical Endocrinologists: *www.aace.com*
- American Diabetes Association: *www.diabetes.org*
- The Endocrine Society: *www.endo-society.org/*
- The Stanford Health Library/Diseases and Disorders/Endocrine System: *http:// healthlibrary.stanford.edu/resources/internet/bodysystems/endocrine_intro.html*

GASTROENTEROLOGY

- American College of Gastroenterology: *www.acg.gi.org/*
- American Gastroenterological Association: *www.gastro.org/*
- American Liver Foundation: *www.liverfoundation.org/*
- HCV Advocate: *www.hcvadvocate.org/*
- Hepatitis C Association: *www.hepcassoc.org/*
- Hepatitis Foundation International: *www.hepfi.org/*

HOSPICE AND PALLIATIVE

- American Academy of Hospice and Palliative Medicine (AAHPM): *www. aahpm.org/*
- American Pain Society: *http://ampainsoc.org/*
- The EPEC Project, Education in Palliative and End-of-Life Care (EPEC): *www. epec.net/EPEC/webpages/index.cfm*
- Center for Palliative Care, Harvard Medical School: *www.hms.harvard.edu/cdi/ pallcare/*
- Hospice and Palliative Nurses Association: *www.hpna.org/*
- National Hospice and Palliative Care Organization: *www.nhpco.org/*

IMMUNOLOGY

- American Academy of Allergy, Asthma, and Immunology: *www.aaaai.org/*
- AIDS info: *www.aidsinfo.nih.gov/*

INFECTIOUS DISEASE AND EPIDEMIOLOGY

- Association for Professionals in Infection Control and Epidemiology: *www.apic.org*
- Centers for Disease Control and Prevention: *www.cdc.gov/*
- HIV Clinical Resource: *www.hivguidelines.org/Content.aspx*
- HIV InSite: *http://hivinsite.ucsf.edu/*

MEDICAL EQUIPMENT

- Allheart: *www.Allheart.com*
- NP Mall: *www.TheMalls.com*

MEN'S HEALTH

- The Stanford Health Library/Men's Health: *http://healthlibrary.stanford.edu/resources/internet/bodysystems/men_intro.html*

MENTAL HEALTH

- American Psychiatric Association: *www.psych.org*
- National Alliance on Mental Illness: *www.nami.org*

MISCELLANEOUS

- Almanacs, Atlas, Encyclopedia, and Dictionary: *www.infoplease.com/*
- American Medical Association: HIPAA updates: *http://www.ama-assn.org/ama/pub/category/4234.html*
- CNN Health News: *www.cnn.com/HEALTH/*
- One Look Dictionary Search: *www.onelook.com/*
- Health on the Net Foundation (HON): *www.hon.ch*
- Map Quest: *www.mapquest.com/*

- The Medem Network, Connecting Physicians and Patients Online (Provides secure e-mail connectivity): *www.medem.com*
- APJ (Advanced Practice Jobs): *www.advancedpracticejobs.com//advertising.php*
- The ePolicy Institute: *www.epolicyinstitute.com/*
- Virginia Commonwealth University (VCU), Internal Medicine: *http://www.intmed.vcu.edu/home/divisions/general.html*
- Yellow Pages: *www.infospace.com/*

NEUROLOGY

- American Council for the Blind: *www.acb.org/index.html*
- The National Eye Institute: *www.nei.gov*

NURSE PRACTITIONER SITES

- ADVANCE for Nurse Practitioners: *www.advanceweb.com*
- American Academy of Nurse Practitioners: *www.aanp.org*
- American College of Nurse Midwives: *www.acnm.org*
- American College of Nurse Practitioners: *www.acnpweb.org*
- American Nurses' Association: *www.nursingworld.org*
- American Nurses Credentialing Center: *www.nursingworld.org/ancc*
- Fitzgerald Health Education: *www.fhea.com*
- HealthyInfo: *www.healthyinfo.com*
- National Association of Nurse Practitioners in Women's Health: *www.npwh.org*
- National Conference of Gerontological Nurse Practitioners: *www.ncgnp.org*
- National Organization of Nurse Practitioner Faculties (NONPF): *www.nonpf.com*
- NP Central: *www.npcentral.net*
- Nurse Practitioner Association for Continuing Education: *www.npace.org*
- Uniformed Nurse Practitioner Association: *www.unpa.org*

OCCUPATIONAL HEALTH

- Occupational Safety and Health Administration (OSHA): *www.osha.gov*
- The National Institute for Occupational Safety and Health: *www.cdc.gov/niosh/homepage.html*

ONCOLOGY

- American Society of Clinical Oncology (ASCO): *www.asco.org*
- National Cancer Institute: *www.cancer.gov*
- OncoLink: *www.oncolink.com*

ORTHOPEDICS

- American Academy or Orthopedic Surgeons: *www.aaos.org*
- American Academy of Physical Medicine and Rehabilitation: *www.aapmr.org*
- American College of Rheumatology: *www.rheumatology.org*
- American College of Sports Medicine: *www.acsm.org*

PATHOLOGY

- College of American Pathologist: *www.cap.org/*

PATIENT SUPPORT LINKS AND EDUCATIONAL RESOURCES FOR THE PRACTITIONER

- Oregon Health Sciences University: Multilingual educational material: *www.ohsu.edu/library/patiented/links.shtml*
- Adam.com: *www.adam.com*
- Drkoop: *www.drkoop.com*
- Healthfinder: *www.healthfinder.gov*

- InteliHealth: *www.intelihealth.com*
- Mayo Clinic Health Oasis: *www.mayohealth.org*
- National Campaign to Prevent Teen Pregnancy: *www.teenpregnancy.org*
- OncoLink: *www.oncolink.com*
- Polycystic Ovarian Syndrome: Soul Cysters support site: *www.soulcysters.com*

PDA RESOURCES

- American Association of Critical Care Nurses: *http://.aacn.pdaorder.com/welcome.xml*
- CollectiveMed: *www.collectivemed.com*
- Dr.Gadget: *www.doctorsgadgets.com*
- Ectopic Brain: *http://.pbrain.hypermart.net*
- Epocrates: *www.epocrates.com*
- Franklin: Book reader software: *www.franklin.com*
- Freeware Home: *www.freewarehome.com*
- Handango: *www.handango.com/home.jsp?siteId=1*
- Handheldmed: *www.handheldmed.com*
- Healthy Palmpilot: *www.healthypalmpilot.com*
- Iscribe: Electronic prescription writing: *www.iscribe.com*
- Medical Pocket PC: *www.medicalpocketpc.com*
- PalmGear: *www.PalmGear.com*
- Palmzone: *www.palmzone.com/software.html*
- Patientkeeper: *www.patientkeeper.com*
- PDA Buyers Guide: *www.pdabuyersguide.com/tips/palm_vs_pocketpc.htm*
- PDA MD: *www.pdamd.com or http://acp.pdaorder.com/welcome.xml*
- PDx Handheld: *www.firstconsult.com/home/framework/fs_main.htm*
- Pocketgear: *www.pocketgear.com*
- Pocket PC Magazine: *www.pocketpcmag.com/*
- Statcoder: *www.statcoder.com*
- Skyscape: *www.skyscape.com*
- Zapmed: Program for point of service billing: *www.zapmed.com*

PEDIATRICS

- American Academy of Pediatrics: *www.aap.org*
- HealthWeb: *http://healthweb.org/*
- Keep Kids Healthy: *www.keepkidshealthy.com/*
- National Association of Pediatric Nurse Practitioners: *www.napnap.org*
- National Center for Missing and Exploited Children: *www.missingkids.org/ missingkids/servlet/PublicHomeServlet?LanguageCountry=en_US*
- National Clearinghouse on Child Abuse and Neglect: *http://nccanch.acf. hhs.gov/*
- The Stanford Health Library: *http://healthlibrary.stanford.edu/resources/internet/ bodysystems/childrenshealth.html*
- UCFF University of California School of Nursing: *http://nurseweb.ucsf.edu/www/ appnres.htm*
- Virtual Pediatric Hospital: *www.vh.org/pediatric/*

PODIATRY

- American Podiatric Medical Association: *www.apma.org*

POLITICAL RESOURCES

- Thomas Legislative Information on the Internet: *http://thomas.loc.gov*
- Michigan Legislature: *www.michiganlegislature.org*
- FirstGov: *www.firstgov.gov/Agencies/Federal/Legislative.shtml*

PRIMARY CARE

- Advance NP Complimentary Care Forum: *www.advancefornp.com/Common/ CompCareForum/Welcome.aspx*
- American Academy of Family Physicians: *www.aafp.org*
- American Academy of Physician Assistants: *www.aapa.org*
- Antibiotic Consult: *www.antibiotic-consult.com*

- Department of Transportation: Safety hotline/teaching tools: *www.nhtsa.dot. gov/hotline*
- Doctor's Guide: *www.docguide.com*
- Journal of the American Academy of Physician Assistants: *www.jaapa.com/ be_core/j/index.jsp*
- Patient Care for the NP: *www.patientcarenp.com/be_core/n/index.jsp*
- Patient Care Best Clinical Practices for Today's Physician: *www.patientcareonline. com/patcare/article/articleDetail.jsp?id=119753*
- Primary Care Internet Guide: *www.uib.no/isf/guide/family.htm*
- MD Consult: *www.mdconsult.com*

PULMONARY

- American Association of Respiratory Therapist: *www.aarc.org*
- American College of Chest Physicians: *www.chestnet.org*
- National Heart Lung Blood Institute: *www.nhlbi.nih.gov/*

RADIOLOGY

- American College of Radiology: *www.acr.org/flash.html*
- Society for Cardiovascular & Interventional Radiology: *www.scvir.org*

RESEARCH SITES

- Agency for Health Care Policy and Research Quality (AHRQ): *www.ahcpr.gov/*
- Centers for Disease Control and Prevention (CDC): *www.cdc.gov*
- Healthy People 2010: *www.healthypeople.gov/*
- Medscape: *www.medscape.com/px/urlinfo*
- National Institute of Health: *http://grants.nih.gov/grants*
- National Institute of Nursing Research: *http://ninr.nih.gov/ninr*
- National Occupational Research Agenda (NORA): *www.cdc.gov/niosh/nora/*
- National Library of Medicine's PUBMED: *www.nlm.nih.gov*

- Sigma Theta Tau International: *www.nursingsociety.org*
- Survey Monkey: Survey tool: *www.surveymonkey.com/home.asp*

SEARCH ENGINES AND SEARCH INFORMATION

- Alltheweb.com: *www.alltheweb.com*
- AOL Search internal: *http://search.aol.com/aolcom/index.jsp*
- Ask Jeeves: *www.askjeeves.com*
- Boston University Medical Center: Search engine guide and tutorial: *http://med-libwww.bu.edu/library/engines.html*
- Dogpile: *www.dogpile.com/*
- Google: *www.google.com*
- HotBot: *www.hotbot.com/*
- Medical Dictionary Meta-Search Engine (CDC, Joslin, NFB, NIDDK, & UL): *http://medical-dictionary-search-engines.com/diabetes/*
- MSN Search: *www.search.msn.com*
- Yahoo: *www.yahoo.com*

UNDERSERVED

- Association for Clinicians for Underserved: *www.clinicians.org*
- National Commission of Correctional Health Care: *www.ncchc.org*

UROLOGY

- Urology Associations/Societies/Foundations: *www.edae.gr/uro-ass.html*

WOMEN'S HEALTH

- Association of Reproductive Health Professionals: *www.arhp.org*
- Breast Feeding Basics: *www.breastfeedingbasics.org*

- Center for Applied Reproductive Science: *www.ivf-et.com*
- Contemporary OB/GYN: *www.contemporaryobgyn.net*
- Contraception Online: *www.contraceptiononline.org/*
- La Leche League: *www.lalecheleague.org/home_intro.html*
- National Association of Nurse Practitioners in Women's Health: *www.npwh.org*
- Obgyn: *www.obgyn.net/*
- National Campaign to Prevent Teen Pregnancy: *www.teenpregnancy.org*
- Polycystic Ovarian Syndrome Association: *www.pcosupport.org*
- The Stanford Health Library: *http://healthlibrary.stanford.edu/resources/internet/bodysystems/womenshealth.html*
- Washington State Midwives Health Care Resources and Web Sites: *www.midwivesofwa.org/online.htm*

From Nagelkerk J: *Starting your practice: a survival guide for nurse practitioners,* St. Louis, 2006, Mosby.

NATIONAL PROVIDER IDENTIFIER (NPI)

What an NP Must Know to Conduct Future HIPAA Standard Electronic Transactions

*T*he National Provider Identifier (NPI) numbers are a new identifier for use in standard electronic health care transactions. NPI will be the single provider identifier and will replace the various identifiers providers currently use for each health care plan with whom they do business. NPI implements a requirement of the Health Insurance Portability and Accountability Act of 1966 (HIPAA) and must be used by most HIPAA covered entities that conduct electronic standard transactions.[1]

The NPI is a 10-digit, intelligence-free number. Intelligence free means that the numbers do not carry information about health care providers. The NPI will replace health care provider identifiers in use today in HIPAA standard transactions such as Unique Physician Identifier Number (UPIN), Online Survey, Certification and Reporting (OSCAR), Personal Indentification Number (PIN), and National Supplier Clearinghouse, or NSC.[2]

An NPI number does not guarantee that a provider is licensed or appropriately credentialed, that payment will be made by a health plan, that a provider will be enrolled in a health plan, or require a provider to conduct HIPAA transactions. However, an NPI does simplify electronic transmission of HIPAA standard transactions, standardize unique identifiers for providers, health plans, and employers, and promotes more efficient coordination of benefits transactions.[2]

Nurse practitioners who conduct electronic standard transactions that fall under HIPAA, such as completing electronic claims, reimbursement remittance, and referral authorizations, will need to obtain an NPI number. Once an NPI number is obtained, a provider's NPI will not change, and the NPI remains with the provider regardless of any work or location changes.[1]

Nurse practitioners can apply for an NPI number in one of three ways:

- By utilizing the CMS web-based process at http://www.cms.hhs.gov and going to the link for the National Plan and Provider Enumeration System (NPPES)

- By filling out a paper NPI Application/Update form and mailing it to the Enumerator. This paper application is available online at: http://www.cms.hhs.gov/NationalProvIdentStand/Downloads/NPIapplication.pdf. See Appendix K for the NPI application/update form.

- By having their NPI application information, along with the application information for many other health care providers, submitted to NPPES on their behalf in an electronic file by an organization. This process is known as "electronic file interchange" (EFI) for bulk enumeration. Providers must give their permission for an organization to do this. This process is not yet available. For more detailed information on EFI, please refer to the EFI web section.[3]

The NPI must be used by HIPAA-covered entities such as health care providers who conduct HIPAA standard transactions and health care clearinghouses by May 23, 2007. Small health plans with less than 5 million dollars in annual revenues must use only the NPI by May 23, 2008.[2]

REFERENCES

1. McClellan M: *Dear Health Care Provider: National Provider Identifier Activities Begin in 2005*, Letter from the Administrator, Center for Medicare and Medicaid Services, May 6, 2006 (website): http://www.cms.hhs.gov/NationalProvIdentStand/Downloads/NPIdearprovider.pdf. Accessed July 20, 2006.
2. Center for Medicare and Medicaid Services: (Jan. 2006). The National Provider Identifier Fact Sheet., January 2006 (website): http://www.cms.hhs.gov/NationalProvIdentStand/downloads/npi_fs_geninfo_010906.pdf. Accessed July 20, 2006.
3. Center for Medicare and Medicaid Services: *National Provider Identifier: how to apply* (website): http://www.cms.hhs.gov/NationalProvIdentStand/03_apply.asp#TopOfPage. Accessed July 21, 2006.

DEPARTMENT OF HEALTH AND HUMAN SERVICES
CENTERS FOR MEDICARE & MEDICAID SERVICES

Form Approved
OMB No. 0938-0931

NATIONAL PROVIDER IDENTIFIER (NPI) APPLICATION/UPDATE FORM

Please PRINT or TYPE all information so it is legible. Do not use pencil. Failure to provide complete and accurate information may cause your application to be returned and delay processing of your application. In addition, you may experience problems being recognized by insurers if the records in their systems do not match the information you have furnished on this form.

SECTION 1 – BASIC INFORMATION

A. Reason For Submittal Of This Form (Check the appropriate box)

1. ❑ Initial Application
2. ❑ Change of Information (See instructions)
   NPI No._____

3. Deactivation NPI No._____
   REASON (Check one of the following)
   ❑ Death   ❑ Business Dissolved
   ❑ Other _____

B. Entity Type (Check the appropriate box)

1. ❑ An individual who renders health care. (Complete Sections 2A, 3, 4A and 5)
2. ❑ An organization that renders health care. (Complete Sections 2B, 3, 4B and 5)

SECTION 2 – IDENTIFYING INFORMATION

A. Individuals

1. Prefix (e.g.,Major, Mrs.)	2. First	3. Middle	4. Last
5. Suffix (e.g., Jr., Sr.)		6. Credential (e.g., M.D., D.O.)	

Other Name Information (If applicable. Use additional sheets of paper if necessary)

7. Prefix (e.g.,Major, Mrs.)	8. First	9. Middle	10. Last
11. Suffix (e.g., Jr., Sr.)		12. Credential (e.g., M.D., D.O.)	

13. Type of other Name
    ❑ Former Name   ❑ Professional Name   ❑ Other (Describe) _____

14. Date of Birth (mm/dd/yyyy)	15. State of Birth (U.S. only)	16. Country of Birth (If other than U.S.)

17. Gender
    ❑ Male   ❑ Female

18. Social Security Number (SSN)	19. IRS Individual Taxpayer Identification Number

B. Organizations and Groups

1. Name (Legal Business Name)	2. Employer Identification Number (EIN) or SSN

3. Other Name (Use additional sheets of paper if necessary)

4. Type of Other Name
   ❑ Former Legal Business Name   ❑ D/B/A Name   ❑ Other (Describe) _____

Form CMS-10114 (02/05) EF (05/2005)

1

SECTION 3 – ADDRESSES AND OTHER INFORMATION

A. Mailing Address Information

1. Mailing Address Line 1 (Street Number and Name or P.O. Box)

2. Mailing Address Line 2 (Address Information; e.g., Suite Number)

3. City	4. State	5. ZIP+4 or Foreign Postal Code

6. Country Name (if outside U.S.)

7. Telephone Number (Include Area Code & Extension)	8. Fax Number (Include Area Code)

B. Practice Location Information

1. Primary Practice Location Address Line 1 (Street Number and Name – P.O. Boxes Not Acceptable)

2. Primary Practice Location Address Line 2 (Address Information; e.g., Suite Number)

3. City	4. State	5. ZIP+4 or Foreign Postal Code

6. Country Name (if outside U.S.)

7. Telephone Number (Include Area Code & Extension)	8. Fax Number (Include Area Code)

C. Other Provider Identification Numbers (Use additional sheets of paper if necessary)

Number Type	Number	State (if applicable)	Issuer (Other type)
UPIN	_____		
Medicare	_____	_____	
Medicaid	_____	_____	
Other	_____	_____	_____
Other	_____	_____	_____

D. Provider Taxonomy Code (Provider Type/Specialty. Enter one or more codes) and License Number Information

Information on provider taxonomy codes is available at *www.wpc-edi.com/taxonomy*. Please see instructions if you plan to submit more than one taxonomy code for a Type 2 (organization) entity.

1. Primary Provider Taxonomy Code or describe your specialty or provider type (e.g., chiropractor, pediatric hospital)

☐☐☐☐☐☐☐☐☐☐

2. License Number	3. State where issued

4. Provider Taxonomy Code or describe your specialty or provider type (e.g., chiropractor, pediatric hospital)

☐☐☐☐☐☐☐☐☐☐

5. License Number	6. State where issued

7. Provider Taxonomy Code or describe your specialty or provider type (e.g., chiropractor, pediatric hospital)

☐☐☐☐☐☐☐☐☐☐

8. License Number	9. State where issued

PENALTIES FOR FALSIFYING INFORMATION ON THE
NATIONAL PROVIDER IDENTIFIER (NPI) APPLICATION/UPDATE FORM

18 U.S.C. 1001 authorizes criminal penalties against an individual who in any matter within the jurisdiction of any department or agency of the United States knowingly and willfully falsifies, conceals or covers up by any trick, scheme or device a material fact, or makes any false, fictitious or fraudulent statements or representations, or makes any false writing or document knowing the same to contain any false, fictitious or fraudulent statement or entry. Individual offenders are subject to fines of up to $250,000 and imprisonment for up to 5 years. Offenders that are organizations are subject to fines of up to $500,000. 18 U.S.C. 3571(d) also authorizes fines of up to twice the gross gain derived by the offender if it is greater than the amount specifically authorized by the sentencing statute.

SECTION 4 – CERTIFICATION STATEMENT

I, the undersigned, certify to the following:
- This form is being completed by, or on behalf of, a health care provider as defined at 45 CFR 160.103.

- I have read the contents of the application and the information contained herein is true, correct and complete. If I become aware that any information in this application is not true, correct, or complete, I agree to notify the NPI Enumerator of this fact immediately.

- I authorize the NPI Enumerator to verify the information contained herein. I agree to notify the NPI Enumerator of any changes in this form within 30 days of the effective date of the change.

- I have read and understand the Penalties for Falsifying Information on the NPI Application/Update Form as printed in this application. I am aware that falsifying information will result in fines and/or imprisonment.

A. Individual Practitioner's Signature

1. Applicant's Signature (First, Middle, Last, Jr., Sr., M.D., D.O., etc.)	2. Date (mm/dd/yyyy)

B. Authorized Official's Information and Signature for the Organization

1. Prefix (e.g.,Major, Mrs.)	2. First	3. Middle	4. Last
5. Suffix (e.g., Jr., Sr.)		6. Credential (e.g., M.D., D.O.)	
7. Title/Position		8. Telephone Number (Area Code & Extension)	
9. Authorized Official's Signature (First, Middle, Last, Jr., Sr., M.D., D.O., etc.)		10. Date (mm/dd/yyyy)	

SECTION 5 – CONTACT PERSON

A. Contact Person's Information

❑ Check here if you are the same person identified in 2A or 4B.
If you checked the box, complete only item 8, e-mail address in this section (Section 5).

1. Prefix (e.g.,Major, Mrs.)	2. First	3. Middle	4. Last
5. Suffix (e.g., Jr., Sr.)		6. Credential (e.g., M.D., D.O.)	
7. Title/Position	8. E-Mail Address		9. Telephone Number

For the most efficient and fast receipt of your NPI, please use the web-based NPI process at the following address: https://nppes.cms.hhs.gov. NPI web is a quick and easy way for you to get your NPI.

Or send the completed application to: NPI Enumerator
P.O. Box 6059
Fargo, ND 58108-6059

According to the Paperwork Reduction Act of 1995, no persons are required to respond to a collection of information unless it displays a valid OMB control number. The valid OMB control number for this information collection is 0938-0931. The time required to complete this information collection is estimated to average 20 minutes per response for new applications and 10 minutes for changes, including the time to review instructions, search existing data resources, gather the data needed, and complete and review the information collection. If you have any comments concerning the accuracy of the time estimate or suggestions for improving this form, please write to: CMS, Attn: Reports Clearance Officer, 7500 Security Boulevard, Baltimore, Maryland 21244-1850. Do not send the applications to this address.

PRIVACY ACT STATEMENT

Section 1173 of the Social Security Act authorizes the adoption of a standard unique health identifier for all health care providers who conduct electronically any standard transaction adopted under 45 CFR 162. The purpose of collecting this information is to assign a standard unique health identifier, the National Provider Identifier (NPI), to each health care provider for use on standard transactions. The NPI will simplify the administrative processing of certain health information. Further, it will improve the efficiency and effectiveness of standard transactions in the Medicare and Medicaid programs and other Federal health programs and private health programs. The information collected will be entered into a new system of records called the National Provider System (NPS), HHS/HCFA/OIS No. 09-70-0008. Institutional providers' data are protected by section 1106 of the Social Security Act and the Freedom of Information Act, while individually identifiable providers' data are protected by the Privacy Act of 1974.

Failure to provide complete and accurate information may cause the application to be returned and delay processing. In addition, you may experience problems being recognized by insurers if the records in their systems do not match the information you furnished on the form. (See the instructions for completing the NPI application/update form to find the information that is voluntary or mandatory.)

Information may be disclosed under specific circumstances to:

1. The entity that contracts with HHS to perform the enumeration functions, and its agents, and the NPS for the purpose of uniquely identifying and assigning NPIs to providers.
2. Entities implementing or maintaining systems and data files necessary for compliance with standards promulgated to comply with title XI, part C, of the Social Security Act.
3. A congressional office, from the record of an individual, in response to an inquiry from the congressional office made at the request of that individual.
4. Another Federal agency for use in processing research and statistical data directly related to the administration of its programs.
5. The Department of Justice, to a court or other tribunal, or to another party before such tribunal, when
   (a) HHS, or any component thereof, or
   (b) Any HHS employee in his or her official capacity; or
   (c) Any HHS employee in his or her individual capacity, where the Department of Justice (or HHS, where it is authorized to do so) has agreed to represent the employee; or
   (d) The United States or any agency thereof where HHS determines that the litigation is likely to affect HHS or any of its components
   is party to litigation or has an interest in such litigation, and HHS determines that the use of such records by the Department of Justice, the tribunal, or the other party is relevant and necessary to the litigation and would help in the effective representation of the governmental party or interest, provided, however, that in each case HHS determines that such disclosure is compatible with the purpose for which the records were collected.
6. An individual or organization for a research, demonstration, evaluation, or epidemiological project related to the prevention of disease or disability, the restoration or maintenance of health, or for the purposes of determining, evaluating and/or assessing cost, effectiveness, and/or the quality of health care services provided.
7. An Agency contractor for the purpose of collating, analyzing, aggregating or otherwise refining or processing records in this system, or for developing, modifying and/or manipulating automated data processing (ADP) software. Data would also be disclosed to contractors incidental to consultation, programming, operation, user assistance, or maintenance for ADP or telecommunications systems containing or supporting records in the system.
8. An agency of a State Government, or established by State law, for purposes of determining, evaluating and/or assessing cost, effectiveness, and/or quality of health care services provided in the State.
9. Another Federal or State agency
   (a) As necessary to enable such agency to fulfill a requirement of a Federal statute or regulation, or a State statute or regulation that implements a program funded in whole or in part with Federal funds.
   (b) For the purpose of identifying health care providers for debt collection under the provisions of the Debt Collection Information Act of 1996 and the Balanced Budget Act.

INSTRUCTIONS FOR COMPLETING
THE NATIONAL PROVIDER IDENTIFIER (NPI) APPLICATION/UPDATE FORM

Please PRINT or TYPE all information so it is legible. Do not use pencil. Failure to provide complete and accurate information may cause your application to be returned and delay processing of your application. In addition, you may experience problems being recognized by insurers if the records in their systems do not match the information you have furnished on this form.

This application is to be completed by, or on behalf of, a health care provider or a subpart seeking to obtain an NPI. (See 45 CFR 162.408 and 162.410 (a) (1).

SECTION 1 – BASIC INFORMATION
This section is to identify the reason for submittal of this form and the type of entity seeking to obtain an NPI.

A. Reason for Submittal of this Form
This section identifies the reason the health care provider is submitting this form. *(Required)*
1. **Initial Application**
   If applying for a NPI for the first time check box #1, and complete appropriate sections as indicated in Section 1B for your entity type.
2. **Change of Information**
   If changing information, check box #2, write your NPI number in the space provided, and provide the new/changed information within the appropriate section. See the instructions in Section 4, then sign and date the certification statement in Section 4A or 4B. All changes must be reported to the NPI enumerator within 30 days of the change. It is not necessary to complete sections that are not being changed; however, please ensure that your NPI number is legible and correct. Complete Section 5 so that we may contact you in the event of problems processing this form.
3. **Deactivation**
   Record the NPI number you want to deactivate and check box #3 indicating the reason. If you check Other, give reason; e.g., Fraudulent Use. Sign and date the certification statement in Section 4A or 4B, as appropriate. See instructions for section 4. Use additional sheets of paper if necessary.

B. Entity Type
Check the box that most applies to you or your organization. *(Required for initial applications)*
1. Individuals who render health care or furnish health care supplies to patients; e.g., physicians, dentists, nurses, chiropractors, pharmacists, physical therapists. Note that incorporated individuals may also obtain NPIs as type 2 organizations.
2. Organizations that render health care services, or furnish health care supplies to patients; e.g., hospitals, home health agencies, ambulance companies, health maintenance organizations, durable medical equipment suppliers, pharmacies.

SECTION 2 – IDENTIFYING INFORMATION

A. Individual
NOTE: An individual may obtain only one NPI, regardless of the number of taxonomies (specialties), licenses, or practice locations he/she may possess.
Name Information
1–6. Provide your full legal name. (Required first and last name) Do not use initials or abbreviations. If you furnish your social security number in block 19, this name must match the name on file with the Social Security Administration (SSA). In addition, the date of birth must match that on file with SSA. You may include multiple credentials. Use additional sheets of paper for multiple credentials if necessary.
Other name information *(Use additional sheets of paper if necessary)*
7-12. If you have used another name, including a maiden name, supply that "Other Name" in this area. (Optional) You may include multiple credentials. Use additional sheets of paper for multiple credentials if necessary.
13. Mark the check box to indicate the type of "Other Name" you used. (Required if 7-12 are completed)
14-16. Provide the date *(Required)*, State *(Required)*, and country *(Required, if other than U.S.)* of your birth. Do not use abbreviations other than United States (U.S.).
17. Indicate your gender. *(Required)*
18. Furnish your Social Security Number (SSN) for purposes of unique identification. *(Optional)* If you furnish your SSN, this name must match the name and date of birth on file with the Social Security Administration (SSA). If you do not furnish your SSN, processing of your application may be delayed because of the difficulty of verifying your identity via other means; you may also have difficulty establishing your proper identity with insurers from whom you receive payments. If you are not eligible for an SSN, see item #19.
19. Furnish your IRS Individual Taxpayer Identification Number (ITIN) if you do not quality for an SSN. *(Required, if the applicant has an ITIN)* You may not use an ITIN if you have an SSN. IRS issues ITINs to foreign nationals and others who have federal tax reporting or filing requirements and do not qualify for SSNs. Examples of individuals who need ITINs include:
   - Non-resident alien filing a U.S. tax return and not eligible for an SSN;
   - U.S. resident alien *(based on days present in the United States)* filing a U.S. tax return and not eligible for an SSN;
   - Dependent or spouse of a U.S. citizen/resident alien; and
   - Dependent or spouse of a non-resident alien visa holder.
   If you do not furnish your SSN or ITIN, you must furnish another proof of identity with this application form: a photocopy of your driver's license, State issued ID, employer ID, passport, or birth certificate.

B. Organizations and Groups
1-2. Provide your organization's or group's name *(legal business name used to file tax returns with the IRS)* and Employer Identification Number *(assigned by the IRS)* or Social Security Number (SSN). *(Required)*
3. If your organization or group uses or previously used another name, supply that "Other Name" in this area. *(Optional)* Use additional sheets of paper if necessary.
4. Mark the check box to indicate the type of "Other Name" used by your organization. *(D/B/A Name=Doing Business As Name.)* *(Required if 3 is completed.)*

SECTION 3 – ADDRESSES AND OTHER INFORMATION

A. Mailing Address Information
This information will assist us in contacting you with any questions we may have regarding your application for an NPI or with other information regarding NPI. You must provide an address and telephone number where we can contact you directly to resolve any issues that may arise during our review of your application. You may also add an e-mail address. *(Required)*

B. Practice Location Information
Provide information on the address of your primary practice location. If you have more than one practice location, select one as the "primary" location. Do not furnish information about additional locations on additional sheets of paper. *(Required)*

C. Other Provider Identification Numbers *(Optional)*
Please list the provider identification number(s) you currently use. This would include Medicare-issued numbers (UPIN, NSC, OSCAR, and PIN numbers), Medicaid-issued number *(show State)*, and numbers issued by other health plans *(give a brief description of issuer)*. If you do not have such numbers, you are not required to obtain them in order to be assigned an NPI.

D. Provider Taxonomy Code *(Provider Type/Specialty) (Required)*
Provide your 10-digit taxonomy code. Information on taxonomy codes is available at www.wpc-edi.com/taxonomy. You may provide a written description instead in the space provided, and we will assign the closest appropriate code.

Furnish the provider's health care license or certificate number(s) (if applicable). If issued by a State, show the State that issued the license/certificate. The following individual practitioners are required to submit a license number *(If you are one of the following and do not have a license or certificate, you must enclose a letter to the Enumerator explaining why not)*:

Psychoanalyst	Clinical Psychologist	Chiropractor
Dentist	Optometrist	Licensed Nurse
Pharmacist	Nurse Practitioner	Physician Assistant
Clinical Nurse Specialist	Podiatrist	Certified Registered Nurse Anesthetist
Physician/Osteopath	Licensed Psychiatric Technician	Psychologist, Psychotherapy
Registered Nurse		

The following organizations are also required to submit a license number. Provide your license number(s) and State(s) where issued:

Home Health Agency	Hospital Unit	Hospital
Clinical Medical Laboratory	Managed Care Organization	Nursing Facility
Pharmacy	Federally Qualified Health Center	

You may use the same license or certificate number for multiple taxonomies; e.g., if you are a physician with several different specialties.
NOTE: A health care provider that is an organization, such as a hospital, may obtain an NPI for itself and for any subparts that it determines need to be assigned NPIs. In some cases, the subparts have Provider Taxonomy Codes that may be different from that of the hospital and of each other, and each subpart may require separate licensing by the State (e.g., General Acute Care Hospital and Psychiatric Unit). If the organization provider chooses to include these multiple Provider Taxonomy Codes in a request for a single NPI, and later determines that the subparts should have been assigned their own NPIs with their associated Provider Taxonomy Codes, the organization provider must delete from its NPS record any Provider Taxonomy Codes that belong to the subparts who will be obtaining their own NPIs. The organization provider must do this by initiating the Change of Information option on this form.

SECTION 4 – CERTIFICATION STATEMENT *(Required)*
This section is intended for the applicant to attest that he/she is aware of the requirements that must be met and maintained in order to obtain and retain an NPI. This section also requires the signature and date of signature of the "Individual" who is the type 1 provider, or the "Authorized Official" of the type 2 organization who can legally bind the provider to the laws and regulations relating to the NPI. See below to determine who within the provider qualifies as an Authorized Official. Review these requirements carefully.

Authorized Official's Information and Signature for the Organization
By his/her signature, the authorized official binds the provider/supplier to all of the requirements listed in the Certification Statement and acknowledges that the provider may be denied a National Provider Identifier if any requirements are not met. All signatures must be original. Stamps, faxed or photocopied signatures are unacceptable. You may include multiple credentials. Use additional sheets of paper for multiple credentials if necessary.

An authorized official is an appointed official with the legal authority to make changes and/or updates to the provider's status (e.g., change of address, etc.) and to commit the provider to fully abide by the laws and regulations relating to the National Provider Identifier. The authorized official must be a general partner, chairman of the board, chief financial officer, chief executive officer, direct owner of 5 percent or more of the provider being enumerated, or must hold a position of similar status and authority within the provider.

Only the authorized official(s) has the authority to sign the application on behalf of the provider.

By signing this application for the National Provider Identifier, the authorized official agrees to immediately notify the NPI Enumerator if any information in the application is not true, correct, or complete. In addition, the authorized official, by his/her signature, agrees to notify the NPI Enumerator of any changes to the information contained in this form within 30 days of the effective date of the change.

SECTION 5 – CONTACT PERSON *(If the contact person is the same person identified in 2A or 4B, complete only item 8, E-mail Address.) (Optional)*
To assist in the timely processing of the NPI application, provide the name and telephone number of an individual who can be reached to answer questions regarding the information furnished in this application. Please note that if a contact person is not provided, all questions about this application will be directed to the authorized official named in Section 4 or the provider named in Section 2, as appropriate. You may include multiple credentials. Use additional sheets of paper for multiple credentials if necessary.

A

AANP. *See* American Academy of Nurse
   Practitioners
Academic nursing centers
   core competencies that affect, 186-187
   definition of, 185
   exemplars, 187-188
   federal funding of, 199
   history of, 186-187
   program planning, 188
   quality of, 187
   services provided in, 185
   vulnerable populations served in, 188
Academic nursing practice
   barriers to, 185
   definition of, 181
   exemplars of, 184-185
   facilitators of, 185
   history of, 182-183
   models of, 183-184
   Penn-Macy Initiative to advance, 182
   success of, 182-183
Acceptance, of employment offer, 13
Accountability, 33b, 237
Accountants, 114
Accounts, chart of, 117, 118f
Accreditation, 47-48
Action plan, 87, 95
Active privileges, 52
Acute care nurse practitioner, 34
ADA. *See* Americans with Disabilities Act
Administrative law, 26
Administrative rules, 41-42
Advanced practice license, 49
Advanced practice nurses, 46
Advertisements, 141-142
Affiliate privileges, 52
Agreements. *See also* Employment contract
   collaborative practice, 10-11, 32, 106
   professional services, 105
   Uniform Commercial Code
      definition of, 13
Allied health professional privileges, 52-53
American Academy of Family Physicians,
   166, 171

American Academy of Nurse Practitioners
   certification by, 6, 7t, 53, 182
   nurse practitioners as defined by, 4
   prescriptive authority advocacy by, 8
   scope of practice, 33b
   standards of practice, 29b-31b
American Association of Colleges of
      Nursing, 212
American Association of Nurse Anesthetists, 48
American Nurses Credential Center
   certification requirements, 6, 7t, 53, 182
   recertification requirements, 6
Americans with Disabilities Act
   description of, 113
   practice space requirements, 152, 156
ANCC. *See* American Nurses Credential Center
Anchor tenant, 159t
Ancillary services, 133
ANCs. *See* Academic nursing centers
"Anti-dumping" statute, 254
Anti-kickback statute, 254-255
Appointments
   group, 231
   scheduling of, 143
   telephone-based, 231
APRNDB. *See* National Practitioner Data Bank
Arizona State University College
      of Nursing, 187
Arkansas, 105-106
Arrest record, 112-113
Asset protection, 108
Assign lease, 159t
Attorney, 114-115
"At-will" employment, 11-12, 16

B

Bankers, 75
Base salary plus percentage, 18
Benchmarks, 85, 117
Benefits
   description of, 18-19, 245-246
   employment manual regarding, 107
Billing. *See also* Fees; Reimbursement
   by business office, 152-153
   of correctional facility, 132

Page numbers followed by f indicate figures; t, tables; b, boxes.

Billing—cont'd
  follow-up after, 116
  Medicaid. *See* Medicaid
  Medicare. *See* Medicare
  outsourcing of, 116
  self-pay, 127
  of sponsoring organization, 132
  third-party, 116, 127, 129-132
Blood transfusions, 250
Bloodborne pathogens, 157
Boards of nursing. *See* State boards of nursing
Bonus formulas, 15-16
Bookkeeping, 114, 152
Boomers, 144
Branding, 140
Breach of contract, 14
Breach of standards of care, 259
Budget, 87, 117
Business. *See also* Practice; Venture
  failure of, 21
  growth of, 175-178
  volatility of, 177
Business hours, 100
Business interruption insurance, 108-109
Business knowledge, 78
Business office, 152-153
Business plan
  core questions answered in, 88-91
  critical success factors described in, 91
  definition of, 83
  description of, 20, 77
  development of, 83-84
  elements of, 91-95, 92t
  evaluation of, 95-96
  executive summary, 96-97
  financing addressed in, 91
  form of, 88
  goal of, 85
  importance of, 84
  managing of, 97
  marketing provisions in, 90
  objectives of, 85-88
  outline of, 93b
  physical setup of practice
    described by, 90
  preparations for, 85
  purpose of, 84
  risk preemption using, 86-87
  steps involved in creating, 91-95
  strategy described in, 94
  summary of, 97-98
  venture description in, 92, 94
Business strategy, 139
Business structures, 100-104, 102t-103t

C

C corporation, 103t
Call system, 120
Capital, 73-75
Capitated practice
  income calculations in, 18
  productivity-based bonus formula in, 15
Capitation, 193
Causation, 259-260
CCNE. *See* Commission on Collegiate
    Nursing Education
Center for Integrated Health Care, 187
Centers for Medicare and Medicaid Services.
    See also Medicaid; Medicare
  certification requirements, 6
  description of, 129
  electronic health record adoption promoted
    by, 171
  *Evaluation and Management Services
    Guide,* 123
  rural health center reimbursement, 215
Certificate of need, 157
Certification. *See also* Credentialing;
    Licensure
  agencies that provide, 6, 7t
  by American Academy of Nurse Practitioners,
    6, 7t, 53, 182
  by American Nurses Credential Center, 6, 7t,
    53, 182
  definition of, 6, 48-49
  eligibility for, 6
  national, 6, 49, 53-54, 57
Certification examinations, 49, 50t, 53-54
Certified nurse midwives, 257
Certified registered nurse assistants, 257
Cervical neoplasia, 227
Cervicography, 227
Chart audit, 119
Chart of accounts, 117, 118f
Chart review and signing, 105
CHEA. *See* Council for Higher Education
    Accreditation
Chief complaint, 124
Civil Rights Act of 1964, 11
Claims, denial of, 134
Clinical Laboratory Improvement Act, 155
Clinical privileges, 52-53
Code of Ethics for Nursing, 28-29
Collaboration
  changes in, 34
  practice guidelines, 32
  principles of, 8, 10
  regulation of, 10, 34
  scope of practice inclusion of, 104

Collaborative agreement
  copies of, 106
  description of, 10-11, 32
  protocols listed in, 106
Collaborative formularies, 41
Collaborative model, of academic nursing
      practice, 183
Collaborative physician
  chart review and signing by, 105
  costs of, 105
  need for, 10, 21
  number of states that require, 246
  oversight of, 41
  prescription writing oversight by, 39, 41, 105
  professional services agreement with, 105
Colleagues, 143
College accreditation, 47-48
Commission on Collegiate Nursing
      Education, 48
Common area maintenance, 159t
Communication
  business, 84
  Health Insurance Portability and
      Accountability Act privacy rule and, 145
  importance of, 67
  during job interview, 112
Community health centers
  description of, 215
  federal funding of, 219
  federally qualified, 216-217
  governance of, 216-217
  history of, 216-217
Community nursing centers, 188
Compensation, 14. See also Salary
Competition
  assessment of, 76, 77f
  mapping of, 76
  understanding of, 139
Complaints, 251-252
Comprehensive examination, 127
Computer backup systems, 170
Computer networks, 166
Computer physician order entry systems, 169
Computer security, 170-171
Confidentiality
  employment contract provisions, 14
  of health records, 252
Conflict of interest, 14
Conflict of laws, 14
Congress, 25, 193
Continuing education, 57
Contract for employment. See Employment
      contract
Controlled substances, 8, 9t-10t

Corporation
  C, 103t
  nonprofit, 101, 104
  S, 103t
Correctional facilities, 132, 197
Cost(s)
  collaborative physician, 105
  depreciation, 120
  direct, 119
  health information technologies
      effect on, 164
  indirect, 119-120
Cost analyses, 119-120
Cost per patient visit, 119-120
Council for Higher Education
      Accreditation, 48
Council on Accreditation of Nurse Anesthesia
      Educational Programs, 48
Courtesy privileges, 52
Covenant not to compete, 15, 246
Covered entities, 168
Credentialing. See also Certification; Licensure
  controversy regarding, 56
  definition of, 5, 49, 52, 134
  history of, 45-46
  for hospital privileges, 49
  International Council of Nurses, 47
  international influences on, 55-56
  Joint Commission on Accreditation of
      Healthcare Organizations and, 5, 48
  for managed care organizations, 49, 51
  reimbursement and, 56
  for staff privileges, 49
  step-by-step approach to, 56-57
  terms associated with, 5
  for third-party payers, 49
Credentialing application, 49, 51b
Credentials, 5, 45
Criminal background checks, 252
Critical success factors, 91
Current Procedural Terminology, 126
Customer segmentation, 141
Customer value pyramid, 139, 139f
Customer value theory, 139-140
Cyber liability insurance, 109

D

Daily operations, 114-115, 120
Damages, 260
DEA. See Drug Enforcement Administration
"Defensive medicine," 256
Degrees, 51
Denial of claims, 134

Department of Health and Human Services, 168, 255
Depreciation costs, 120
Designated record set, 169
Detailed examination, 127
Dictation, 154
Direct costs, 119
Direct practice
  definition of, 204
  exemplars of, 204-210
Disallowance, 132
Discharge against medical advice, 251
Discounted fee-for-service program, 129-130
Discrimination, in employment, 11
Dishonesty insurance, 109
Dispute resolution, 14
Division of Nursing. *See* Federal Division of Nursing
Doctor of Nursing Practice, 203, 210-212
Doctor of Nursing Science, 212
Doctor of Philosophy, 212
Doctoral education, 195-196
Drug Enforcement Administration, 8, 57, 134
Duty of care, 259

E

Economic Opportunity Act of 1964, 216
Education. *See* Nursing education
Educational programs. *See also* Nursing education
  accreditation of, 47-48, 56
  description of, 39-40
EEOC. *See* Equal Employment Opportunity Commission
EHRs. *See* Electronic health records
Elder abuse, 256
Elder care, 194
Elective termination of pregnancy, 251
Electronic data transfers, 171
Electronic health records
  adoption of, 163-165, 171-172
  barriers to use, 164
  considerations before using, 165-166
  Health Insurance Portability and Accountability Act protections, 168
  incentives to use, 171
  information resources regarding, 166
  interoperability of, 171
  vendors of, 165
E-mail, 228, 231
Emergency care, 250
Emergency Medical Treatment and Labor Act, 254

Employees. *See also* Staff
  business growth and, 177
  criminal background checks, 252
  dishonesty by, 109, 114
  employment manuals for, 107
  empowerment of, 177
  federal, 247
  hiring of, 109-114
  job interview. *See* Job interview
  non-compete clauses, 15, 246
  payroll taxes, 115-116
  safety of, 156-157
Employer, 17
Employment
  "at-will," 11-12, 16
  discriminatory practices in, 11
  formal offer of, 13
  by government, 246
  independent contractor, 12-13
Employment contract
  benefits, 246
  binding nature of, 12-13
  bonus formulas in, 15-16
  considerations before signing, 16-18
  definition of, 12, 246
  elements of, 12-15
  formation of, 13
  negotiation of, 246
  parties of, 13
  restrictive covenants in, 15, 246
  salary determinations in, 17
  termination-without-cause clause in, 16
Employment manual, 107
Employment practices liability insurance, 109
End-of-life decisions, 249
Entrepreneurial model, of academic nursing practice, 183-184
Entrepreneurs
  lifestyle, 68
  motivation of, 64-65
  multitasking by, 64
  personal characteristics of, 62-64
Entrepreneurship
  family effects, 66
  fear and, 65-66, 67f
Equal Employment Opportunity Commission, 11
Error-back propagation, 212
Escalation clause, 160t
Evaluation/management services, 126-127
Evidence-based practice, 212
Examination. *See* Physical examination
Exclusionary formularies, 41
Exclusivity provision, 159t

Executive summary, 96-97
Exit plan, 66
Expanded problem-focused examination, 127
Expenses
  benchmarks for, 117
  estimating of, 74f
  in financial plan, 87-88
  overhead, 17
  personal, 72f, 73
  tracking of, 117
  worksheet for detailing of, 72f
Express contract, 13

F

Faculty full-time equivalent, 204
Faculty practice
  benefits of, 204
  challenges to, 210
  definition of, 181
  Doctor of Nursing Practice, 203, 210-212
  exemplars of, 204-210
  history of, 194
  models, 203
  nursing school emphasis on, 194
  payment models, 207
Faculty practice plans
  description of, 203
  at Purdue School of Nursing. *See* Purdue
    School of Nursing
  universities that offer, 203-204
  at University of Texas—Houston, 208
  at University of Wisconsin—Madison,
    208-210
Failure, fear of, 65
Family
  communication with, 67
  entrepreneurship effects on, 66
  in planning, 68
  startup capital from, 73-74
  support from, 61-62, 66-67
Family Health Clinic of Carroll County, 205
Family history, 125, 128b
Fast growth of business, 176-177
Fear, 65-66, 67f
Feasibility, 71
Federal Division of Nursing
  description of, 192-193
  doctoral education support by, 195-196
  nursing clinics funded by, 195
Federal employees, 247
Federal Insurance Contributions Act, 115
Federal laws, 253-265
Federal Tort Claims Act, 101, 217, 220

Federal unemployment taxes, 115
Federally qualified health center look-alikes, 218
Federally qualified health centers,
    101, 216-217
Fee-for-service program, by Medicare, 129-130
Fees. *See also* Billing; Reimbursement
  gross collection rate, 133
  net collection rate, 133
  reducing of, 133
FICA tax, 115
Finances
  business plan description of, 91
  capital, 73-75
  fast business growth and, 177
  fears regarding, 66
  feasibility and, relationship between, 71
  quality of care and, 238
  recommendations regarding, 73
Financial plan, 87-88, 95
Fiscal intermediary, 215
Force majeure, 14
Ford, Loretta C., 46, 53-54
Formal offer, 13
Formularies, 41
FQHCs. *See* Federally qualified health centers
Fraud and abuse/billing errors and omissions
    insurance, 109
Free clinics, 219-220
"Front office." *See* Business office

G

General partnerships, 100-101, 102t
Georgia, 105
Geriatric care nurse practitioner, 34
Gerontologic nurse practitioner, 194
Goals
  action plan to achieve, 87
  lifestyle, 68
  productivity, 117
  self-assessment of, 65, 65f
Government employment, 246
Gross collection rate, 133
Gross lease, 159t
Group appointments, 231

H

HCFA. *See* Health Care Financing
    Administration
Health care
  access to, 230-232
  alternative pathways to, 231
  federal laws, 253-265

Health care—cont'd
labor-intensive nature of, 230
operational effectiveness and, 231-232
patient needs and, 231
quality of. *See* Quality of care
state laws, 248-253
Health care consumers, 149-150.
See also Patient
Health Care Financing Administration
Common Procedure Coding
System code, 131
rural health clinics, 218
Health care power of attorney, 249
Health centers
community. *See* Community health centers
migrant, 217-218
Health Centers Consolidated Care Act of
1996, 217
Health Centers Consolidation Act, 216
Health information
Health Insurance Portability and
Accountability Act privacy rule effects on,
144-145
protected, 168-169
Health Information and Management Systems
Society ambulatory electronic health
record selector, 166
Health information technologies
adoption of, 164-165
barriers to use of, 164
cost savings associated with, 164
integration of, 165
vendors of, 165-166
"Wired for Health Care Quality Act" effect on,
163-165
Health Insurance Portability and
Accountability Act
compliance with, 169-170
covered entities, 168
definition of, 144, 167
description of, 55, 130
designated record set, 169
electronic data concerns, 167-171
electronic health records and, 168
marketing and, 144-145
noncompliance with, 255
personal digital assistant concerns, 167
privacy rule, 144-145, 167-169, 255
protected health information, 168-169
security compliance with, 170-171
standards, 255
violations of, 255-256
Wi-Fi requirements, 167
workplace requirements, 169

Health maintenance organizations.
See also Managed care organizations
Medicare, 130
reimbursements by, 133
Health Professional Shortage Area, 219
Health Professions Education Partnerships
Act of 1998, 199
Health records
accuracy of, 153
amending of, 169
confidentiality of, 252
electronic. *See* Electronic health records
patient's right to, 169
retention requirements, 252
storage of, 153
transfer of, 143
Health Resources and Services Administration,
198, 217
Heating and air conditioning, 160t
Henry, O. Marie, 195
HIPAA. *See* Health Insurance Portability and
Accountability Act
History of present illness, 124t,
124-125, 128b
HITs. *See* Health information
technologies
HMOs. *See* Health maintenance
organizations
Homeless population, 197
Honorary privileges, 52
Hours of operation, 100
House privileges, 52

I

Improvements, in lease, 160t
Incident reporting, 258
Incident-to-services, 130-131
Income
benchmarks for, 117
in capitated practice, 18
estimating of, 73f
generation of, 18
Indemnification, 14
Indemnity insurance companies,
131-132
Independent contractor, 12-13
Indian Self-Determination Act, 217
Indirect care, 207
Indirect costs, 119-120
Informatics, 229-230
Information technologies, 163-164
Informed consent, 249-251
Initiatives, 89

Institute of Medicine
 description of, 163, 186
 health care system improvements as
   recommended by, 230
 quality of care as defined by, 234-235
Insurance
 business interruption, 108-109
 cyber liability, 109
 dishonesty, 109
 employment practices liability, 109
 fraud and abuse/billing errors and
   omissions, 109
 lessor requirements, 160t
 liability, 79, 108
 loss of income protection, 108-109
 malpractice, 108
 medical. *See* Medical insurance
 property, 108
 worker's compensation, 108
Insurance card, 123
Integrative model, of academic nursing
   practice, 183
International Council of Nurses, 47
IOM. *See* Institute of Medicine

J

Job interview
 communication during, 112
 environment for, 112
 fair treatment of candidates during, 111
 information gathering during, 110-111
 preparing for, 110
 professional behavior during, 111
 questions not allowed in, 112-114
 respect and courtesy during, 112
Joint Commission on Accreditation of
   Healthcare Organizations
 credentialing requirements, 5
 criminal background checks, 252
 mission of, 48
Judicial law, 26

L

Laboratory, 151, 154-155
LAN. *See* Local area network
Law(s). *See also* Nursing regulation
 changes in, 40-42, 106
 compliance with, 105
 federal, 253-265
 prescription writing and, 40-42
 understanding of, 105

Lawsuits
 description of, 79
 malpractice. *See* Malpractice lawsuits
 negligence, 259-260
Lay healers, 45
Leasing, of practice space, 158-159,
   159t-160t
Legal authority, 14
Legal business structure, 100-104, 102t-103t
Legal surrogacy, 249
Legend drugs, 37, 38f, 41
Legislation
 medical administration review, 251
 Nurse Practice Act, 26, 27f
Liability insurance, 79, 108
Licensed independent providers
 clinical privileges, 52
 definition of, 46
Licensure. *See also* Certification; Credentialing
 definition of, 5, 52
 history of, 46
 purpose of, 5
 state boards of nursing, 26, 53, 57
 state requirements, 247
Limited liability partnerships, 101
Limited partnerships, 101
Litigation, 258-260
Living wills, 249
Local area network, 166
Location, 99-100
Loss of income protection insurance, 108-109
Lost productivity, 117, 119

M

Malpractice lawsuits
 damages for, 260
 elements required for, 259-260
 insurance against, 108
 prevention of, 257, 257t
 reasons for, 258
 release of medical information, 252
 reporting to National Practitioner
   Data Bank, 253
 risks for, 256-257
 state-defined parameters for, 259
 statute of limitations, 259
Managed care organizations. *See also* Health
   maintenance organizations
 credentialing for, 49, 51
 manuals for, 107
 Medicaid and, 131
 reimbursement by, 131-132
 types of, 131

Mandatory reporting, 253
Manuals
 employment, 107
 office policy, 107
 policies and procedure, 106-108
 types of, 107-108
Market
 description of, 89-90
 specialty types of, 143-144
Market research, 137-138, 140-141
Marketing
 description of, 90
 Health Insurance Portability and
  Accountability Act and, 144-145
 principles of, 137
 quality services as part of, 141
 resources for, 141
 strategies for, 141-142, 146
 target, 141
Marketing mix, 138
Marketing strategies, 138
Martindale-Hubbell Law Dictionary, 115
Master's degree, 33b, 40, 51
MCOs. *See* Managed care organizations
Medicaid
 billing and reimbursement
  for federally qualified health centers, 101
  methodologies, 132
  of rural health centers, 104
 description of, 131
Medical administration, legislative review of,
 251-252
Medical Group Management Association, 117
Medical insurance
 denial of claims, 134
 services not covered by, 127
Medical office building, 151
Medical record. *See* Health records
Medical therapeutics, 40
Medicare
 billing and reimbursement
  for federally qualified health centers, 101
  fee percentages, 129
  incident-to-services, 130-131
  methodologies, 132
  of rural health centers, 104
 description of, 129
 discounted fee-for-service program,
  129-130
 health maintenance organization, 130
 programs offered by, 129
 Stark Law regarding, 255
Medicare provider number, 54-55, 57
Michigan Academic Consortium, 187

Midwest Nursing Center Consortium
 Research Network, 210
Migrant health centers, 217-218
Minors, 250
Missouri Telemedicine Network, 226-227
Modular designs, of practice space, 151
Motivation, 64-65
Move-in and delivery requirements, 160t
Mutual agreement, 13
Mystery shopper, 143

N

NARHC. *See* National Association of Rural
 Health Clinics
National Advisory Committee on Rural Health
 and Social Services, 220-221
National Advisory Council on Nurse Education
 and Practice, 197-198
National Association of Community Health
 Centers, 216
National Association of Free Clinics, 220
National Association of Rural Health
 Clinics, 219
National Center for Farmworker Health, 218
National certification, 6, 49, 53-54, 57
National Certification Board of Pediatric Nurse
 Practitioners and Nurses, 7t
National Certification Corporation for the
 Women's Health, Obstetric, and
 Neonatal Nursing Specialties, 7t
National Commission for Certifying
 Agencies, 49
National Committee for Quality Assurance, 5
National Council of State Boards of Nursing
 examination offered by, 51
 regulation as viewed by, 52
National League for Nursing Accrediting
 Commission, 48
National Organization of Nurse Practitioner
 Faculties, 181
National Plan and Provider Enumeration
 System, 55
National Practitioner Data Bank, 253-254
National provider identifier, 55
National Rural Health Association, 220
NCLEX examination, 51
Negative formularies, 41
Negligence lawsuits, 259-260
Net collection rate, 133
Niche, 75, 178
Nightingale Training School of Nurses, 46
NLNAC. *See* National League for Nursing
 Accrediting Commission

Noncompetition covenant, 15, 246
Nondisturbance clause, 159t
NONPF. *See* National Organization of Nurse
    Practitioner Faculties
Nonprofit corporation, 101, 104
North American Nursing Diagnosis
    Association, 228
NRHA. *See* National Rural Health Association
Nurse Education Amendments of 1985,
    197-198
Nurse practice acts
  amendments to, for prescriptive
      authority, 41
  copies of, 28
  description of, 26
  purpose of, 53
  scope of practice in, 7, 25-26
Nurse practitioners
  characteristics of, 4
  definition of, 4, 25
  shortage of, 193
  specialization of, 4
  statistics, 245
  studies of, 193
  title recognition for, 40-41
Nurse Reinvestment Act of 2004, 199
Nurse station, 153-155
Nurse Training Act
  of 1964
    benefits of, 192-193
    Division of Nursing, 193
    elements of, 191-192
    modifications to, 192
    monies allocated, 192
    Professional Nurse Traineeship
        Program, 191
  of 1975, 194
Nurse-managed centers
  community involvement, 198, 200
  evolution of, 196-198
  funding of, 197
  growth of, 195
  location of, 198
  primary care services offered by, 196
  role of, 198
  services provided by, 198-199
Nursing boards. *See* State boards
    of nursing
Nursing Center for Family Health, 204
Nursing centers
  academic. *See* Academic nursing centers
  community, 188
  definition of, 185
  federal funding for, 195

Nursing education. *See also* Educational programs
  American Academy of Nurse Practitioners
      requirements, 33b
  amount of, 51
  continuing, 57
  degrees obtained, 51
  Doctor of Nursing Practice, 203, 210-212
  doctoral, 195-196
  faculty practice and, 194-195
  federal funding of, 198-200
  horizontal integration of, 204
  vertical integration of, 204
Nursing informatics, 229-230
Nursing practice. *See* Practice
Nursing regulation. *See also* Law(s)
  description of, 247
  federal, 247
  history of, 45-46
  National Council of State Boards of Nursing
      views on, 52
Nursing Special Projects, 197

O

Objectives, of business plan
  action plan to achieve, 87
  description of, 85-88
Occupational health nurse practitioner
    programs, 195
Occupational Safety and Health Act, 11
Occupational Safety and Health Administration,
    156-157
Office. *See* Practice space
Office of Civil Rights, 255-256
Office of Rural Health Policy Outreach Grant
    Program, 219
Office of the National Coordinator of Health
    Information Technologies, 164
Office policy manual, 107
Off-service hours, 100
Open formularies, 41
Organizational chart, 121
OSHA. *See* Occupational Safety and Health
    Administration
Outpatient privileges, 52
Outsourcing, 115-116
Overhead expenses, 17

P

Partnerships
  general, 100-101, 102t
  limited, 101
  limited liability, 101

Past history, 124, 128b
Patient
    difficult types of, 143
    first impressions by, 150
    refusal of treatment by, 250
    responsibility to, 69
    satisfaction of, 149
    self-payment by, 127
    staff handling of, 142-143
Patient education area, in practice space, 152
Patient encounter
    chief complaint, 124
    description of, 123-124
    documentation of, 126-127, 128b
    history of present illness, 124t, 124-125, 128b
    personalizing of, 142
    physical examination, 125-126, 128b
    review of systems, 125, 128b
Patient satisfaction-based bonus formula, 16
Patient-centered access to care, 230
Patients Bill of Rights, 250
Payroll service, 115
Payroll taxes, 115-116
PDAs. See Personal digital assistants
Peer review, 257
Penn Nursing Network, 184-185, 228
Penn-Macy Initiative to Advance Academic
        Nursing Practice, 182
"People skills," 79
Percentage lease, 159t
Percentage salary, 18
Performance evaluation, 19-20
Performance measures
    characteristics of, 239-241
    data collection, 240
    development of, 242
    existing, 241
    improvement-based focus of, 239
    interpretable nature of, 240
    overview of, 238
    problems commonly encountered with, 241
    reliability of, 240
    risk-adjusted, 240
    sensitivity and specificity of, 239-240
    usefulness of, 239
    validity of, 239
Personal digital assistants, 167, 169, 228-229
Personal expenses, 72f, 73
PHSA. See Public Health Service Act
Physical comfort, of practice space, 150
Physical examination
    description of, 125-126, 128b
    rooms for, 153-154
Physical space. See Practice space

Physician
    collaborative. See Collaborative physician
    consultation with, 17
    states that require, 246
Planning. See also Business plan
    family involvement in, 68
    outline of practice, 76
    practice space, 150-151
    of resources, 87
PNN. See Penn Nursing Network
Policies and procedure manuals, 106-108
Population-based models, 207
Power of attorney, health care-related, 249
Practice. See also Business; Venture
    advantages and disadvantages of, 21
    barriers for, 21
    collaboration in, 8, 10-11
    considerations before beginning,
        20-21, 61-62
    designing of, 79-80
    faculty. See Faculty practice
    fear associated with, 65-66
    growth of, 175-178
    how to find, 246-247
    income estimating, 73f
    initiatives for, 89
    legal environment for, 25
    lifestyle changes associated with, 68
    location of, 149
    market for, 89-90
    outlining of, 76
    personal considerations, 62-69
    promoting of, 90
    readiness for, 77-78
    responsibility to, 69
    scope of. See Scope of practice
    services offered by, 89
    standards of. See Standards of practice
    strategy for, 85
    types of, 4, 245
Practice guidelines, 31
Practice management
    business plan description of, 91
    computerized systems for, 119
    tips for, 120-121
Practice space
    Americans with Disabilities Act
        requirements, 152, 156
    business office, 152-153
    business plan description of, 90
    certificate of need, 157
    codes, 155-157
    consumer needs regarding, 150
    examination rooms, 153-154

Practice space—cont'd
first impressions of, 150
functions of, 151
laboratory location, 151, 154-155
leasing of, 158-159, 159t-160t
modular design of, 151
nurse station, 153-155
patient education area, 152
physical comfort of, 150
planning of, 150-151
reception area, 152
safety regulation, 155-157
seating arrangements, 150
social contact in, 150
storage, 155
symbolic meaning associated with, 150
toilets, 151-152, 156
treatment room, 154
wayfinding considerations, 150
workroom, 155
Pregnancy termination, 251
Prescribing patterns
legal development of, 39, 41-42
scope of practice as basis for, 37-39
Prescriptive authority
description of, 8
formularies, 41
growth of, 39
information needed regarding, 42-43
legal changes needed for, 40-42
legend drugs, 37, 38f, 41
patterns for, 41
physician involvement, 105
state laws regarding, 249
states that allow, 35f, 38f
Primary care, 196
Privacy rule, of Health Insurance Portability and
Accountability Act, 144-145, 167-168, 255
Privileges
categories of, 52-53
clinical, 52-53
definition of, 5
Privileging
clinical, 52
definition of, 5
tips for, 57
Problem-focused examination, 126
Procrastination, 64
Productivity
bonus formula based on, 15
employment contract provisions regarding, 17
goal setting, 117
lost, 117, 119
maximizing of, 119

Professional boards, complaints to, 251-252
Professional image, 79
Professional Nurse Traineeship Program, 191
Professional service corporations, 101
Professional services agreement, 105
Profit-based bonus formula, 16
Property insurance, 108
Protected health information, 168-169
Protocols, 106
Public Health Service Act
Nursing Special Projects, 197
rural health center funding under, 215
Title VIII, 101, 191, 193-194, 197, 199-200
Punitive damages. *See* Damages
Purdue School of Nursing
clinics and contracts, 205-206
community partners, 206
consultation models, 207
Doctor of Nursing program at, 211
indirect care, 207
population-based models, 207
Trinity Nursing Center for Infant Health, 206

Q

Qualitative strategies, for marketing, 138, 138t
Quality improvement, 236
Quality management, 233
Quality of care
accountability for, 237
description of, 233-234
finances and, 238
Institute of Medicine definition of, 234-235
managing of, 234-238
measuring of, 236-238
objectivity in evaluation of, 237-238
research evidence and, 234-235
subjective nature of, 236
Quality-based bonus formula, 15
Quantitative strategies, for marketing, 138, 138t

R

Reception area, 152
Recertification, 6
Record. *See* Health records
Referrals
importance of, 143
insurance approval of, 123
Refusal of treatment, 250
Regulation. *See* Nursing regulation
Reimbursement. *See also* Billing; Fees
credentialing and, 56
denied claims, 134

Reimbursement—cont'd
  for e-mail consultations, 231
  health maintenance organizations, 133
  indemnity insurance companies, 131-132
  managed care organizations, 131-132
  methodologies for, 132-133
  to non-physician health care providers, 56
Relative value unit, 132
Reliability, of performance measures, 240
Relocation, 246-247
Renewal option, 160t
Renovations and repairs, 160t
Reporting
  incident, 258
  mandatory, 253
Research
  evidence obtained through, 234
  importance of, 75-76
  reasons for, 76
Resources
  estimating of, 87
  marketing, 141
Responsibility, 33b
Restrictions on use, 160t
Restrictive covenants, 15
Revenue
  business growth and, 176
  projections regarding, 88
Revenue collections, 115-116
Revenue loss
  areas of, 116
  lost productivity as cause of, 117, 119
Review of systems, 125, 128b
RHCs. *See* Rural health centers; Rural
    health clinics
Right of first refusal, 159t
Risk assessment, 86-87
Risk management
  behaviors to support, 257t
  employment contract, 246-247
  high-risk areas, 256-258
  incident reporting, 258
  malpractice lawsuit prevention, 257, 257t
Rural areas
  business plan description of, 90
  residents in, 215
  telehealth in, 226-227, 252-253
Rural health centers
  definition of, 104
  description of, 101
  federal reimbursement of, 215
  Medicare and Medicaid reimbursement of, 104
  Public Health Service Act funding
      provisions, 215

Rural health centers—cont'd
  purpose of, 104
  services offered by, 215
Rural health clinics, 218-219

S

S corporation, 103t
Salary
  base salary plus percentage, 18
  employment contract provisions
      regarding, 17
  negotiating of, 18
  percentage, 18
  straight, 17-18
Scheduling of appointments, 143
Scope of practice
  American Academy of Nurse Practitioners,
      33b
  breach of, 32, 34
  challenges, 32, 34
  collaboration requirement in, 104
  description of, 6-8, 104
  in Nurse Practice Act, 7, 25-26
  prescribing patterns based on, 37-39, 43
  professional agencies' role in, 28
  protocols for establishing, 106
  state boards of nursing influence
      on, 26, 28
  state laws regarding, 249
  variations in, 53
Self-defeating behaviors, 63
Self-pay, 127
Seniors, 144
Sensitivity, of performance measure, 239-240
Service
  marketing and, 142
  quality of, 142-143
Severability, 14
Small Business Administration, 20, 62, 76, 78
Small business development centers, 77
Social contact, in practice space, 150
Social history, 125, 128b
Sole proprietorships, 100-101, 102t
Specialty markets, 143-144
Specificity, of performance measure, 239-240
Staff. *See also* Employees
  fast business growth effects on, 176
  handling of patients by, 142-143
  interactions with colleagues, 143
  telephone etiquette by, 142-143
Stakeholders
  core questions by, 88-91
  quality of care measurements and, 236

Standards of care
  breach of, 259
  description of, 31-32
Standards of practice
  American Academy of Nurse Practitioners,
    29b-31b
  definition of, 28
  history of, 28-29
  legal implications of, 31
Stark Law, 255
Startup capital, 73-75
State boards of nursing
  description of, 26, 28
  licensure, 26, 53, 57
  prescriptive authority rules developed by,
    41-42
  responsibilities of, 53
State legislatures, 25
State statutes, 247-248
*Statistics Report on Medical and Dental Income
    and Expense Averages*, 117
Statute of limitations, 259
Statutory duty to report, 253
Statutory law, 26
Storage space, 155, 160t
Straight salary, 17-18
Strategic planning, 140
Strategic thinking, 85
Strategy
  action plan for, 87, 95
  business, 139
  developing of, 94
  identifying of, 85-86
  implementation of, 87
  operationalizing of, 95
Strengths, 61, 63
Sublet, 159t-160t
Subrogation, 14
"Super-leader trap," 89
Supply chain, 90
Support professionals, 78-79
Surrogacy, 249
SWOT analysis, 94

T

Target marketing, 141
Target markets, 138
Taxes, payroll, 115-116
Telecolposcopy, 227
Telehealth
  advancement of, 247
  definition of, 225
  history of, 225-226

Telehealth—cont'd
  nurse practitioner use of, 228
  patient outcome benefits of, 226
  remote diagnosis abilities of, 227
  rural health care and, 226-227, 252-253
Telemedicine, 252-253
Telephone
  appointments performed through, 231
  etiquette in using, 142-143
Tennessee, 105
Termination of lease, 160t
Termination-without-cause clause, 16
Third-party payers. *See also specific payer*
  billing of, 116, 127, 129-132
  contracting with, 119
  credentialing requirements, 134
  description of, 49
  documentation of services required by, 126
  manuals for, 107
Title VIII, of Public Health Service Act, 101,
    193-194, 197, 199-200
Toilets, 151-152, 156
Tort reform, 260
Treatment refusal, 250
Treatment room, 154
Trinity Nursing Center for Infant Health, 206
Triple net lease, 159t

U

Unification model, of academic nursing
    practice, 183
Unit cost analysis, 119
United States Department of Education, 47
Universal provider identifying number, 54-55
Universities
  accreditation of, 47-48
  small business development centers at, 77
University of Lowell, 194
University of Maryland School of Nursing,
    187-188
University of Rochester, 194
University of Texas—Houston, 208
University of Wisconsin—Madison, 208-210
University of Wisconsin-Milwaukee School of
    Nursing, 188
UPIN. *See* Universal provider identifying
    number

V

Value, 139
Vanderbilt University School of Nursing, 184
Variance analysis, 117

Venture. *See also* Business; Practice
  business plan description of, 92, 94
  critical success factors for, 91
  key players in, 88-89
  stakeholder questions, 88-91
Volatility, 177
Vulnerable adult abuse, 256
VUSN. *See* Vanderbilt University School
  of Nursing

W

WAN. *See* Wide area network
Weaknesses, 61, 63

West Virginia Rural Health Education
  Partnership Program, 184
"What-if?" scenarios, 86-87
Wide area network, 166
Wi-Fi, 166-167
"Wired for Health Care Quality Act,"
  163-165
Wireless networks, 166-167
Work habits, 64
Worker's compensation insurance, 108
Workroom, 155
WVRHEP. *See* West Virginia
  Rural Health Education
  Partnership Program

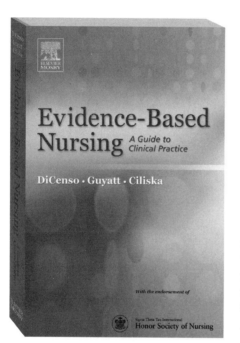